The Complete
Weight-Loss
Surgery
Guide & Diet Program

Includes 150 Delicious & Nutritious Recipes

Sue Ekserci, RD
with Dr. Laz Klein, MD

ROSE

617.43 EKS
Ekserci, Sue
The complete weight-loss
    surgery guide & diet
    program

$24.95

CENTRAL   31994014694514

For complete cataloguing information, see page 343.

Disclaimer
This book is a general guide only and should never be considered a substitute for the skill, knowledge and
experience of a qualified medical professional dealing with the facts, circumstances and symptoms of a
particular case.

The nutritional, medical and health information presented in this book is based on the research,
training and professional experience of the author and is true and complete to the best of her knowledge.
However, this book is intended only as an informative guide for those wishing to know more about health,
nutrition and medicine; it is not intended to replace or countermand advice given by the reader's personal
physician. Because each person and situation is unique, the author and the publisher urge the reader to
check with a qualified health-care professional before using any procedure when there is a question as to
its appropriateness. A physician should be consulted before beginning any exercise program. The author
and the publisher are not responsible for any adverse effects or consequences resulting from the use of
the information in this book. It is the responsibility of the reader to consult a physician or other qualified
health-care professional regarding his or her personal care.

This book contains references to products that may not be available everywhere. The intent of
the information provided is to be helpful; however, there is no guarantee of results associated with the
information provided. Use of brand names is for educational purposes only and does not imply endorsement.

The recipes in this book have been carefully tested by our kitchen and our tasters. To the best of our
knowledge, they are safe and nutritious for ordinary use and users. For those people with food or other
allergies or who have special food requirements or health issues, please read the suggested contents of each
recipe carefully and determine whether or not they may create a problem for you. All recipes are used at the
risk of the consumer. We cannot be responsible for any hazards, loss or damage that may occur as a result of
any recipe use. For those with special needs, allergies, requirements or health problems, in the event of any
doubt, please contact your medical adviser prior to the use of any recipe.

Design and Production: Kevin Cockburn/PageWave Graphics Inc.
Editors: Bob Hilderley, Senior Editor, Health, and Sue Sumeraj and Jennifer MacKenzie, Recipes
Proofreader: Sheila Wawanash
Indexer: Gillian Watts
Illustrations: Kveta/Three in a Box
Cover photograph: © istockphoto.com/Lilyana Vynogradova

We acknowledge the financial support of the Government of Canada through the Book Publishing Industry
Development Program (BPIDP) for our publishing activities.

Published by Robert Rose Inc.
120 Eglinton Avenue East, Suite 800, Toronto, Ontario, Canada M4P 1E2
Tel: (416) 322-6552 Fax: (416) 322-6936
www.robertrose.ca

Printed and bound in Canada

1 2 3 4 5 6 7 8 9 MP 19 18 17 16 15 14 13 12 11

Contents

Introduction

Weight-loss surgery, also known as bariatric surgery, is a procedure designed to help you decrease your food intake and change the way your body handles food, with the intention of promoting significant weight loss. Several types of weight-loss surgery are well studied and have been shown to promote achievable and sustainable weight loss for people who are obese, with a body mass index above 35 (BMI is a standard measure of healthy and unhealthy weight).

The most successful procedures allow you to eat less, which leads to weight loss. All procedures can be performed laparoscopically, by surgical instruments inserted through very small incisions.

Weight-loss surgery has become quite common and successful during the past two decades. In North America approximately 222,000 surgeries are performed each year. Most are considered to be successful in the long term.

Did you know?

The key to success is not only the surgery itself but also lifestyle changes, including healthy and mindful eating and active living, which are not always easy to establish and maintain.

Should You Consider Weight-Loss Surgery?

Several criteria need to be met in order for you to be considered a suitable candidate for bariatric surgery. The selection criteria for adults have been established by several medical associations, including the American Association of Clinical Endocrinologists (AACE), the Obesity Society (TOS) and the American Society for Metabolic and Bariatric Surgery (ASMBS). The selection criteria help determine who is most likely to benefit from surgery. These guidelines change with advances in research; for example, new research shows that people with diabetes whose BMI is 30 or more may benefit from some types of bariatric surgery.

Bariatric surgery is generally limited to people between 18 and 60 years of age. However, both younger and older patients may be candidates for surgery depending on their individual circumstances. Age does not directly determine someone's eligibility for bariatric surgery, but it is an important factor in choosing the best procedure and weighing risk versus benefit for a patient. Surgery is contraindicated in people who have a severe psychiatric illness that is uncontrolled, and for those who are currently abusing drugs or alcohol. Other exclusion criteria include some endocrine disorders that cause obesity, such as hypothyroidism or Cushing's syndrome. If present, these disorders should be treated before considering surgery.

▶ Selection criteria for weight-loss surgery

Factor	Criteria
Weight	• Body mass index (BMI) of 40 or more with no co-morbidities of obesity • BMI of 35 or more with co-morbidities of obesity
Weight-loss history	• Tried and failed previous nonsurgical attempts at weight loss
Commitment	• Expected to adhere to postoperative care requirements, including follow-up visits with health-care team • Will take recommended nutritional supplements • Will follow recommended medical management, including any pertinent procedures or tests
Comprehension	• Ability to comprehend the nature of the surgery, associated risk, and dietary and lifestyle modifications needed to achieve an acceptable level of health

To help you make the decision whether or not weight-loss surgery is for you, start asking yourself the following questions. If you can answer yes to these questions without hesitation, you may be ready for bariatric surgery. If not, read on. This book is designed to answer questions and allay any concerns you may have about this method of losing weight.

• Do I qualify for bariatric surgery?
• Have I exhausted nonsurgical methods for weight loss?
• Do I understand what weight-loss surgery is?
• Do I understand the risks and benefits of weight-loss surgery?
• Do I understand the life-changing effects of weight-loss surgery?
• Am I prepared to deal with excess skin?
• Am I prepared to make a lifestyle change?
• Do I have a good support system in place?
• Have I discussed this option with my health-care team?
• Have I talked to others who have had weight-loss surgery?
• Do I know the cost of weight-loss surgery and can I afford it?

Frequently Asked Questions

Will my health insurance plan cover the costs of bariatric surgery?

Coverage varies from country to country, from province to province and from policy to policy. Read your insurance policy carefully.

In the United States, insurance coverage varies, based on several factors. You will likely need to consult with your insurance company to get details on how to apply for coverage. You should expect to provide the insurance company with letters and documentation to support your individual need for bariatric surgery, including

- your height, weight history and BMI
- a description of your obesity-related health conditions and treatments
- documentation and receipts related to your weight-loss efforts and exercise programs
- nutrition consultation and psychological evaluation

Insurance may partially or completely cover some procedures but not others. Most insurance companies are now realizing the long-term health benefits and cost savings associated with weight-loss surgery.

In Canada, coverage for gastric bypass surgery is government funded, but other procedures are covered on a case-by-case basis. In most provinces the laparoscopic adjustable gastric band (LAGB) procedure is not covered; you can expect to pay more than CAN$17,000, depending on where you have the procedure done. In some provinces limited funding has become available for the LAGB.

In the United Kingdom, all procedures (including the LAGB) are covered by the public health service. In the private sector, private insurance does not cover any procedures, so patients must pay by themselves.

The weight-loss surgery health-care team

If you qualify for weight-loss surgery, you will be cared for by a team of health-care professionals, including some or all of these specialists:

- Anesthetist
- Clinical nurse specialist
- Dentist

- Endocrinologist
- Family physician/general practitioner
- Insurance specialist
- Medical internist
- Medical specialist
- Nurse
- Nurse practitioner
- Ophthalmologist
- Personal support worker
- Pharmacist
- Physical therapist
- Physician
- Physiotherapist
- Program manager or coordinator
- Psychiatrist
- Psychologist
- Registered dietitian
- Registered social worker
- Respiratory therapist
- Rheumatologist
- Surgeon
- Wellness coach

Top 5 Tips for Lifelong Success

1. Follow the bariatric diet program for mindful eating.
2. Practice the principles of active living.
3. Change what you eat, how you eat and why you eat.
4. Take the required vitamins and minerals for life to prevent deficiencies.
5. Cooperate with your health-care team and join or create support groups.

Part 1

Obesity and Weight-Loss Surgery

What Is Obesity?

The World Health Organization defines health as a state of complete physical, mental and social well-being and not merely the absence of disease or infirmity. It can be argued that achieving complete health is next to impossible, but we can strive to achieve and maintain an overall healthy lifestyle, which encompasses a combination of physical, mental and social well-being. Measures of success for attaining health traditionally include reducing health risk factors, preventing medical conditions and decreasing reliance on medications.

Achieving and maintaining a healthy weight through balanced diet and moderate exercise reduces health risks significantly, whereas severe overweight, or obesity, and a sedentary lifestyle are associated with progressive, serious, debilitating disease. Obesity is the leading preventable cause of death worldwide. Treating obesity not only addresses immediate health concerns such as stroke or diabetes but also prevents possible problems years later. Successful weight management also has important side effects — improvement in your quality of life, development of a positive self-image and a feeling of general well-being.

Measuring Obesity

Obesity is defined as the accumulation of an excessive amount of adipose (fatty) tissue, but how much adipose tissue is unhealthy? There are several different ways to measure body fat. You can compare your weight to an ideal weight for your gender, age and stature, using published charts such as the Metropolitan Life tables (available on the Internet). If you are 20% above your ideal body weight, you are considered to be obese. This method is not always accurate because the ideal weight charts are based on a specific population that is not representative of the current general population as a whole.

Body fat percentage

You can also estimate the percentage of your total body weight that is fatty tissue. In general, women whose body fat is greater than 30% and men whose body fat is greater than 25% are considered obese. You can calculate body fat content by using calipers to measure skin-fold thickness on the back of the upper arm and at other sites. This method requires specialized equipment and specialized administration. The most accurate way of measuring body fat involves immersing a person in water and measuring the relative displacement, but this method is somewhat impractical. The most widely used means of calculating healthy weight, underweight, overweight or obesity is called the body mass index (BMI), even though it does not measure body fat directly.

Body mass index

BMI is a tool used to assess, classify and monitor changes in body weight. A BMI greater than 30 is considered to indicate obesity.

BMI is calculated as follows:

Imperial units

BMI = weight in pounds x 703 ÷ (height in inches)^2

International (metric) units

BMI = weight in kilograms ÷ (height in meters)^2

For example, if you weigh 265 pounds and are 65 inches tall, your BMI is (265 x 703) ÷ (65 x 65) = 186,295 ÷ 4,225 = 44.1. Now use the chart to classify your actual BMI.

▶ BMI Classifications

BMI Category (kg/m2)	Classification	Risk of developing health problems
< 18.5	underweight	increased
18.5 – 24.9	normal weight	least
25.0 – 29.9	overweight	increased
30.0 – 34.9	obese class I	high
35.0 – 39.9	obese class II	very high
≥ 40	obese class III	extremely high

BODY MASS INDEX TABLE

BMI	19	20	21	22	23	24	25	26	27	28	29	30	31	32	33	34	35	36
Height (inches)	Body Weight (pounds)																	
	NORMAL						OVERWEIGHT					OBESE						
58	91	96	100	105	110	115	119	124	129	134	138	143	148	153	158	162	167	172
59	94	99	104	109	114	119	124	128	133	138	143	148	153	158	163	168	173	178
60	97	102	107	112	118	123	128	133	138	143	148	153	158	163	168	174	179	184
61	100	106	111	116	122	127	132	137	143	148	153	158	164	169	174	180	185	190
62	104	109	115	120	126	131	136	142	147	153	158	164	169	175	180	186	191	196
63	107	113	118	124	130	135	141	146	152	158	163	169	175	180	186	191	197	203
64	110	116	122	128	134	140	145	151	157	163	169	174	180	186	192	197	204	209
65	114	120	126	132	138	144	150	156	162	168	174	180	186	192	198	204	210	216
66	118	124	130	136	142	148	155	161	167	173	179	186	192	198	204	210	216	223
67	121	127	134	140	146	153	159	166	172	178	185	191	198	204	211	217	223	230
68	125	131	138	144	151	158	164	171	177	184	190	197	203	210	216	223	230	236
69	128	135	142	149	155	162	169	176	182	189	196	203	209	216	223	230	236	243
70	132	139	146	153	160	167	174	181	188	195	202	209	216	222	229	236	243	250
71	136	143	150	157	165	172	179	186	193	200	208	215	222	229	236	243	250	257
72	140	147	154	162	169	177	184	191	199	206	213	221	228	235	242	250	258	265
73	144	151	159	166	174	182	189	197	204	212	219	227	235	242	250	257	265	272
74	148	155	163	171	179	186	194	202	210	218	225	233	241	249	256	264	272	280
75	152	160	168	176	184	192	200	208	216	224	232	240	248	256	264	272	279	287
76	156	164	172	180	189	197	205	213	221	230	238	246	254	263	271	279	287	295

SOURCE: Adapted from *Clinical Guidelines on the Identification, Evaluation, and Treatment of Overweight and Obesity in Adults: The Evidence Report.*

Did you know?

BMI and life expectancy

Life expectancy is reduced by two to four years if your BMI is between 30 and 35. It is reduced by eight to ten years if your BMI is between 40 and 45.

Use the BMI tables above to find your ideal body weight range. For example, if you are 65 inches tall, your ideal body weight range is 114 to 144 pounds. Determining your ideal weight using BMI may not apply to you if you were never within a healthy weight range during adolescence or early adulthood. You may need to speak to your health-care provider to determine a realistic ideal weight for you. And bear in mind that the BMI does not take into account body composition or fat distribution, and thus does not differentiate between muscle mass and fat. Many muscular people and short, stocky people have a high BMI but are not necessarily at higher health risk.

Waist circumference and waist-to-hip ratio

Waist circumference is an important indicator of health risk for type 2 diabetes, hypertension and coronary heart disease. Considered at risk are men with a waist circumference greater than 40 inches (102 cm) and women with a waist circumference greater than 35 inches (88 cm).

BODY MASS INDEX TABLE

BMI	37	38	39	40	41	42	43	44	45	46	47	48	49	50	51	52	53	54
Height (inches)	Body Weight (pounds)																	
	OBESE			EXTREME OBESITY														
58	177	181	186	191	196	201	205	210	215	220	224	229	234	239	244	248	253	258
59	183	188	193	198	203	208	212	217	222	227	232	237	242	247	252	257	262	267
60	189	194	199	204	209	215	220	225	230	235	240	245	250	255	261	266	271	276
61	195	201	206	211	217	222	227	232	238	243	248	254	259	264	269	275	280	285
62	202	207	213	218	224	229	235	240	246	251	256	262	267	273	278	284	289	295
63	208	214	220	225	231	237	242	248	254	259	265	270	278	282	287	293	299	304
64	215	221	227	232	238	244	250	256	262	267	273	279	285	291	296	302	308	314
65	222	228	234	240	246	252	258	264	270	276	282	288	294	300	306	312	318	324
66	229	235	241	247	253	260	266	272	278	284	291	297	303	309	315	322	328	334
67	236	242	249	255	261	268	274	280	287	293	299	306	312	319	325	331	338	344
68	243	249	256	262	269	276	282	289	295	302	308	315	322	328	335	341	348	354
69	250	257	263	270	277	284	291	297	304	311	318	324	331	338	345	351	358	365
70	257	264	271	278	285	292	299	306	313	320	327	334	341	348	355	362	369	376
71	265	272	279	286	293	301	308	315	322	329	338	343	351	358	365	372	379	386
72	272	279	287	294	302	309	316	324	331	338	346	353	361	368	375	383	390	397
73	280	288	295	302	310	318	325	333	340	348	355	363	371	378	386	393	401	408
74	287	295	303	311	319	326	334	342	350	358	365	373	381	389	396	404	412	420
75	295	303	311	319	327	335	343	351	359	367	375	383	391	399	407	415	423	431
76	304	312	320	328	336	344	353	361	369	377	385	394	402	410	418	426	435	443

Waist-to-hip ratio is another method of determining health risk. This is calculated by dividing the circumference of the waist by the circumference of the hips. A normal waist-to-hip ratio for males is 0.95 or less and for females 0.85 or less. A high waist-to-hip ratio is associated with a three-fold increase in risk for a heart attack.

Causes of Obesity

North Americans have become increasingly sedentary during the past century or so. Mass transportation, processed convenience foods and electronic technology have made life easier, but not without consequences. Consider the days when we walked rather than drove to work, which burned calories rather than gasoline. The result is a sedentary society that is one factor in the rise of obesity. But there are many other, complex reasons why someone may become obese.

Factors causing obesity

- Genetic or hereditary factors. Research involving twins has shown that there are genetic factors at play in obesity. Weight regulation involves hormones that are genetically determined, as are the number and size of fat cells and how body fat is distributed.
- Changes in the food environment. Larger portion sizes and the availability of a wide variety of foods are associated with an increase in the number of calories consumed.
- Level of physical activity. With decreasing levels of physical activity there is an associated decrease in the number of calories used.
- Diet and exercise habits of family, friends and acquaintances. The poor eating and exercise habits of others can influence people adversely.
- Psychological factors. Some people may have a form of disordered eating, such as binge eating or night-eating syndrome, that leads to obesity.
- Medical treatments. Medications such as steroids and antidepressants can cause weight gain and retention.

All causes of obesity lead to eating more calories than needed. When more calories are taken in than are used, the body stores the calories as fat, and over time this leads to weight gain.

Did you know?

Sitting and eating too much

A survey completed in 1998 showed that 46% of American adults reported insufficient activity and 29% reported no physical activity. Only 25% of adult Americans engaged in recommended levels of physical activity. National health and nutrition surveys over the years have also shown an increase in calories consumed. The total average energy intake in 1978 was 1,969 calories. This increased to 2,200 calories in 1990.

Frequently Asked Questions

What hormones are involved in weight regulation?

Several hormones and chemicals that the body produces are involved in eating. For example, ghrelin is a hormone produced primarily by the stomach. Ghrelin tells the hypothalamus (an area in the brain) to start eating. It also slows down metabolism and the breakdown of fat. It is still unclear whether higher levels of ghrelin are associated with obesity or whether obesity cause ghrelin levels to increase.

Another hormone involved with eating is called leptin. This hormone is secreted by fat tissue. Its job is to make you feel full, which is known as satiety. Other chemicals, such as serotonin, neuropeptide Y and endorphins, are also involved in behavior related to eating. Decreases in serotonin and increases in neuropeptide Y have been shown to increase carbohydrate appetite. Neuropeptide Y increases during times of food deprivation and may be a reason why people who diet have increased appetite and food cravings.

BMI of 47

Anne is 28 years old and has a BMI of 47. She currently smokes about one package of cigarettes a day. She came to our clinic complaining that she was tired of being fat and feeling unattractive. She is afraid to quit smoking for fear of gaining more weight, because whenever she quits smoking, she tends to eat more. She has no medical conditions but says she is afraid of developing diabetes and having to inject herself with insulin.

Anne recently got married and plans to have children, but she told us she wants to lose weight and quit smoking before she starts trying to conceive a baby. Her nutritional assessment revealed that she skips breakfast almost daily and has a lot of evening snacks, usually while watching TV with her husband at night. She feels that she is at a loss and at times that there is no point in living. She told the health-care team that she is depressed. When asked about her feelings of not wanting to live, she commented that she has no intentions of or plans for suicide but just feels down. During the assessments she became quite teary on several occasions.

We recommended that she consult with the team psychiatrist regarding her mental well-being, enroll in a smoking-cessation program, become better educated about bariatric procedures, and work with the team counselors regarding her problematic eating behaviors. These concerns need to be addressed before Anne can be considered for weight-loss surgery. Anne has been brought back for further assessments and to monitor her progress while she continues to work on making positive changes to better prepare her for weight-loss surgery.

Disordered eating

Disordered eating refers to a wide range of abnormal eating behaviors, including clinical eating disorders such as anorexia and bulimia; chronic restriction; and habitual or compulsive eating. Disordered eating usually involves irregular, chaotic eating patterns, and oftentimes hunger and fullness cues are ignored.

Binge eating

About one in five obese people engage in binge eating, which refers to eating excessive amounts of food at one sitting, possibly while feeling out of control. Common reasons for binging include being hungry in response to dieting, restricting food in some way or overeating as a means of soothing oneself, avoiding uncomfortable situations or numbing feelings.

Binge-eating symptoms

- Eating large amounts of food frequently and at one sitting
- Feeling out of control and unable to stop eating
- Eating quickly
- Eating in secret or privately
- Feeling uncomfortably full after eating
- Feeling guilty and ashamed

Night-eating syndrome

With night-eating syndrome, people tend to restrict or limit their food intake during the day and then eat at night to compensate. This pattern of behavior usually causes problems with sleep.

Night-eating syndrome symptoms

- Little to no appetite for breakfast
- Eating more than half of one's food intake after dinner, with this behavior continuing for at least three months
- Feelings of tension, anxiety or guilt while eating
- Difficulty falling asleep or staying asleep
- Continually eating in the evening
- Feelings of guilt and shame from eating

Negative body image

Body image is the mental picture you have of yourself and your feelings about that picture. Body image is defined as how you perceive your appearance. Oftentimes people who are overweight or obese have a poor body image, although people who are underweight or within a healthy body-weight range may also have poor body image. Self-esteem, which is how you value yourself as a person, is closely linked to body image.

Consequences of negative body image

- Depression
- Disturbances in interpersonal functions
- Impaired sexual relationships
- Poor self-esteem
- Diminished quality of life

People have different body shapes, sizes and types. No matter how much you weigh, your body type is difficult to change. Learning to recognize your body type can help you build a positive self-image and accept your natural physique no matter what the scale says. There are three main categories of body types:

▶ Categories of body types

Endomorph	Mesomorph	Ectomorph
• broad and soft • heavy • rounded • shoulders narrower than hips • pear-shaped or apple-shaped	• muscular and blocky • broad shoulders • weight concentrated in upper body	• slender and linear • tall • small frame • narrow shoulders and hips

How do you know if you have body image issues?
• You avoid social gatherings.
• You avoid looking in the mirror.
• You avoid having your picture taken.
• You wear clothing that hides certain areas of your body

Accepting your natural curves and body shape is important for building a healthy sense of self. Be aware of the messages you send yourself. When someone compliments you, be sure to pause, take a deep breath and accept the compliment. This is an important step toward building a healthy body image.

Obesity-Related Health Problems

Obesity contributes to numerous health conditions and problems, which are known as co-morbidities. Chief among these are metabolic syndrome, which increases the risk of heart disease, stroke and diabetes.

Metabolic syndrome

The health conditions associated with obesity and metabolic syndrome include glucose intolerance, insulin resistance, hyperlipidemia (high cholesterol) and hypertension (high blood pressure). These are strongly linked to abdominal obesity.

In insulin resistance, the cells become resistant to the effects of insulin, a hormone that helps to transport glucose (sugar) into the cells. Think about it this way: imagine that insulin knocks on the doors of cells. When the cells hear the knock, they open up and let glucose in to be used. However, with insulin resistance the cells do not hear the knock clearly, so the pancreas is notified that it needs to make more insulin. Increasing the level of insulin in the blood makes the knock

Did you know?

Diabetes risk
Obesity is one of the leading factors in heart disease and stroke, as well as in type 2 diabetes. Type 2 diabetes is five times more common among obese people.

louder. Eventually the pancreas is producing more insulin than normal but the cells are still resisting the knock. Once the pancreas is not able to keep up with the demand for insulin, glucose levels in the blood rise, resulting in type 2 diabetes.

Common obesity co-morbidities

- type 2 diabetes
- impaired glucose tolerance
- gallbladder disease
- hypertension (high blood pressure)
- heart disease
- degenerative arthritis of weight-bearing joints, such as knees, and low back pain
- dyslipidemia (abnormal levels of cholesterol, lipids or fat in the blood)
- stroke
- angina (chest pain caused when the heart does not get enough blood and oxygen)
- sleep apnea (long pauses in breathing or shallow breathing while asleep)
- fatty liver disease
- gout (a disease affecting the joints)
- asthma
- some forms of cancer, especially of the breast and prostate
- impaired mobility (difficulty walking)
- poor tolerance for exercise or activity
- reproductive and fertility problems
- psychological and social effects
- depression
- varicose veins (abnormally thick, twisted or enlarged veins)
- gastroesophageal reflux disease (GERD), in which acid backs up from stomach into the esophagus

Standard Treatments for Obesity

Obesity treatments include diet therapies, physical activity, behavior modification, pharmacotherapy (drug treatment) and weight-loss surgery. The first approach to treating obesity includes any combination of diet, activity and behavior modification. The next step may include some type of drug treatment, usually in combination with a weight-loss program. If these fail, then weight-loss surgery is considered.

Obesity treatments

- diet therapies
- physical activity

- behavior modification
- pharmacotherapy (weight-loss medication)
- weight-loss surgery

Dieting

Millions of dollars are spent each year in search of the perfect weight-loss diet, and more than $33 billion is spent annually on weight-reduction products and services. Many of these diets become popular instantly, but they often do not result in permanent weight loss. Fad diets may even be dangerous. Dieting does not give you the freedom to trust your inner signals of hunger, appetite and satiety. You need to be able to trust your own feelings of fullness and satiety and to become more mindful of your eating.

Yo-yo dieting

Fad diets typically guarantee that you will lose a significant amount of weight if you follow the prescribed program, but in most cases any weight lost is soon regained. So you try again. You lose weight, then you gain weight — and maybe you end up heavier than your starting weight. This is yo-yo dieting, and yo-yo dieting leads to frustration. The diet mentality sets you up for failure time and time again. For chronic dieters, dieting is like an addiction. When they start a diet, they feel euphoric, but when the diet fails, they may experience deflated self-worth, disappointment and frustration.

<aside>
Did you know?

Regaining weight
People usually regain one-third to two-thirds of the weight lost through fad diets within one year, and almost all of the weight within five years.
</aside>

▶ Dangers of fad diets and dieting

Physical	Psychological
• inadequate nutrition • fatigue • weakness • cardiac issues • gallstone formation • hypertension • reduced bone mass • alterations in metabolism • alterations in body-fat distribution • increased risk of cardiovascular disease	• heightened responsiveness to external food cues • weight obsession • poor self-image • disordered eating patterns • excessive or inadequate exercise • increased incidence of eating disorders • sense of failure • financial burden • increased pressure to conform to society

Physical activity

Physical activity is effective in promoting and maintaining weight loss, as well as decreasing abdominal fat and improving heart function. One of the major setbacks for people who are severely obese is that physical activity can be difficult, strenuous and, for some, especially those with arthritis, painful. This makes incorporating physical activity into the weight-loss equation almost impossible until some weight loss has been achieved and activity becomes more tolerable.

Behavior modification

Behavior modification provides patients with tools for overcoming barriers to achieving successful weight loss. Examples of some strategies include

- self-monitoring eating habits and activity
- managing stress
- problem solving and planning
- rewarding specific actions
- providing a social support network

Behavior modification programs work best in combination with decreased caloric intake and increased activity.

Pharmacotherapy

Pharmacotherapy is the use of prescription medications, in this case medications designed to promote weight loss. Over the years several weight-loss medications have come on and off the market. There are different classes of weight-loss drugs, depending on how they work. Some work by suppressing the appetite, while others work by blocking the absorption of fat. Drugs are best used in combination with diet and physical activity programs.

What Is Weight-Loss Surgery?

Weight-loss surgery, also known as bariatric surgery, promotes significant and long-lasting weight loss by decreasing food intake and changing the way the body handles food.

"Bariatric" is a term for the branch of medicine that deals with the causes, prevention and treatment of obesity. *Bar-* is from the Greek root word meaning weight; *-iatr* refers to treatment; and *-ic* means pertaining to. The first reported bariatric procedure was performed in 1952 by Victor Henrickson of Norway, who removed a substantial portion of the small bowel to cause malabsorption of food ingested. There were many complications with this type of surgery, however, and during the next three decades a variety of gastric bypass surgeries were developed. In the 1990s minimally invasive laparoscopic procedures replaced open surgery. There are now several types of weight-loss surgery that have been shown to promote achievable and sustainable weight loss for people who are obese.

The Anatomy of Digestion

To understand how bariatric surgeries work, we need to review the anatomy of the digestive system, where ingestion and absorption of food occurs. It extends from the mouth and esophagus through the stomach and into the small intestine and colon. Bariatric surgery is performed on the stomach, and in some cases the small intestine, and this changes how food is digested and how nutrients are absorbed.

Components of the digestive system

The digestive system has two components: the alimentary canal and the accessory organs. The alimentary canal is also known as the digestive tract or the gut. The muscles in the walls of the digestive system move the food along from top to bottom. During this process, food is broken down into increasingly smaller particles, called nutrients. These include macronutrients (carbohydrates, proteins and fats) and micronutrients (vitamins and minerals). They move through the walls of the intestine and are absorbed into

Did you know?

Mortality
Canadian research has shown that in a five-year period, obese patients who did not have weight-loss surgery were 10 times more likely to die from any cause than patients who did have the operation.

Did you know?

Long gut
The digestive system, or gut, is 30 feet (9 m) long, which is about five times the average height of a human, or about half the length of a bowling lane.

the bloodstream, where the blood distributes the nutrients to the rest of the body to be used for its various functions. Waste — the parts of the food that the body does not use — is passed out of the body as feces. The accessory organs include the liver, pancreas and gallbladder, which work together with the gut to help in the digestion of food.

Anatomy of the Digestive Tract

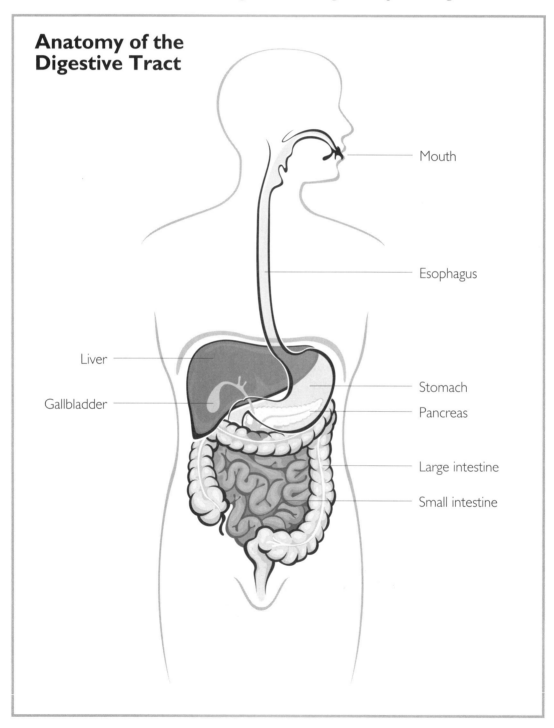

Mouth

Esophagus

Liver

Stomach

Gallbladder

Pancreas

Large intestine

Small intestine

The digestive process

Digestion begins in the mouth with the action of chewing food: an enzyme in the saliva starts to break down starches. Digestive enzymes are substances that the body produces to help break down larger pieces of food into smaller, more absorbable particles, or nutrients.

Now that the food is moist with saliva and chewed into smaller pieces, the muscle movements of the tongue and mouth carry it down the throat and into the esophagus. Waves of muscle contractions, called peristalsis, force the food down the esophagus and into the stomach.

Stomach

The stomach churns and mixes the food with acids and enzymes, breaking it down into even smaller, more digestible particles. At the bottom of the stomach is a valve called the pyloric sphincter (a sphincter is a strong, ring-like muscle that opens and closes), which is connected to the duodenum, the first part of the small intestine. The pyloric sphincter controls the rate at which digested food moves from the stomach into the intestine. Once the processed food moves into the small intestine, further digestion occurs and the nutrients begin to be absorbed.

Did you know?

Stomach capacity
The average shape and size of the stomach varies from person to person and even from one meal to the next. In general, the average stomach can expand to hold about 32 to 48 ounces (1 to 1.5 L).

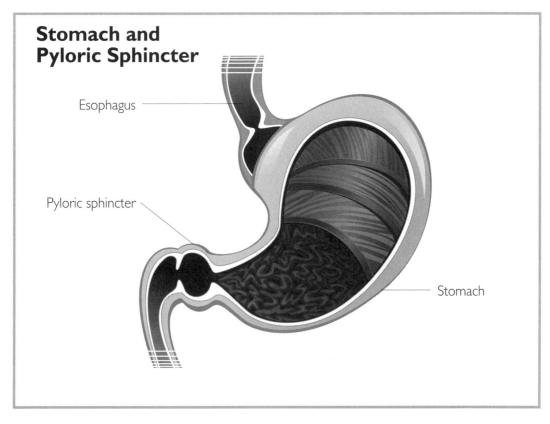

Stomach and Pyloric Sphincter

Esophagus

Pyloric sphincter

Stomach

Stomach functions

- Holds food coming from the esophagus and releases it into the duodenum
- Breaks down food mechanically using muscles that squeeze and churn
- Breaks down food chemically using acids and enzymes such as hydrochloric acid and pepsin
- Produces intrinsic factor, a substance required for the absorption of vitamin B_{12}
- Produces hormones responsible for hunger, such as ghrelin

Small intestine

The small intestine is made up of the three parts: duodenum, jejunum and ileum. The liver and pancreas, both important organs for digestion, are connected to the small intestine at the duodenum by ducts. The liver produces bile, which is responsible for helping the body absorb fat; the bile is stored in the gallbladder until needed. The pancreas produces digestive juices and enzymes that help digest proteins, fats and carbohydrates. Broken-down food meets these digestive juices and enzymes in the duodenum, where the absorption of nutrients begins, and the process continues along the entire small intestine. The walls of the intestines are covered with villi and microvilli, microscopic, finger-like projections

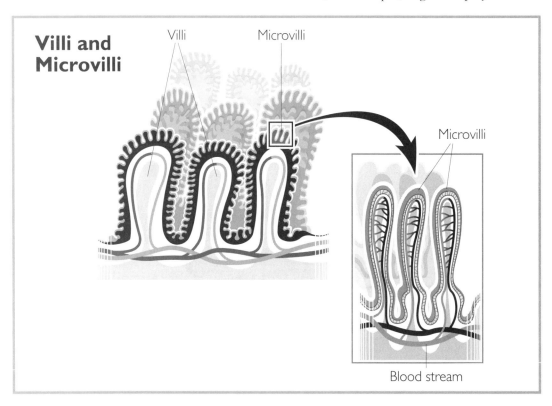

Villi and Microvilli

Villi

Microvilli

Microvilli

Blood stream

where nutrients are transported from the inside of the gut to the bloodstream. Different nutrients are primarily absorbed in specific sections of the small intestine.

▶ Common sites of nutrient absorption in the small intestine

Duodenum	Jejunum	Ileum
• iron	• iron	• vitamin B_{12}
• calcium	• zinc	• vitamin C
• magnesium	• chromium	• folate
• phosphorus	• calcium	• vitamins D and K
• copper	• phosphorus	• magnesium
• selenium	• manganese	
• vitamins A, D, E and K	• molybdenum	
• several B vitamins, including thiamine, biotin and folate	• several B vitamins	
	• vitamins A, D, E and K	
	• vitamin C	

Large intestine

By the time food reaches the last part of the alimentary canal, the large intestine, the work of absorbing nutrients is nearly finished. The large intestine removes water from the undigested matter and forms waste that is excreted as feces.

Frequently Asked Questions

I had my gallbladder removed recently. How will this affect how I digest food?

Having your gallbladder removed, also known as a cholecystectomy, is a surgical technique used to treat gallstone disease. The liver makes bile (which helps the body absorb fat) and the gallbladder stores and secretes it. When the gallbladder is removed, the liver secretes bile directly into the small intestine. Over time the body adapts: the tube that connects the liver to the small intestine expands. Food continues to be digested normally.

Bariatric Surgery Procedures

Some weight-loss procedures are restrictive in nature, meaning that the surgical procedure restricts the quantity of food that can be eaten and the rate at which the food is ingested. This limits how many calories are consumed, and weight loss will follow. Other procedures involve bypassing part of the stomach and small intestines to reduce nutrient intake and change the way the body handles digestion.

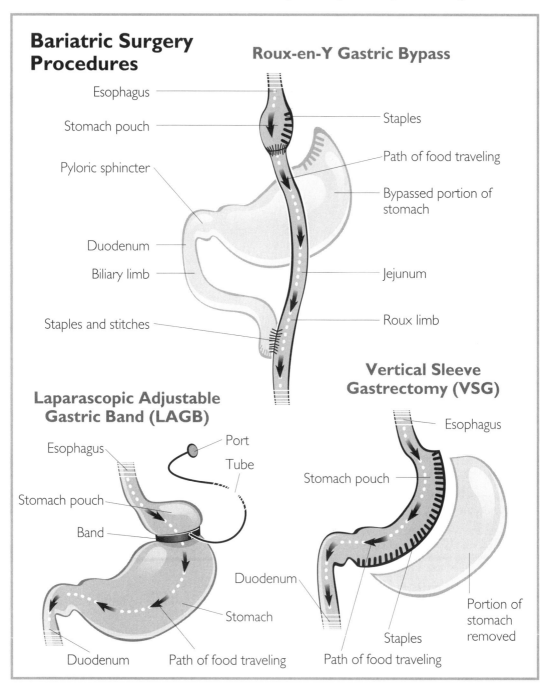

Bariatric Surgery Procedures

Roux-en-Y Gastric Bypass

Esophagus

Stomach pouch

Pyloric sphincter

Staples

Path of food traveling

Bypassed portion of stomach

Duodenum

Biliary limb

Jejunum

Staples and stitches

Roux limb

Laparascopic Adjustable Gastric Band (LAGB)

Vertical Sleeve Gastrectomy (VSG)

Esophagus

Port

Tube

Esophagus

Stomach pouch

Stomach pouch

Band

Duodenum

Stomach

Portion of stomach removed

Duodenum

Staples

Path of food traveling

Path of food traveling

Laparoscopic adjustable gastric band

The laparoscopic adjustable gastric band (LAGB) surgical procedure works by restriction. An adjustable band is implanted around the stomach under a general anesthetic, using laparoscopic surgical techniques. The band is placed around the uppermost part of the stomach, dividing it into two portions, one smaller and one larger. The band contains a small balloon in its inner diameter that can be adjusted in size by using a small port located under the skin of the abdominal wall.

The upper part of the stomach — the pouch — fills up quickly when food is eaten, which means that a smaller portion of food will cause a feeling of fullness. It is thought that stretch receptors in the upper stomach send a message to the brain that the person is satiated. The passage of food through the upper stomach into the lower occurs at a controlled rate, so most patients feel full faster. The feeling of satiety helps to control the feelings of hunger that are common in dieters. Food digestion then progresses through the normal digestive process.

Weight-loss potential

Most studies show that about 30% to 50% of excess weight is lost in the first year after LAGB surgery. Long-term weight loss is generally less than with gastric bypass surgery.

Frequently Asked Questions

How is the band adjustable?

The gastric band contains a small balloon on its inner surface. Patients with a gastric band have a small port under the skin of the abdomen that is used to make adjustments. A special needle is inserted through the skin and into this port. When fluid is added, the balloon inflates and tightens slightly around the stomach, which produces more restriction. If there is too much restriction, fluid can be removed by the same technique.

Advantages of LAGB

- The amount of food that can be consumed at a meal is restricted.
- A feeling of satiety (fullness) is produced.
- Food consumed passes through the digestive tract according to the usual processes, allowing nutrients to be fully absorbed by the body.

- It is the least invasive procedure — no stapling, cutting or intestinal rerouting is necessary.
- The treatment is adjustable and can be customized to the patient's needs.
- The operation time is shorter than for other bariatric surgeries.
- The patient can return to work within a week.
- The procedure is reversible — if the band is unsuccessful or poorly tolerated, it can be removed.
- It has the lowest short-term complication and mortality rates compared with other weight-loss operations.

Disadvantages of LAGB
- The slower rate of weight loss may not suit some people.
- The long-term durability of gastric banding is unknown — as time passes, the rates of band failure increase.
- Complications such as band erosion, slippage or looseness, dilation of the pouch, obstruction of the outlet, or nausea and vomiting may occur. These problems often require removal of the band.

CASE HISTORY
Ready for surgery

Mary is 55 years old and has a BMI of 42, type 2 diabetes and back pain. She works full-time as a real estate agent. She is financially stable and has a wonderful, supportive family. Mary has tried dieting, weight-loss regimes and exercise programs over the years, but she complains that it is difficult to be active because of her back pain. She usually eats three well-balanced meals each day. She is following a diabetes meal plan but finds it somewhat difficult to have her lunch on time if she is out with a client. She feels that the time has come to slow down her life. Her daughter is expecting her first child, and Mary wants to decrease her hours of work so she can be there to help care for her new grandchild.

   Mary came to our bariatric clinic inquiring about LAGB surgery. She met with the surgeon and various members of the health-care team for assessments and attended several educational workshops and seminars. Given her history and based on the team's assessments, they decided that she was ready for LAGB surgery.

Laparoscopic Roux-en-Y gastric bypass
In the Roux-en-Y procedure, the upper portion of the stomach is stapled, creating a small pouch that is less than an ounce (15 to 20 mL) in volume. The remainder of the stomach is not removed but is stapled completely shut and

separated from the pouch. The outlet from the newly formed stomach pouch empties directly into the lower portion of the jejunum, thus delivering food rapidly to a point farther along the digestive tract than normal. The connection is made by dividing the small intestine 20 to 30 inches (50 to 75 cm) along, just beyond the duodenum, bringing up one end (the Roux limb) and stitching or stapling it to the newly formed stomach pouch. The end still attached to the old stomach (the biliary limb) is stitched or stapled to the small intestine farther along, creating the Y shape that gives the technique its name. Each stitched or stapled connection is called an anastomosis.

The stomach pouch is about the size of your thumb and the opening between the pouch and the small intestine is about the size of a dime. This small opening is known as a gastrojejunostomy. The length of the biliary limb is usually about 20 inches (50 cm) and the length of the Roux limb is about 60 inches (150 cm); however, these lengths vary depending on the surgeon and the bariatric clinic. The length of either segment of the intestine can be increased to start digestion farther along the digestive tract.

After gastric bypass, food arrives in the small intestine much more quickly and mixes with digestive juices much farther along the digestive tract. The result is an early sense of fullness combined with a sense of satisfaction that reduces the desire to eat.

Weight-loss potential

One year after gastric bypass surgery, weight loss averages about 75% of excess body weight.

Studies show that after 10 to 14 years, a loss of 55% to 75% of excess body weight has been maintained by most patients.

Advantages of gastric bypass

- The amount of food that can be eaten at once is restricted.
- The small pouch produces a feeling of fullness.
- Bypassing the upper digestive tract has a profound beneficial effect on metabolic conditions such as diabetes, high blood pressure and high cholesterol.
- Quick and dramatic weight loss results.
- Health problems associated with obesity improve.
- Mobility and quality of life are improved.
- Average weight loss after the gastric bypass procedure is generally higher for a compliant patient than with restrictive procedures.

Did you know?

Gold standard

According to the American Society for Metabolic and Bariatric Surgery and the National Institutes of Health, the Roux-en-Y gastric bypass is the most frequently performed weight-loss surgery in the United States. This type of gastric bypass is also the most commonly performed bariatric surgery in Canada, and it is considered the gold standard of weight-loss surgeries.

Disadvantages of gastric bypass

- The patient requires lifelong supplementation with vitamins and minerals.
- The procedure is difficult to reverse and should be considered permanent.
- Dumping syndrome — rapid gastric emptying — leads to unpleasant symptoms ranging from fainting to nausea, vomiting and diarrhea.
- There is a risk of medical complications.
- Rapid weight loss may cause increased risk of gallstones.
- Hair loss and loss of bone density may be caused by a rapid decrease in weight.

Laparoscopic vertical sleeve gastrectomy

In vertical sleeve gastrectomy (VSG), the stomach is stapled vertically, leaving about 15% of it shaped like a sleeve or a banana. The larger portion of the stomach is then removed. With inflammation and swelling present, the remaining sleeve, or pouch, holds about 4 to 6 ounces (125 to 175 mL). This procedure is restrictive in that it controls how much can be eaten before you feel full. With only 15% of the stomach remaining, fewer hunger hormones are produced in the stomach.

VSG is a relatively new weight-loss surgery. It was initially used as the first step in a two-stage procedure for patients who had a very high BMI or were too unhealthy to have full gastric bypass or duodenal switch surgery as their first procedure. Many of these patients lost enough weight after their VSG that they did not require the second surgery. This fact has increased interest in VSG as a sole procedure for morbidly obese patients. Its main advantage is that it is generally simpler to perform than a gastric bypass and avoids the risk of the malabsorption and dumping syndrome that can occur with gastric bypass.

Advantages of VSG

- Reduced stomach volume increases feelings of fullness.
- The stomach functions relatively normally.
- Most foods are tolerated, but in smaller amounts.
- The portion of the stomach that produces hunger hormones (ghrelin) is removed.
- No dumping syndrome results.
- No intestinal bypass, with its associated risks, is required.
- The procedure is simpler than a gastric bypass.
- Patients who do not lose enough weight can go on to have a gastric bypass.

Did you know?

Metabolic surgery

"Metabolic surgery" is the term that has been coined for the future of bariatric surgery. Emerging techniques, such as VSG, duodenal-jejunal bypass and endoluminal sleeves, have shown promising results for treating metabolic syndrome and diabetes.

- Less time is required in surgery and the hospital stay is shorter.

Disadvantages of VSG

- Risks may be higher for inadequate weight loss or weight regain compared to gastric bypass surgery.
- The procedure is irreversible.
- Some surgeons and insurance companies consider the procedure investigational.
- There is potential for stretching (dilation) of the sleeve pouch.
- Heartburn can develop or become worse.
- Leaks from the staple line can take a very long time to heal.
- Long-term effectiveness data are not yet available.

Duodenal switch

The duodenal switch is another operation used for weight loss in some bariatric clinics. It involves some restriction but mostly relies on a profound bypass of the digestive tract. The stomach is reduced in size, creating a sleeve, as in VSG. More than half the small intestine is then bypassed and the smaller stomach is reconnected to the shortened small intestine. This operation has the advantage of the greatest amount of weight loss but is also associated with the highest rate of short- and long-term complications, so it is not widely used.

Intragastric balloon

In the intragastric balloon procedure, an inflatable balloon is inserted into the stomach and then filled with sterile water (saline solution). The balloon floats around in the stomach, taking up space and restricting how much can be eaten. The balloon can remain in the stomach for only about six months. This procedure is gaining popularity in Canada and the United States, but it does not have the same effects as metabolic surgeries. In the United Kingdom the intragastric balloon is used primarily to help patients with a very high BMI lose some weight to reduce their operative risk for gastric bypass surgery. In the private sector some people pay for this surgery as a stand-alone method for weight loss.

Testing and screening

Your doctor may request a series of tests to check for other conditions before going ahead with your bariatric surgery. Note that bariatric clinics may have different criteria for pre-operative testing.

Did you know?

Choosing the right surgical procedure
Several studies have shown that the most successful bariatric procedure in terms of percentage of long-term weight loss is the Roux-en-Y gastric bypass. However, your doctor will recommend the best procedure for you, weighing the advantages and disadvantages and bearing in mind your medical history.

▶ Some common tests and procedures

Test	Reason
Sleep study	to help with airway management during surgery and prevent lung complications after surgery
Cardiac tests (EKG, ECG, stress test)	if clinically indicated by a doctor
Laboratory blood work	to look for metabolic abnormalities, including vitamin and mineral deficiencies
Dental exam	to ensure that good dentition exists so the patient can properly chew food
Gastroscopy	if surgeon is concerned about anatomy of the gastrointestinal tract or if patient has gastrointestinal symptoms necessitating investigation
Chest X-ray	if clinically indicated
Psychological evaluation	if there is concern that psychological issues exist
Bone density scan	to serve as a baseline

CASE HISTORY

Can't lose weight

George is 45 years old, with a BMI of 55, and he has sleep apnea, type 2 diabetes, hypertension and high cholesterol. During college he started to gain a significant amount of weight. By the time he graduated, his BMI had reached 50. He tried several fad diets in his late 20s. During the past five years, under the care of his physician and his diabetes health-care team, he has been able to maintain his weight and control his blood sugars. However, he cannot seem to lose weight.

After discussions with his family, George decided it was time to take things more seriously, so he consulted with his physician about being referred to a bariatric program to be considered for weight-loss surgery. While awaiting initial consultation with the bariatric team, he began researching and learning about the various procedures. He is seriously considering having a gastric bypass. When he met with the surgeon and members of the health-care team for various assessments, he was advised to attend several educational workshops and seminars. Given George's history and based on their assessments, they decided gastric bypass surgery would be an effective answer to his need to lose excess weight.

Laparoscopic versus open surgery

The various bariatric surgeries can now be performed laparoscopically instead of making a large incision to allow the surgeon access inside the patient. Laparoscopic surgery is video-assisted and uses a number of tiny incisions (keyholes) — typically about $\frac{1}{4}$ to $\frac{1}{2}$ inch (5 to 12 mm) long — through the patient's abdominal wall. One incision is used for a video camera and the rest are for the long, slender instruments the surgeon needs to perform the surgery, which are inserted through tubes called trocars, or ports.

Most bariatric procedures use between four and five trocars. Usually the port for the camera is near the umbilicus (belly button). Two ports are used by the surgeon (one for each hand), one port is used by his or her assistant and one is used to hold the left end of the liver out of the way.

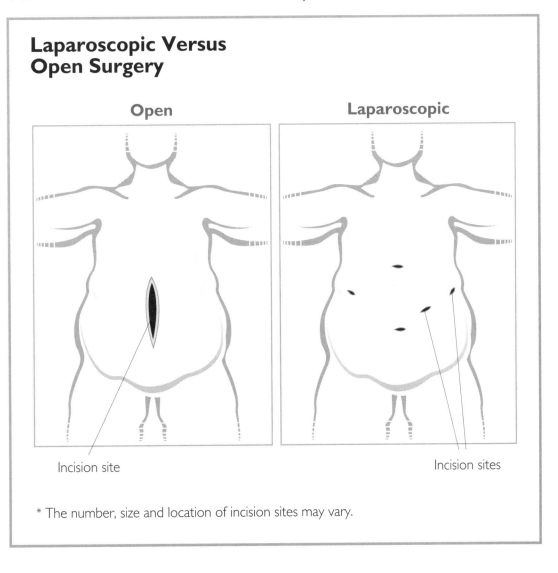

Laparoscopic Versus Open Surgery

Open

Laparoscopic

Incision site

Incision sites

* The number, size and location of incision sites may vary.

Laparoscopic surgery generally allows a procedure inside the abdomen to be performed with much less injury to the patient. This usually translates into much less pain, fewer complications, a quicker recovery and a better cosmetic result.

Frequently Asked Questions

How long does each surgical procedure take if it is done laparoscopically?

Depending on the experience of the surgical team, a gastric bypass takes an average of one to two hours. LAGB and VSG procedures take a little less time, on average a half-hour to one hour.

Risks and Benefits of Surgery

Now that you have an understanding of how bariatric surgery works to reduce weight, you can consult with your doctor to weigh the risks and benefits of each procedure.

Risks of weight-loss surgery

All weight-loss surgeries come with some risk, including serious complications. Each surgical procedure also has its own individual risk factors.

Some possible complications of weight-loss surgery

- blood loss requiring a transfusion
- blood clots in the legs or lungs
- heart attack or stroke
- kidney failure
- complications from anesthetic
- infection at one or more of the incisions (rare with laparoscopy)
- blockage of the bowel because of scar tissue
- hernia
- pneumonia
- bladder infection
- ulcers in the stomach or intestine
- gallstones that may require the gallbladder to be surgically removed
- death

Risks of Roux-en-Y gastric bypass surgery

Early complications of gastric bypass surgery include leaks at one of the anastomoses (the stapled or stitched connections). Stomach and intestinal contents may leak into the abdomen, which can lead to infection and possibly further surgery. This is a serious complication, even if it is detected early. Later complications can include (among others) bowel obstruction, nutritional deficiency, anastomotic stricture (narrowing caused by scarring) and changes in pouch size. A gastric bypass is difficult to reverse and the procedure should be considered permanent.

Gastric bypass risks

- leakage of digestive contents around staples and stitches, leading to infection, which can be life threatening
- blood clots in the legs
- damage to adjacent organs
- stricture, or narrowing of the opening between the stomach and the intestine
- dumping syndrome, which can lead to hypoglycemia (low blood sugars)
- abdominal hernia (rare with laparoscopy)
- gallstones
- dehydration
- gastric or intestinal ulcers
- abscess (accumulation of pus caused by infection)
- malabsorption of nutrients

Malabsorption of nutrients

When the duodenum is bypassed, absorption of micronutrients is decreased. Iron is absorbed primarily in the duodenum, so there is a greater risk of iron-deficiency anemia. This is of particular concern for patients who experience chronic blood loss from excessive menstrual flow or bleeding hemorrhoids, and for those who have difficulty ingesting enough iron-rich food.

Did you know?

Blood clots
Blood clots in the legs may be prevented by walking as soon as possible after surgery and, if recommended by your physician, by taking a prescribed anticoagulant (a medication that stops blood from clotting) such as tinzaparin (Innohep) injections or warfarin (Coumadin) orally.

Did you know?

Bone density
With any type of weight-loss surgery, it is generally recommended that you have a baseline bone density scan before the operation, and then every two years thereafter.

Did you know?

Difficult to detect
The bypassed portions of the stomach, duodenum and small intestine cannot be easily viewed by using X-rays or endoscopy. If problems such as ulcers, bleeding or malignancy should occur, they may be difficult to detect.

Calcium is also absorbed in the duodenum, and bypassing of the duodenum brings an increased risk of osteoporosis or other metabolic bone disease, resulting in bone pain, loss of height, a humped back and fractures of the ribs and hipbones. People who are already at risk for osteoporosis should be aware of the potential for greater bone calcium loss.

Chronic anemia caused by vitamin B_{12} deficiency can also occur, but this problem can usually be managed by taking a vitamin B_{12} supplement. Thiamine (vitamin B_1) can become depleted quickly, especially in the case of excessive vomiting, which can result in neurological problems. Routine bone density screening and laboratory assessments, including blood work and urinalysis, are vital in the prevention and treatment of these risks.

Dumping syndrome

A condition known as dumping syndrome can occur as a result of rapid emptying of the stomach contents into the small intestine. Dumping syndrome is triggered when too much sugar and possibly fat are consumed. While generally not considered to be a serious risk to your health, the results can be extremely unpleasant — nausea, weakness, sweating, faintness, vomiting and diarrhea, and, in some cases, low blood sugar (hypoglycemia). This can be avoided by adhering to dietary recommendations.

Risks of the laparoscopic adjustable gastric band

The LAGB procedure has its own unique complications, as well as some complications in common with gastric bypass surgery.

LAGB risks

- gastric perforation, or tearing in the stomach wall, which could require further surgery (this is rare)
- breaks in the balloon, causing leakage of saline
- leakage or twisting of the access port, possibly requiring an additional operation
- scar tissue buildup around the band, causing blockages and possibly infection
- infection
- bleeding

- band erosion (wear), migration or slippage
- outlet obstruction, in which the narrowed opening of the stomach may get blocked
- lack of satisfaction after eating (a feeling that one has not had enough to eat)
- nausea and vomiting
- pouch dilation
- failure to lose weight
- esophageal reflux (regurgitation or heartburn), especially in the evening, which is a sign that the lap band may have slipped

Risks of vertical sleeve gastrectomy

The risks associated with vertical sleeve gastrectomy are similar to gastric bypass and LAGB procedures. However, leakage is more serious in VSG procedures.

VSG risks
- blood clots
- damage to adjacent organs
- leakage of digestive contents from staple line, leading to infection
- abscess
- reflux

Benefits of weight-loss surgery

Many positive health benefits can be attributed to weight-loss surgery. The ultimate goal of all bariatric surgeries is to help you live a healthier and longer life. The benefits may outweigh the risks.

Possible benefits of weight-loss surgery for pre-existing health conditions
- resolved or improved high blood pressure
- improved lipid (cholesterol) levels
- improvement or cure of type 2 diabetes
- reduced risk of heart disease
- resolved or improved sleep apnea
- less joint or back pain, as well as less degenerative disk and joint disease
- increased mobility (ability to move around and walk)
- increased tolerance for activity or exercise
- improved quality of life

Recovery from Surgery

After surgery you will need to take time to recover and heal. The process is challenging both physically and psychologically, as your body is going through changes and your life is changing too. Things will be different, and sometimes change can be difficult. Having someone to support you during the recovery stage is helpful.

Tips for a safe recovery

- To prevent blood clots and promote blood circulation, avoid sitting or standing without moving for long periods of time.
- Climbing stairs is safe and is actually encouraged.
- Avoid driving until you are off prescription pain medications and feeling alert enough (usually about a week). Be sure to get clearance from your surgeon or physician first.

Frequently Asked Questions

How long will I stay in the hospital or clinic? And what is the average recovery time?

Gastric bypass and VSG patients generally require a hospital stay of two to four nights, although this can vary slightly from center to center. Recovery time is usually between four and six weeks. Most people can comfortably resume the normal activities of daily living by that time. The LAGB procedure can be done as day surgery; if all goes well the patient goes home the same day (some centers recommend a two-hour stay). Recovery time for the LAGB is about one week.

Hygiene

Keeping yourself clean after surgery helps to prevent infections. Wash your hands frequently, especially before and after eating or drinking and using the restroom. Shower as soon as you are able to, washing your entire body well with mild soap and water (avoid scrubbing incision sites). Rinse thoroughly and pat the incision sites dry with a clean towel.

Wound care

If your surgery was done laparoscopically, you will have sutures (stitches) at the incision sites with tape over them. The sutures are usually the kind that dissolve on their own, and the tape that covers them usually falls off on its own as well. If you required surgical staples to close the incision site, the surgeon will usually remove them around the 10th day after surgery. If you think that an incision site may be infected, contact your health-care professional as soon as possible.

Normal symptoms after weight-loss surgery
- mild swelling and bruising at incision sites
- numbness at incision sites
- itching at incision sites as the skin and nerve ends heal
- pain and discomfort that is relieved by pain medication and not getting worse
- redness of scars (the red, dark pink or purplish scars can take about a year to fade)

Signs and symptoms of incision site infection
- redness and swelling
- leakage of pus
- red streaks
- yellowish or greenish purulent drainage, with or without smell
- cloudy drainage
- soreness
- fever over 100.4°F (38°C)

▶ **Pain medication after weight-loss surgery**

Recommended		Not Recommended	
• acetaminophen (Tylenol) • oxycodone + acetaminophen (Percocet)	• narcotic pain patches • morphine (MS Contin) • codeine	non-steroidal anti-inflammatory drugs (NSAIDs) such as • ibuprofen (Advil, Motrin) • naproxen (Naprosyn, Aleve)	salicylates such as • acetylsalicylic acid (ASA) • Aspirin

Medical concerns
Seek immediate medical attention if you experience one or more of the following:

- fever over 100.4°F (38°C) or shaking chills
- increase in pulse rate while at rest
- pain in the legs, especially if the pain is only on one side and the leg is swollen or red, which are signs of a blood clot
- chest pain with shortness of breath
- pain in the upper back, chest or left shoulder

All narcotics, such as morphine and codeine, can cause constipation and should be taken under medical supervision. NSAIDs can cause ulcers. If you must take them, they should be used in combination with a proton-pump inhibitor medication.

- pain that is unrelieved by pain medication
- difficulty breathing
- increased pain at any incision site
- drainage from an incision site that is cloudy, smelly or pus-like
- persistent pain, nausea or vomiting after eating
- severe swelling and bruising at the incision sites
- prolonged periods of diarrhea
- signs of bladder infection, such as urinating more often than usual, burning, pain, bleeding or hesitancy when urinating
- persistent hiccups
- depression that worsens or unusual fatigue
- changes in mental status, such as disorientation or forgetfulness
- inability to pass a bowel movement and abdominal swelling and discomfort

Frequently Asked Questions

If I have a stricture, what can be done?

If a stricture is suspected, you will need to undergo a gastroscopy or an x-ray swallow study. This involves drinking a liquid that will show up on an X-ray, indicating flows in the stomach and small intestine. The test can show if there is narrowing in the gut (stricture) or any ulceration or inflammation. A stricture can occur between the stomach and small intestine after gastric bypass surgery and may require stretching (dilation) using a balloon. The surgeon inserts a gastroscope into the esophagus and stomach, with a balloon attached that can be inflated to open up the stricture. This procedure is usually a day operation and is not usually done until four to six weeks after surgery.

What can happen to me if I have a leak?

The usual symptoms of leakage include an increase in pulse rate while at rest, decreased blood pressure, low blood hemoglobin levels and/or a feeling of impending doom. A CT scan can be done to determine if a leak if present. The surgical team will investigate either laparoscopically or with open surgery to find and repair the cause. Depending on the situation, you may or may not require drainage tubes to be inserted to collect infected fluids.

Measures of Success

Loss of weight is one measure of success for any bariatric procedure, but there are other important measures, including resolution or improvement of health conditions and an increased quality of life.

As time progresses after surgery, the rate of weight loss starts to slow down. The general goal is not to plateau, or stop losing weight, in the first year after surgery. Some patients do experience a short temporary plateau and then start to lose again. Temporary short plateaus are normal.

Calculating percent excess weight loss

Weight loss is typically calculated as percent excess weight loss to measure how much the surgery has helped. This measure is often used in the medical literature, and your health-care team will use it to determine if you are on track with expected weight loss. This is calculated by determining how much you need to lose, which is your excess weight. The amount of weight lost at a given time, divided by the excess weight and multiplied by 100, gives the percent excess weight loss.

For example, say you weighed 300 pounds (136 kg) at the time of your surgery and your ideal weight is 140 pounds (63.5 kg). Your excess weight is your starting weight less your ideal weight: 300 pounds – 140 pounds = 160 pounds (72.5 kg).

Let's say that one year after weight-loss surgery, you have lost 110 pounds (50 kg). Now divide the weight you've lost by your excess weight and multiply by 100 to get a percentage: 110 pounds / 160 pounds x 100 = 69%. This is your percent excess weight loss.

Gastric bypass success

After gastric bypass surgery, a percent excess weight loss of 60% to 70% at one year is considered ideal. Another target that some health-care professionals use is the loss of 100 pounds (45 kg) in the first year. During the initial few months, a weight loss of about 4 to 7 pounds (1.8 to 3 kg) per week can be expected, depending on the starting BMI. A higher BMI at the beginning usually results in a quicker rate of weight loss. After the first few months, weight loss will slow down to about 1 to 2 pounds (0.5 to 1 kg) per week.

LAGB success

Patients who undergo LAGB procedures generally achieve a percent excess weight loss of approximately 50%, but this can vary. The usual rate of weight loss is about 1 to 2 pounds (0.5 to 1 kg) each week, once the band has been adjusted to the optimum level of restriction for the individual (which can take time), but it can be quicker in the case of a higher BMI.

VSG success

Early reports suggest that patients can lose about 65% of excess weight within two years of the VSG procedure. The rate of weight loss is slower than after a gastric bypass.

Emotional changes

After weight-loss surgery, patients undergo a period of emotional and psychological change. It is important for you to realize that weight loss will not solve all your problems in life. Be sure not to undermine any emotional changes you experience during this journey, and do seek support.

Body image

Having a healthy body image means feeling at home in your body and accepting yourself for who you are. After weight-loss surgery, as you lose weight you may find it difficult to accept your new reflection in the mirror. You may feel as if the person in the mirror is not you. Some patients do not really see their new reflection, still perceiving themselves as they were when they were obese. Feelings of self-worth and self-esteem come from your inner being. An improved appearance may help you feel better, but you are still the same person inside.

If you have been battling your weight for as long as you can remember, looking at yourself in the mirror may be a very different experience for you after surgery. You may not recognize the person looking back at you. Remember that you are still the same inside. Seeing someone in the mirror who looks so different may encourage you to be more outgoing, more social; on the other hand, you may be uncomfortable with the weight loss and become more quiet or shy. Getting accustomed to the new you will take time. It will be a time of both excitement and worry, joy and sadness. It may feel as if you are saying goodbye to who you used to be — a new chapter of your life is beginning.

Tips to promote a healthy body image

- Change your self-talk. Send yourself positive messages such as I have an inviting smile; I have nice eyes; I am

Did you know?

Reclaiming your life
When people who want to have weight-loss surgery first meet with their health-care team, they are often asked, Why do you want surgery? They may respond that they want their life back, or that they want an improved quality of life. Your reasons for wanting to lose weight should not be forgotten.

intelligent; I am fun. Decrease your negative self-messages such as I am ugly; I have thick ankles; I am worthless.

- Learn to accept compliments from others and practice saying thank you.
- Acknowledge your accomplishments and successes — and review them frequently.
- Learn to laugh.
- Develop affirmations that focus on a new attitude about your body.
- Ditch the scale.
- Exercise for fitness rather than appearance.
- Avoid comparisons.
- Talk to a health-care professional.
- Take pictures of yourself monthly or weekly and compare the way you look.
- Try on clothes in different sizes.
- Hug yourself.
- Treat yourself to a massage.
- Nurture your body and your senses with scented body creams, perfume or cologne.
- Practice yoga.
- Tape written compliments to your bathroom mirror.

Excess skin

After weight loss you will have excess skin. Some people can afford plastic surgery and some can't. If you cannot afford the surgery, you will have to think of ways to come to terms with the excess skin, such as hiding it by dressing differently. Some feel that the benefits of weight loss outweigh the bother of excess skin. Learning to love yourself from the inside out is what truly healthy self-esteem is built on. Living as we do in a society that places so much emphasis on physical beauty, learning to feel comfortable in one's own body can be difficult. Work on building your self-esteem and becoming content with who you are.

Replacement addictions

Many people have emotional eating habits, meaning that they use food for reasons other than true physiological need. We encourage addressing emotional eating tendencies prior to having surgery, to help prevent developing replacement addictions afterward. If you are used to turning to food for comfort or to deal with certain emotions or difficult situations, after surgery you may not be able to do so. Life goes on after surgery, and you will still have to confront upsetting, stressful events. If you have not conquered your

> ### Did you know?
>
> **Cosmetic surgery**
> Body image may sometimes improve following significant weight loss, but research has shown that about two-thirds of patients who have undergone weight-loss surgery report dissatisfaction with their body because of sagging excess skin on the breasts, thighs and abdomen. Some people may become depressed as a result. This leads many bariatric patients to desire plastic surgery, which is not always possible.

emotional eating tendencies, you may be tempted to turn to other measures, such as smoking, gambling, excessive shopping, alcohol or drug abuse, or other replacement addictions. Learn what triggers your addictive behaviors and get help to develop coping mechanisms.

Frequently Asked Questions

When can I become pregnant after surgery?

Pregnancy should be avoided for the first one to two years after surgery, depending on the type of surgery and the center's or surgeon's recommendation. Pregnancy during this time could cause complications and nutritional deficiencies for you and your baby, possibly resulting in birth defects. You need to take precautions to prevent pregnancy, even if you had difficulty getting pregnant before the surgery. Rapid weight loss increases fertility, so you must be more careful.

If you do become pregnant, close monitoring by your health-care team is important to check for nutrient deficiencies and to ensure that you are gaining an appropriate amount of weight and following a well-balanced diet. You will need to take a special prenatal vitamin and mineral supplement that is higher in certain nutrients that are important during pregnancy, such as folic acid and iron. You will also need to continue taking your other vitamin and mineral supplements. Your registered dietitian can help ensure that you are taking the correct supplements and following a healthy, well-balanced diet, while also providing you with suggestions for dealing with pregnancy-related symptoms that may hinder your nutritional intake. For more information about pregnancy after weight-loss surgery, speak to your health-care professional.

Part 2

Nutritional Needs Before and After Surgery

Healthy Eating

In the days prior to your weight-loss surgery and thereafter, you will need to change your eating habits — not only what you eat but also how you eat. You will need to keep up your energy levels and nutritional health by strategically eating a balanced diet of nutrient-rich foods. Eating strategies will include adapting standard food guides to your needs, avoiding some foods and supplementing with vitamins and minerals as recommended.

Food Guides

Studying the chief national food guides — the United States Department of Agriculture (USDA) MyPyramid diet and exercise guide, Eating Well with Canada's Food Guide and the Eatwell Plate from the United Kingdom — is the best place to start getting a handle on healthy eating. These guides classify food according to common groups, recommend how much to eat from each food group daily to maintain good health and caution against eating too many servings of specific foods, such as those with a high sugar, fat or salt content.

While classification of foods into groups is helpful for understanding the basics of good nutrition, the amount of food that you consume after surgery will be significantly less than for the average population, so the recommended serving sizes will not be helpful for you. Instead you will need to follow the recommendations for number of daily servings and portion sizes given in this book and by your health-care team.

The value of healthy eating

- Intake of adequate nutrients for good health, including vitamins and minerals important for growth and development
- Lowered risk of diseases such as type 2 diabetes, heart disease and certain types of cancer
- Achievement and maintenance of a healthy body weight
- Increased energy levels
- Stronger muscles and bones
- Improved overall health and well-being
- Enhanced quality of life

Did you know?

Mindful eating
Although your food choices can significantly affect your overall health and well-being, consideration must also be given to why you choose to eat. Are you physically hungry, or are you choosing to eat because you have a craving? Do you seek emotional comfort from food? Mindful eating is an important concept that will help you become more aware of your physical hunger and satiety cues to guide your decisions to begin and to stop eating.

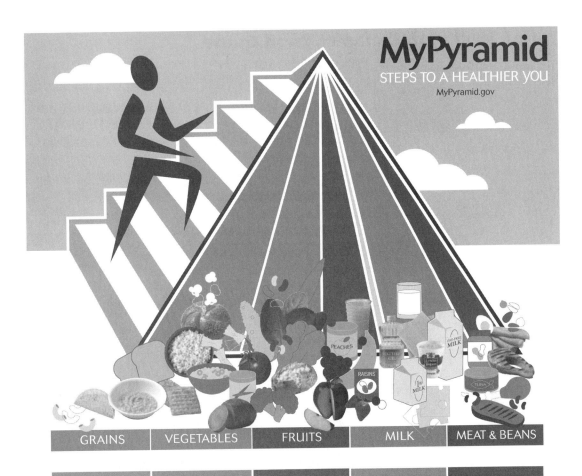

MyPyramid
STEPS TO A HEALTHIER YOU
MyPyramid.gov

GRAINS	VEGETABLES	FRUITS	MILK	MEAT & BEANS

GRAINS Make half your grains whole	VEGETABLES Vary your veggies	FRUITS Focus on fruits	MILK Get your calcium-rich foods	MEAT & BEANS Go lean with protein
Eat at least 3 oz. of whole-grain cereals, breads, crackers, rice, or pasta every day 1 oz. is about 1 slice of bread, about 1 cup of breakfast cereal, or ½ cup of cooked rice, cereal, or pasta	Eat more dark-green veggies like broccoli, spinach, and other dark leafy greens Eat more orange vegetables like carrots and sweetpotatoes Eat more dry beans and peas like pinto beans, kidney beans, and lentils	Eat a variety of fruit Choose fresh, frozen, canned, or dried fruit Go easy on fruit juices	Go low-fat or fat-free when you choose milk, yogurt, and other milk products If you don't or can't consume milk, choose lactose-free products or other calcium sources such as fortified foods and beverages	Choose low-fat or lean meats and poultry Bake it, broil it, or grill it Vary your protein routine — choose more fish, beans, peas, nuts, and seeds

For a 2,000-calorie diet, you need the amounts below from each food group. To find the amounts that are right for you, go to MyPyramid.gov.

Eat 6 oz. every day	Eat 2½ cups every day	Eat 2 cups every day	Get 3 cups every day; for kids aged 2 to 8, it's 2	Eat 5½ oz. every day

Find your balance between food and physical activity
- Be sure to stay within your daily calorie needs.
- Be physically active for at least 30 minutes most days of the week.
- About 60 minutes a day of physical activity may be needed to prevent weight gain.
- For sustaining weight loss, at least 60 to 90 minutes a day of physical activity may be required.
- Children and teenagers should be physically active for 60 minutes every day, or most days.

Know the limits on fats, sugars, and salt (sodium)
- Make most of your fat sources from fish, nuts, and vegetable oils.
- Limit solid fats like butter, stick margarine, shortening, and lard, as well as foods that contain these.
- Check the Nutrition Facts label to keep saturated fats, trans fats, and sodium low.
- Choose food and beverages low in added sugars. Added sugars contribute calories with few, if any, nutrients.

MyPyramid.gov
STEPS TO A HEALTHIER YOU

U.S. Department of Agriculture
Center for Nutrition Policy and Promotion
April 2005
CNPP-15

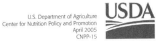

Eating Well with Canada's Food Guide

Recommended Number of *Food Guide Servings* per Day

	Children			Teens		Adults			
Age in Years	2-3	4-8	9-13	14-18		19-50		51+	
Sex	Girls and Boys			Females	Males	Females	Males	Females	Males
Vegetables and Fruit	4	5	6	7	8	7-8	8-10	7	7
Grain Products	3	4	6	6	7	6-7	8	6	7
Milk and Alternatives	2	2	3-4	3-4	3-4	2	2	3	3
Meat and Alternatives	1	1	1-2	2	3	2	3	2	3

What is One Food Guide Serving?
Look at the examples below.

Fresh, frozen or canned vegetables
125 mL (½ cup)

Bread
1 slice (35 g)

Bagel
½ bagel (45 g)

Milk or powdered milk (reconstituted)
250 mL (1 cup)

Cooked fish, shellfish, poultry, lean meat
75 g (2 ½ oz.)/125 mL (½ cup)

The chart above shows how many Food Guide Servings you need from each of the four food groups every day.

Having the amount and type of food recommended and following the tips in *Canada's Food Guide* will help:

• Meet your needs for vitamins, minerals and other nutrients.
• Reduce your risk of obesity, type 2 diabetes, heart disease, certain types of cancer and osteoporosis.
• Contribute to your overall health and vitality.

For the full guide, please contact Health Canada or visit their website.

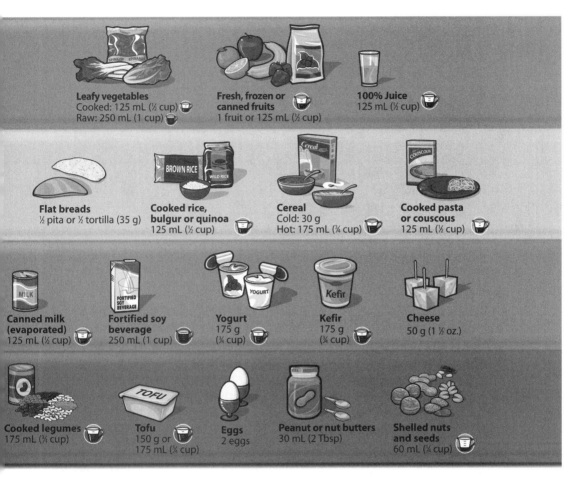

Leafy vegetables
Cooked: 125 mL (½ cup)
Raw: 250 mL (1 cup)

Fresh, frozen or canned fruits
1 fruit or 125 mL (½ cup)

100% Juice
125 mL (½ cup)

Flat breads
½ pita or ½ tortilla (35 g)

Cooked rice, bulgur or quinoa
125 mL (½ cup)

Cereal
Cold: 30 g
Hot: 175 mL (¾ cup)

Cooked pasta or couscous
125 mL (½ cup)

Canned milk (evaporated)
125 mL (½ cup)

Fortified soy beverage
250 mL (1 cup)

Yogurt
175 g
(¾ cup)

Kefir
175 g
(¾ cup)

Cheese
50 g (1 ½ oz.)

Cooked legumes
175 mL (¾ cup)

Tofu
150 g or
175 mL (¾ cup)

Eggs
2 eggs

Peanut or nut butters
30 mL (2 Tbsp)

Shelled nuts and seeds
60 mL (¼ cup)

Oils and Fats

- Include a small amount – 30 to 45 mL (2 to 3 Tbsp) – of unsaturated fat each day. This includes oil used for cooking, salad dressings, margarine and mayonnaise.
- Use vegetable oils such as canola, olive and soybean.
- Choose soft margarines that are low in saturated and trans fats.
- Limit butter, hard margarine, lard and shortening.

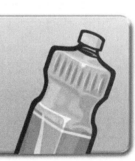

The eatwell plate

Use the eatwell plate to help you get the balance right. It shows how much of what you eat should come from each food group.

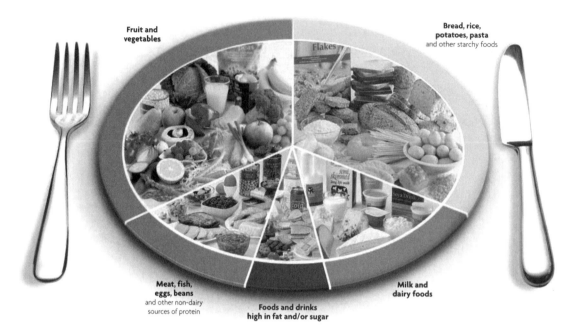

Fruit and vegetables

Bread, rice, potatoes, pasta
and other starchy foods

Meat, fish, eggs, beans
and other non-dairy
sources of protein

Foods and drinks
high in fat and/or sugar

Milk and
dairy foods

Glossary of nutrition terms

The language of nutrition can be complicated. Here is a brief glossary of some of the more difficult terms.

Antioxidants are substances that prevent or slow oxidative damage to the body. When cells use oxygen, they make free radicals, which can cause damage. Antioxidants act as free-radical scavengers, repairing the damage done by free radicals and enhancing the immune system. They are abundant in vegetables and fruit and are also found in grains, teas, legumes and nuts. The most common antioxidants are vitamin C, vitamin E, lycopene, coenzyme Q10 and beta-carotene.

Fatty acids are produced when fat breaks down in the body. They are needed for many important functions in the body, including cell membrane function and transportation of oxygen. **Essential fatty acids** are fatty acids that the body needs but cannot make on its own. For example, omega-3 fatty acids are essential fatty acids. Omega-3 must be obtained from food or supplements. **Eicosapentaenoic acid (EPA)** and **docasahexaenoic acid (DHA)** are omega-3 fatty acids that are used by the body for heart health and for the development of the brain and eyes.

Iron helps to carry oxygen to all parts of your body. **Heme iron**, found in meat, fish and poultry, is well absorbed by the body. **Non-heme iron**, found in beans and lentils, whole grains, vegetables, nuts and seeds and eggs is not so well absorbed. Combining a non-heme-iron food with a food rich in vitamin C, such as citrus fruit, helps to increase the absorption of non-heme iron. Combining a non-heme-iron food with a food rich in heme iron also helps to increase absorption.

Units of measure usually used for nutrients include the gram (g), milligram (mg), microgram (mcg) and international unit (IU).

Food groups

Food guides classify various food items into food groups according to their nutritional profile.

Vegetables and fruit

Vegetables and fruit contain a substantial amount of the vitamins, minerals, fiber and antioxidants essential to good health. Choose a variety of colorful vegetables and fruits daily, especially dark green and dark orange ones, and prepare them with little or no added fat, sugar or salt. Enjoy vegetables steamed, baked or stir-fried instead of deep-fried or with added sauces, fats and gravy.

Limit juice, as it is high in sugar. Even if the label says 100% unsweetened, juice is full of natural sugars. Eat fresh fruit (with the peel, when possible) rather than juice, because the fruit contains fiber and is more filling.

Grain products

Grain products, especially whole grains, provide energy-rich carbohydrates, many B vitamins (thiamin, riboflavin, niacin and folic acid), iron, zinc, magnesium and fiber. Choose whole-grain varieties such as barley, brown rice, oats, quinoa, wild rice, whole-grain bread and whole wheat pasta, because they contain more nutritional value, including higher amounts of fiber. Choose grain-based products that are low in fat and added sugars.

Milk, milk products and milk alternatives

Milk, milk products and milk alternatives provide protein, calcium, vitamin A, vitamin D, riboflavin, vitamin B_{12}, zinc, magnesium and potassium. Choose lower-fat milks such as skim or 1%, or fortified unsweetened soy beverages. When choosing lower-fat milk alternatives, read the Nutrition Facts label on the package for information that will help you make a healthier choice. Yogurts should be low in fat and sugar, and aim for less than 15% milk fat when choosing cheeses. Limit cream cheese, ice cream, coffee (18%) cream, whipping (35%) cream and sour cream, because these foods are high in fat and calories.

Frequently Asked Questions

Is goat's milk a healthy alternative to cow's milk? What about almond milk?

Many countries primarily use goat's milk, and it is gaining popularity as an alternative to cow's milk in North America. The nutrient content of milk varies based on several factors, including the breed and the diet of the animal producing the milk. On average there are only minor differences in micronutrient composition between cow's milk and goat's milk. The protein and fat in goat's milk may be a bit easier to digest. The lactose content is slightly lower. If you choose to drink goat's milk instead of cow's milk, ensure that it is low in fat and fortified with folic acid and vitamins A and D.

Almond milk is not comparable to cow's milk in terms of overall nutrient profile. It is low in protein, providing only 1 gram of protein in 8 ounces (250 mL), compared to cow's milk, which provides 8 grams of protein in the same quantity. Almond milk is also lower in calcium and vitamin D, although it is still an excellent source of calcium and vitamins D and E and a good source of vitamin A. It also contains some iron and is lactose-free. Although almond milk is different from cow's milk, it can still be enjoyed as a beverage if you purchase an unsweetened, fortified variety, but it should not replace cow's milk or fortified soy milk.

Meat and meat alternatives

Meat and meat alternatives are high in protein, iron, zinc, magnesium and B vitamins (thiamin, riboflavin, vitamin B_6 and vitamin B_{12}). When choosing meat, look for lean varieties and use lower-fat cooking methods such as roasting, baking and poaching. Lean cuts of red meat include eye of round roast, top round steak, bottom round roast and top sirloin steak. Meat alternatives such as beans, lentils and fortified tofu are excellent choices because they are low in saturated fat yet provide quality protein and are often high in fiber. Fish is another healthy choice because it contains the omega-3 fatty acids EPA and DHA.

▶ Sources of DHA and EPA

Sources	DHA and EPA Content
Salmon, 2½ oz (75 g)	1,600 mg
Rainbow trout, 2½ oz (75 g)	900 mg
Tuna, 2½ oz (75 g)	250 mg
1 egg, enriched with DHA	130 mg
Milk, enriched with DHA, 1 cup (250 mL)	70 mg

Frequently Asked Questions

Are soy foods such as tofu a good source of protein?

A good healthy protein choice is tofu, made from soybeans. Made by curdling hot fresh soy milk with a coagulant (a substance that makes things stick or gel together), it is bland and picks up the flavors of the ingredients with which it is cooked. Tofu is high in protein and B vitamins, is an excellent source of calcium, and also contains iron and zinc. It does not contain any cholesterol or saturated fats but does have healthier unsaturated fats. Given that it is an excellent source of high-quality protein without the saturated fat and also contains micronutrients similar to those in meat, tofu can be used to replace meat. One of the drawbacks is that the iron in tofu is non-heme whereas the iron in meat is heme, which is absorbed better. The U.S. Food and Drug Administration (FDA) recommends eating at least 25 grams of soy protein a day. Four ounces (115 g) of firm tofu provides 13 grams of soy protein.

Did you know?

Omega-3 benefits

Eicosapentaenoic acid (EPA) and docasahexaenoic acid (DHA) are omega-3 fatty acids essential for heart health and for the development of the brain and eyes. The main sources of EPA and DHA are oily fish such as salmon, tuna, mackerel, herring and trout. Many health professionals and organizations recommend eating fish at least twice a week. Omega-3 fatty acids are under-consumed in the average diet. The recommended intake of DHA and EPA is 500 mg each day for prevention benefits and 900 mg each day if you have coronary artery disease. If you can achieve that intake through food, you do not need to take a supplement. However, if you struggle to take in enough, a supplement of DHA and EPA may be helpful.

Energy Needs

Our bodies require energy not only when we are active but also when we are at rest, even while we are sleeping. Energy is measured in calories. Excess calories are stored in the body as fat (adipose tissue). The average total calories a person needs each day varies according to their body type, height, weight, age, gender, activity level and other factors. It is estimated that on average a woman needs about 2,000 calories and a man about 2,500 calories a day to maintain weight. It is important to note that these numbers are averages. Predictive equations can help you determine how many calories you need in a day, but again, these numbers are estimates.

The sources of energy are the three macronutrients — carbohydrates, proteins and fats.

Macronutrients

Macronutrients include carbohydrates, proteins and fats. They provide the body with energy, assisted by micronutrients, including vitamins and minerals.

Carbohydrates

Carbohydrates are the body's preferred source of energy. When you eat carbohydrates, the body breaks them down into simple sugars. These sugars are absorbed into the bloodstream. As the sugar level in your blood rises, the pancreas releases a hormone called insulin. Insulin is needed to move sugar from the blood into the cells, where it can be used as a source of energy. When this process happens quickly, as it does with simple sugars, you are more likely to feel hunger again soon. When the process occurs slowly, as with whole grains and complex carbohydrates, you will be satisfied longer and have energy over a greater period of time.

Simple and complex carbohydrates

Simple carbohydrates include corn syrup, honey, lollipops and other candy, and white sugar. Your body does not need to work hard to break them down into smaller particles because they are already small and easily absorbable from your blood into your cells. Complex carbohydrates have larger particles that require more work, which means it takes longer for your body to break them down. Examples of complex carbohydrates include whole-grain starches, oatmeal, bran and barley.

Glycemic index

The glycemic index is a scale used to rank carbohydrate foods by how much they raise blood glucose levels in comparison to glucose or white bread. Choose whole-grain products and grains with a lower glycemic index to keep you feeling fuller longer and help control blood sugar levels. Eating food with a low glycemic index may help you control your blood glucose and cholesterol levels. Eating foods with a lower glycemic index may also help control your appetite.

Low glycemic-index foods

- 100% stone-ground whole wheat, mixed-grain or pumpernickel bread
- oat bran, bran flakes
- barley, bulgur, pasta and noodles, parboiled (Converted) rice
- sweet potatoes and yams
- legumes (lentils, chickpeas, kidney beans, split peas, soybeans, baked beans)

Fiber

Fiber is the indigestible part of plant food, and it provides many health benefits. Fiber is naturally found in fruits, vegetables and grains, but not in meat or dairy products, though the food industry is adding certain types of fiber to dairy products such as cottage cheese, other cheeses and yogurts. Eating high-fiber foods may help you feel full for a longer time, which may help with weight control.

Insoluble and soluble fiber

Fiber can be insoluble or soluble. Insoluble fiber, also known as roughage, cannot be broken down by digestive enzymes. Because it cannot be broken down, it adds bulk to your stool. Soluble fiber may be fermented by friendly bacteria in the large intestine. It can form a sticky or gummy texture like cooked oatmeal.

Soluble fiber helps to lower blood cholesterol levels and control blood sugar levels. An adult woman should aim for 25 grams of fiber every day and an adult man should aim for 38 grams. There is no upper limit for fiber intake.

When reading food labels, aim for at least 2 grams of dietary fiber or 15% of daily value per serving. When increasing the fiber in your diet, you should do so slowly, to prevent discomfort. Increase your water intake along with your fiber intake.

Carbohydrate scare
With the popularity of low-carb diets, people have become afraid to eat carbohydrates. Carbohydrates are good for you. They provide you with nutrition that your body needs — every gram of carbohydrate provides you with 4 calories of energy. Your brain requires about 130 grams of carbohydrates every day; studies have shown that a diet very low in carbohydrates alters brain function. It is important to choose healthier forms of carbohydrates more often.

▶ Dietary sources of fiber

Insoluble fiber	Soluble fiber
• brown and wild rice • whole wheat bread and cereals • whole-grain breads and cereals • wheat bran • rye flour • skins of fruits (apples, pears) • skins of vegetables (eggplant, tomatoes, corn kernels) • flax seeds • seeds of fruits and vegetables (tomato, cucumber, kiwi)	• oats, oat bran • barley • blueberries, strawberries, apples • legumes (chickpeas, lentils, beans) • pectin • inulin • psyllium fiber • okra • applesauce, bananas

Did you know?

Food coloring

Pumpernickel and rye bread are not considered whole-grain breads because they are made mainly with enriched white flour. The brown color comes from caramel or food coloring. Whole-grain rye is available; you need to read the label to make sure what you are getting.

Protein

The main function of protein is to build, maintain and repair body tissue, including muscle, organs, skin and hair. Protein is made up of building blocks called amino acids — the body needs 20 amino acids to make proteins. While it can manufacture most of those amino acids, some cannot be made and come only from the food we eat. Eating a variety of protein-rich foods throughout the day helps ensure that you are getting a balanced combination of the amino acids your body needs. Protein can also be used a source of energy when carbohydrate and fat stores are in short supply. If you eat more protein than your body needs, it tends to get broken down and stored as fat (not protein) or excreted.

After your surgery, protein is very important to promote healing and weight loss. Aim for at least 60 to 80 grams or more of protein every day. Speak to your dietitian or doctor about your individual protein needs.

Fats

Dietary fat has several important functions, including energy storage, carrying fat-soluble vitamins and making important hormones. Different types of fats in foods affect the fat in your blood differently. Unsaturated (monounsaturated and polyunsaturated) fats are all considered healthier fats. These good fats provide many health benefits, including heart health, skin health and brain development. Fat carries the fat-soluble vitamins A, D, E and K to be used by the body.

▶ Good fat sources

Monounsaturated fats	Polyunsaturated fats
• olive oil	• flax seeds and flaxseed oil
• canola oil	• safflower oil
• peanut oil	• sunflower seeds and oil
• non-hydrogenated margarine	• sesame seeds
• avocados	• fish and fish oil
• soybean oil	• walnuts

Functions of fat in the body

- Lubricates body surfaces
- Forms a component of cell membranes
- Makes important hormones
- Stores energy
- Insulates the body from the cold
- Carries the fat-soluble vitamins A, D, E and K

Lower-fat cooking

Using a variety of lower-fat cooking methods can significantly reduce the fat content of the dishes you prepare. Try these cooking methods:

- steaming
- stir-frying
- grilling or barbecuing
- poaching
- baking or roasting

When you are baking, use nonstick pans or line pans with parchment paper to avoid having to grease them. You can also substitute applesauce for butter or shortening in many recipes.

If you must use oils or fats for cooking, try to use healthier versions. Good cooking oils include

- canola oil
- olive oil
- peanut oil
- non-hydrogenated margarine
- safflower oil
- sunflower oil
- corn oil

It is best to avoid frying foods, but if you do choose to fry occasionally, use corn, safflower, soy or canola oil, as these

Did you know?

Saturated and trans fat cautions
Saturated and trans fats, found mainly in animal products and processed foods, are considered less healthy fats because they can negatively affect your blood fat levels. Saturated and trans fats are found in animal fat (butter, lard), dairy products, egg yolks, tropical oils, deep-fried foods, cakes and pastries and shortening. Instead, include healthier sources of fat in your diet, in moderation. Restricting the fat in your diet completely is not a good idea, as fat is needed for good health.

oils have a higher smoke point. Do not use olive, hempseed or flaxseed oils for frying. If you are adding oil to food after it has been cooked, such as on vegetables, or if you are making a salad dressing, try using flaxseed or hempseed oil, both of which provide beneficial omega fats.

Try to avoid oils and fats that are high in saturated and trans fats, such as

- vegetable shortening
- hard margarine
- butter
- palm or palm kernel oil
- coconut oil

Foods to Limit or Eliminate

Many foods and drinks are considered unhealthy and do not provide you with nutritional benefits. Some of these foods are referred to as empty calories because they have many calories but little nutritional value. Foods that are high in sugar, high in unhealthy types of fat or high in sodium (salt) should be limited. What does limited mean? Restrict how often you consume these foods or drinks on a weekly basis, and control portions when you do have them. Aim to manage not only how rarely you have these foods or drinks but also the amount you consume, by using as smaller bowl or glass.

▶ **Foods to limit**

Foods and drinks to limit	Try instead
Cakes and pastries	• Baked apple or pear sprinkled with cinnamon
Ice cream and frozen desserts	• Frozen yogurt (low-fat and low-sugar)
Chocolate candy	• Small portion of high-quality dark chocolate
Candy	• Small portion of sugar-free candy • Fruit salad
Donuts and muffins	• Homemade high-fiber, low-sugar muffins (add fruit for sweetness) • Smaller portions, such as mini muffins

Foods and drinks to limit	Try instead
French fries	• Homemade baked sweet potato strips • Oven-roasted potatoes with herbs and seasoning
Chips and nachos	• Rice crackers • Homemade baked whole wheat pita crisps • Air-popped popcorn
Fruit-flavored drinks, soda pop, sports drinks	• Water flavored with lemon, lime or cucumber slices • Diet fruit-flavored drinks
Specialty coffee drinks (lattes, mochas)	• Decaffeinated latte made with low-fat milk and unsweetened
Hot chocolate (sweetened)	• Homemade light hot chocolate with low-fat milk and diet hot chocolate or cocoa

Micronutrients

Micronutrients are substances the body cannot make but are vital to good health, and in some cases to life itself. Micronutrients include both vitamins and minerals.

Dietary reference intake

The amount of micronutrients we need to ingest daily in our food to maintain good health is referred to as a dietary reference intake, or DRI. DRIs comprise several other nutrient measures, notably the recommended dietary allowance (RDA), which establishes the minimum intake required to maintain good health.

Recommended dietary allowance

The RDA is the average daily dietary intake level sufficient to meet the nutrient requirements of nearly all (97% to 98%) healthy individuals in a particular life-stage and gender group. The RDA is the goal for an individual's usual intake. For example, the RDA for vitamin C is 75 to 90 mg, which is equivalent to one fresh orange. If there is not enough scientific evidence to calculate an RDA, an Adequate Intake (AI) amount is used.

Nutrient deficiencies

After weight-loss surgery, nutrient deficiencies are quite common. The reasons may include malabsorption of nutrients, reduced intake, and loss of nutrients caused by vomiting. A wide variety of micronutrient deficiencies have been reported.

Iron deficiency

Iron-deficiency anemia is quite common after weight-loss surgery, especially after a gastric bypass procedure. The duodenum is the primary site for iron absorption, and this area of the intestine is completely bypassed. Symptoms of iron deficiency include feeling very tired, looking pale and having a poor appetite. Koilonychia — thin, concave nails with raised ridges — is a symptom of iron deficiency.

Vitamin B_{12} and folate deficiency

Vitamin B_{12} and folate deficiency can lead to abnormally large red blood cells and a condition called megaloblastic anemia. Vitamin B_{12} deficiency can also lead to neurological problems such as nerve damage, problems with coordination and walking, and cognitive impairments. Folate deficiency presents with a wide variety of symptoms, including diarrhea, weakness, decreased appetite, headaches and behavioral changes. Folate deficiency in women who are pregnant is associated with neural tube defects in the fetus.

Vitamin B_1 deficiency

Beriberi results from vitamin B_1 (thiamin) deficiency. The symptoms include confusion, edema (swelling), neuropathy (nerve damage) and increased heart rate. People with a vitamin B_1 deficiency may show signs of Wernicke-Korsakoff syndrome, which can range from mild confusion to coma. Early signs of vitamin B_1 deficiency may include a pins and needles feeling or numbness in the legs, heaviness and weakness of the legs or increased heart rate and palpitations.

▶ Micronutrient DRIs, functions and sources

Micronutrient	Functions	Sources
Vitamins (daily)		
Vitamin A RDA: 700 to 900 mcg	• eye health • keeps skin and membranes smooth and supple • involved in growth • involved in health of bones and teeth • antioxidant • immune booster	liver, kidney, milk, egg yolks, yellow and dark green leafy vegetables, apricots, cantaloupe, peaches
Vitamin B_1 (thiamine) RDA: 1.1 to 1.2 mg	• helps enzymes work for carbohydrate digestion • essential for growth, appetite, digestion and healthy nerves • involved in heart function	whole-grain and enriched cereals and bread, wheat germ, brewer's yeast, potatoes, legumes, brown rice
Vitamin B_2 (riboflavin) RDA: 1.1 to 1.3 mg	• essential for growth • helps enzymes work • helps body use other B vitamins • metabolism of protein, fat, carbohydrate • skin health	dairy products, eggs, green leafy vegetables, enriched breads and cereals, soybeans, meat and poultry
Vitamin B_3 (niacin) RDA: 14 to 16 mg	• helps body use protein, fat, carbohydrate to make energy • helps enzymes work	fish, liver, meat, poultry, grains, eggs, peanuts, milk, legumes
Vitamin B_6 (pyridoxine) RDA: 1.3 to 1.7 mg	• helps enzymes work • essential for growth • helps form hemoglobin	pork, bran cereal, milk, egg yolks, oatmeal, legumes
Vitamin B_{12} (cobalamin) RDA: 2.4 mcg	• makes healthy red blood cells • protects myelin (sheath part of nerves)	liver, kidney, dairy products, meat, eggs, fortified soy products

Ranges are provided for RDAs and AIs because they are gender- and age-specific recommendations.

Micronutrient	Functions	Sources
Pantothenic acid (B vitamin) AI: 5 mg	• involved in metabolism	all plant and animal foods, especially eggs, kidney, liver, salmon, yeast
Folate (folic acid) (B vitamin) RDA: 400 mcg	• helps make red blood cells and prevent anemia • involved in making new cells and tissues and in wound healing	green leafy vegetables, liver, beef, wheat, eggs, fish, dried beans, lentils, asparagus, broccoli, collard greens, yeast
Biotin (B vitamin) AI: 30 mcg	• involved in metabolism • energy production	liver, mushrooms, peanuts, yeast, milk, meat, egg yolks, most vegetables, bananas, grapefruit, watermelon, strawberries, tomatoes
Vitamin C RDA: 75 to 90 mg	• involved in collagen production (found in skin and bones) • important for wound healing • keeps gums healthy • helps absorb iron • antioxidant (protects cells from damage) • immune booster • involved in making hormones	citrus fruits, tomatoes, melon, peppers, guava, strawberries, pineapple, potatoes, kiwis, cauliflower
Vitamin D RDA: 15 mcg or 600 IU	• essential for growth and development • formation and maintenance of healthy bones and teeth • increases amount of phosphorus and calcium the body absorbs • boosts immunity	• salmon, tuna, sardines, fortified milk, liver, egg yolks • sunlight
Vitamin E RDA: 15 mg	• nerve and muscle health • antioxidant	wheat germ, vegetable oils, green leafy vegetables, milk fat, egg yolks, nuts

Ranges are provided for RDAs and AIs because they are gender- and age-specific recommendations.

Micronutrient	Functions	Sources
Vitamin K AI: 90 to 120 mcg	• involved in making proteins for blood, bones, kidneys • aids clotting of blood	liver, soybean oil, vegetable oils, green leafy vegetables, wheat bran
Minerals (daily)		
Calcium RDA: 1,000 to 1,200 mg	• essential for strong bones and teeth • regulates fluid balance • helps cells send messages to each other • keeps muscles working properly (including heart)	dairy products, sardines, canned salmon with bones, clams, oysters, kale, turnip greens, mustard greens, calcium-set tofu
Chromium AI: 20 to 35 mcg	• glucose metabolism	corn oil, clams, whole-grain cereals, brewer's yeast, meat
Copper RDA: 900 mcg	• antioxidant (protects cells from damage) • promotes growth of strong bones • protects nerve tissue	liver, shellfish, whole grains, cherries, legumes, kidney, poultry, oysters, chocolate, nuts
Fluoride AI: 3 to 4 mg	• reduces dental cavities • helps form strong bones and teeth	fluoridated drinking water, rice, soybeans, spinach, onions, lettuce
Iodine RDA: 150 mcg	• aids in thyroid gland function • prevents goiter	iodized salt, seafood, water
Iron RDA: 8 to 18 mg	• brings oxygen to your body tissues • prevents you from feeling tired	meat, fish, poultry, firm tofu, beans and peas (soybeans, chickpeas, split peas, lentils), nuts and seeds, organ meats (liver, heart), egg yolks, whole or enriched greens, dark green vegetables, blackstrap molasses, shrimp, oysters

Ranges are provided for RDAs and AIs because they are gender- and age-specific recommendations.

Micronutrient	Functions	Sources
Magnesium RDA: 310 to 420 mg	• helps move nutrients in and out of cells • keeps nerves and muscles strong • involved in bone development	whole-grain cereals, tofu, nuts, meat, milk, green vegetables, legumes, chocolate
Manganese AI: 1.8 to 2.3 mg	• part of enzyme systems	beet greens, blueberries, whole grains, nuts, legumes, fruit, tea
Molybdenum RDA: 45 mcg	• part of enzyme systems	legumes, cereal grains, dark green leafy vegetables, organ meats
Potassium AI: 4,700 mg	• keeps fluids balanced • helps control blood pressure • allows nerves and muscles to work together	bananas, papayas, sweet potatoes, dark green leafy vegetables, tomatoes, orange juice
Selenium RDA: 55 mcg	• involved in fat metabolism • antioxidant (protects cells from damage)	grains, onions, meats, milk
Phosphorus RDA: 700 mg	• essential for strong bones and teeth	cheese, egg yolks, milk, meat, fish, poultry, whole-grain cereals
Sulfate RDA: not established	• part of protein	meat, fish, poultry, eggs, milk, cheese, legumes, nuts
Zinc RDA: 8 to 11 mg	• needed for growth and development • protects nerve and brain tissue • immune booster • involved in sense of taste	meat, poultry, fish, oysters, shellfish, liver, beans (adzuki, kidney, navy, pinto, soybeans), lentils, pumpkin and sunflower seeds, milk, wheat bran

Ranges are provided for RDAs and AIs because they are gender- and age-specific recommendations.

How do I determine if the food I'm eating is providing me with enough vitamins and minerals?

Oftentimes after weight-loss surgery, people worry that they are not getting enough vitamins and minerals. When you eat well-balanced, nutritious meals and snacks and a variety of food from all the food groups, along with taking the recommended nutritional supplements, your chances of nutrient deficiencies decrease. However, with any type of weight-loss surgery, nutrient deficiencies are inevitable; routine nutritional blood work will help screen for them. If you feel that something is different with your body or the way you feel, this may be a sign of a nutrient deficiency. For example, feeling weak or tired may be a sign of iron deficiency, and numbness and tingling in your extremities may be a sign of vitamin B_1 (thiamin) deficiency. It is best to speak to your health-care provider if you think you have a nutrient deficiency, and ask to have your blood work checked routinely.

Vegetarian and vegan concerns

Following a vegetarian or vegan diet requires extra care and planning to ensure that you meet all your nutrient needs. Vegetarians eat no meat but do eat eggs and dairy products, while vegans eat a strictly vegetable-based diet. Both groups can be deficient in the specific nutrients that others derive from meat; in addition, vegans may be deficient in nutrients derived from egg and dairy products. If you choose a vegetarian or vegan diet, take extra care to eat foods with adequate protein, iron, zinc, calcium, vitamin D, vitamin B_{12} and omega-3 fats.

▶ Vegetarian and vegan special nutrient concerns and food sources

Possible nutrient deficiency	Food sources
Protein	• Soy, soy products, tofu, fortified soy drinks • Meat alternatives such as veggie burgers and texturized vegetable protein (TVP) • Grains, nuts and seeds • Dried beans, peas and lentils

Possible nutrient deficiency	Food sources
Iron	• Soy, soy products (firm and extra-firm tofu), fortified soy drinks • Meat alternatives such as veggie burgers and texturized vegetable protein (TVP) • Fortified grain products • Nuts and seeds • Dried beans, peas and lentils • Prunes, raisins, apricots • Dark green vegetables such as collard greens, okra, bok choy • Blackstrap molasses
Vitamin B_{12}	• Nutritional yeast with added B_{12} • Fortified soy products • Fortified non-dairy drinks • Meat alternatives such as veggie burgers and texturized vegetable protein (TVP)
Vitamin D	• Fortified soy products • Fortified non-dairy drinks • Soft margarine
Calcium	• Fortified soy drinks, soy yogurts, calcium-set tofu • Soybeans, navy beans, white beans • Nuts, almonds, almond butter • Calcium-fortified juices • Figs • Bok choy, okra, collard greens, turnip greens • Seeds and seed products, such as sesame seeds and tahini • Blackstrap molasses
Zinc	• Soybeans and soy products • Dried beans, peas and lentils • Nuts and seeds such as peanuts, peanut butter, sesame seeds, tahini, pecans, cashews, pumpkin seeds and flax seeds • Whole grains, fortified cereals
Omega-3 fats	• Canola, flaxseed, walnut and soybean oils • Ground flax seed • Soybeans and tofu • Walnuts

Hydration

Water is fundamental to most bodily functions. If possible, make water your beverage of choice and avoid or limit beverages that contain caffeine, such as coffee, tea, colas and energy drinks. Caffeine has a diuretic effect that can affect your digestion adversely by flushing fluid out of your body. Also avoid beverages that contain an excessive amount of sugar, because they add extra calories to your diet without providing much nutritional benefit. High-sugar beverage sources include soft drinks, sports drinks, energy drinks, fruit drinks, iced tea, lemonade, punches and other sweetened beverages, both hot and cold.

Functions of fluid in the body

- Controls body temperature
- Carries nutrients around the body
- Cushions and protects organs and joints
- Gets rid of waste products
- Keeps your bowels regular

Did you know?

Water-dependent
Humans are totally dependent on water. You can survive for weeks without food but only days without water. The human body is made up of about 55% to 60% water.

Frequently Asked Questions

Is bottled water better than tap water?

Treated water and bottled water that meet safety standards are both safe. The choice depends on your preference and needs. The tap water distributed by municipalities is regulated for safety, and bottled water is regulated at the federal level. Not all bottled water is the same. If it comes from a spring or an underground source, it is usually labeled as spring or mineral water. Bottled water that is not so labeled may come from any source and is treated to make it safe for human consumption. Sources can include municipal water, which may undergo further treatment to lower its mineral content. Bottled water may be ozonated during the bottling process, which disinfects it and changes the flavor and odor. One major drawback of bottled water is the environmental impact of using plastic bottles. Some people use filtering devices in their homes to further treat municipal water. Consider purchasing a reusable wide-necked stainless steel canteen that can be washed and refilled with the water of your choice.

Caffeine

Caffeine is a natural ingredient found in the leaves, seeds or fruits of various plants such as coffee, tea and cocoa. It is also manufactured and added to some drinks and drugs. Caffeine acts as a diuretic and a stimulant. Caffeine has many adverse effects on the body, including

- increased heart rate and blood pressure
- anxiety, mood changes, changes in attentiveness
- muscle tremors, nausea, irritability
- reduced bone density, increasing risk of fracture
- reduced fertility
- potential linkage to cancer

Health Canada recommends no more than 400 mg of caffeine per day for the average adult. This translates to about 3 cups (750 mL) of brewed coffee. For women of childbearing age, no more than 300 mg of caffeine a day — a little over 2 cups (500 mL) of coffee — are recommended.

▶ Caffeine content of various drinks

Source	Caffeine content
Brewed coffee, 1 cup (8 oz/250 mL)	135 mg
Instant coffee, 1 cup (8 oz/250 mL)	76–106 mg
Decaffeinated coffee, 1 cup (8 oz/250 mL)	3 mg
Espresso, 1 shot (1½ oz/45 mL)	77–96 mg
Tea, black, 1 cup (8 oz/250 mL)	43 mg
Tea, green tea, 1 cup (8 oz/250 mL)	30 mg
Cola, diet, 1 can (12 oz/355 mL)	36–46 mg
Cola, regular, 1 can (12 oz/355 mL)	39–50 mg
Mello Yello or Mountain Dew, 1 can (12 oz/355 mL)	52–54 mg
Energy drinks, 1 can (8 oz/250 mL)	80 mg (varies by brand)
Chocolate milk, 1 cup (8 oz/250 mL)	8 mg

Alcohol

After weight-loss surgery, special attention must be paid to limiting alcohol intake. Alcoholic beverages contain empty calories. When you mix alcoholic drinks with other beverages or mixes, you are adding even more calories. These extra calories do not provide nutritional benefit.

Over time, too much alcohol can cause a number of health problems, including

- heart problems
- liver disease
- vitamin deficiencies
- sexual impotence
- cancer
- menstrual problems
- difficulty maintaining a healthy weight
- addiction

▶ Approximate calories in alcoholic drinks

Source	Calories
Light beer (4%), 1 bottle (12 oz/341 mL)	100 cal
Regular beer (5%), 1 bottle (12 oz/341 mL)	140 cal
Non-alcoholic beer (0.5%), 1 can (12 oz/341 mL)	210 cal
Daiquiri, 7 oz (210 mL)	260 cal
Pina colada, 4½ oz (135 mL)	245 cal
Vodka, 1½ oz (45 mL)	100 cal
Wine (11.5%), 5 oz (150 mL)	100 cal
Liqueurs, 1½ oz (45 mL)	160–190 cal
Regular cooler, 1 bottle (12 oz/341 mL)	310 cal

▶ Alcoholic beverage equivalencies

Each of the following servings of drinks provides approximately the same amount of alcohol:

Beverage	Alcohol Content	Serving Size
Regular beer	5%	12 oz (341 mL)
Wine	12%	5 oz (150 mL)
Fortified wine (sherry, port, vermouth)	16–18%	3 oz (90 mL)
Spirits, liquors (rum, vodka)	40%	1½ oz (45 mL)

Alcohol guidelines

If you do drink alcohol, several organizations have developed programs to help avoid problems with drinking. The Centre for Addiction and Mental Health in Toronto offers the following guidelines for low-risk drinking:

- If you don't already drink, don't start.
- If you do drink, avoid getting intoxicated or drunk.
- Wait at least one hour between drinks.
- Have something to eat.
- Drink non-alcoholic beverages instead, such as water, soft drinks or fruit juice.

These guidelines do not apply if you

- have health problems such as liver disease or mental illness
- are taking medications such as sedatives, painkillers or sleeping pills
- have a personal or family history of drinking problems
- have a family history of cancer or other risk factors for cancer
- are pregnant, trying to get pregnant or breastfeeding
- will be operating a vehicle such as a car, truck, motorcycle, boat, snowmobile, all-terrain vehicle or bicycle
- need to be alert (for example, if you will be operating machinery or working with farm implements or other dangerous equipment)
- will be playing sports or doing other physical activities where you need to be in control

- are responsible for the safety of others at work or at home
- have been told not to drink for legal, medical or other reasons

If you are concerned about how drinking may affect your health, check with your doctor.

Reading Food Labels

Reading food labels is an easy way to help you make better food choices, once you know what you are looking for. Regulatory agencies in Canada and the United States have now made it mandatory that products have a Nutrition Facts table and ingredients list. In the United Kingdom, nutrition information on a food label is mandatory only if a health claim — such as low in fat — is being made.

Nutrient facts

The amounts of common nutrients in a serving of food are listed in the Nutrition Facts table. The table provides you with information on the calorie content and 13 core nutrients: fat, saturated and trans fats, cholesterol, sodium, carbohydrate, fiber and sugars, protein, vitamin A, vitamin C, calcium and iron.

The % Daily Value (% DV) on the Nutrition Facts table shows you at a glance whether there is a lot or a little of a nutrient in the specified serving. More than 15% DV is considered a lot of that nutrient, and less than 5% DV is considered a little of that nutrient. For example, if the Nutrition Facts table states that the food has 25% DV of calcium, that means that every serving contains 25% of your daily calcium needs, which is a lot of that nutrient.

Sample Nutrition Facts Label

Nutrition Facts

Serving Size 2 tortillas (51 g)
Servings Per Container 6

Amount Per Serving

Calories 110	Calories from Fat 10

	% Daily Value
Total Fat 1 g	**2%**
Saturated Fat 0 g	**0%**
Trans Fat 0 g	
Cholesterol 0 mg	**6%**
Sodium 30 mg	**1%**
Total Carbohydrate 22 g	**7%**
Dietary Fiber 2 g	**9%**
Sugars 0 g	
Protein 2 g	

Vitamin A 0%	Vitamin C 0%
Calcium 2%	Iron 4%

*Percent Daily Values are based on a 2,000 calorie diet. Your daily values may be higher or lower depending on your calorie needs:

	Calories	2,000	2,500
Total Fat	Less than	65 g	80 g
Saturdated Fat	Less than	20 g	25 g
Cholesterol	Less than	300 mg	300 mg
Sodium	Less than	2,400 mg	2,400 mg
Total Carbohydrate		300 g	375 g
Dietary Fiber		25 g	30 g

Calories per gram Fat 9 Carbohydrate 4 Protein 4

Nutrient content and health claims

Claims about the nutrient content and health benefits of a food may also appear on its label. The nutrient content claims highlight whether a food is high or low in certain nutrients such as sodium, fat or fiber — for example, a good source of fiber. Health claims describe the potential health benefits of a food or the nutrients it contains. An example might be *A healthy diet containing foods high in potassium and low in sodium may reduce the risk of high blood pressure, a risk factor for stroke and heart disease.*

Using food labels to make wise food choices

Aim for little or low amounts (5% DV or less) of the following nutrients:

- fat
- saturated fat
- trans fat
- cholesterol (U.S. labels only)
- sodium

Aim for a lot or high amounts (20% DV or more) of

- calcium
- iron
- fiber
- vitamin A
- vitamin C

▶ Common health claims made on labels in Canada

Source of fiber	contains at least 2 grams
High source of fiber	contains at least 4 grams
Very high source of fiber	contains at least 6 grams
Low-fat	no more than 3 grams
Low in saturated fat	less than 2 grams
Cholesterol-free	less than 2 mg and also low in saturated and trans fat
Sodium-free	less than 5 mg
Light*	reduced in fat or energy (calories)

* Light can also be used to describe the sensory characteristics of a food, for example, light-tasting or light-colored.

Food labels in the United Kingdom

In the United Kingdom, a number of manufacturers use traffic light colors on food labels to help consumers make quick healthier food choices. The amounts of fat, saturated fat, sugar and salt are color-coded depending on whether they are present in high, medium or low amounts.

▶ Traffic light food labeling system

Per 100-gram serving	Red (high amounts)	Amber (medium amounts)	Green (low amounts)
Fat	> 20 grams	3– 20 grams	< 3 grams
Saturated fat	> 5 grams	1.5–5 grams	< 1.5 grams
Salt	> 1.5 grams	0.3–1.5 grams	< 0.3 grams
Sodium	> 0.6 grams	0.1–0.6 grams	< 0.1 grams
Sugar	> 15 grams	5–15 grams	< 5 grams

Getting Ready for Surgery

Now that you have an understanding of the digestive system, bariatric surgical procedures and healthy eating basics, you can start making final preparations for surgery. Planning ahead now will help save energy after surgery, while you are recovering. Physically preparing for surgery also helps you to prepare mentally.

Make sure you have scheduled the necessary time off work for surgery and recovery. Start putting together a support team of friends and relatives to help with household chores, child care and travel to and from the hospital. If you need to stay near the bariatric center for some time after surgery, make sure you have arranged the necessary accommodations. Prepare a shopping list of safe, nutritious foods you will need, especially during the first month after surgery. To start, follow the preoperative diet that your health-care providers recommend, and stock up on the nutritional supplements you will need immediately after surgery.

Planning for weight-loss surgery

Make a checklist of the things you need to do in a journal or notebook, or use this book to help you get and stay organized. Shop ahead of time for the foods and drinks you will need on hand after weight-loss surgery.

Pre-surgery checklist

❏ Learn about the digestive system, good nutrition and weight-loss surgery.
❏ Complete all required medical tests.
❏ Practice mindful eating, chewing food well and eating slowly.
❏ Engage in healthy coping mechanisms such as hobbies.
❏ Address emotional eating tendencies.
❏ Start making healthier food choices.
❏ Start making healthier beverage choices.
❏ Start eating out less often.
❏ Prepare and freeze food to have on hand after surgery (use this cookbook for great ideas).
❏ Cut back on caffeine.

❏ Try the recommended protein supplements.
❏ Start taking a regular multivitamin and mineral supplement, and other supplements if recommended by your health-care team.
❏ Start some type of physical activity, just to get into the habit or routine.
❏ Quit smoking.
❏ Seek support, both professional and personal.
❏ Go grocery shopping for needed supplies.
❏ Make arrangements for travel and accommodations if necessary.
❏ Schedule time off work for surgery and recovery.
❏ Make arrangements for child care.
❏ Assign household chores to friends or family.
❏ Save money for the financial costs of surgery.
❏ Speak to your pharmacist and doctor about your medications. Which ones will need to be put on hold or changed?
❏ Start the preoperative diet recommended by your health-care team.

Shopping list

❏ Applesauce or other unsweetened fruit sauce
❏ Baby food (strained)
❏ Beans
❏ Beverages (decaffeinated tea, sugar-free flavored drinks, tomato juice)
❏ Broth or bouillon cubes for making broth (reduced-sodium)
❏ Canned fruit (packed in water)
❏ Canned chicken (in water)
❏ Cream of wheat (plain)
❏ Creamed soups (low-fat, condensed)
❏ Cottage cheese (low-fat)
❏ Egg substitutes (liquid)
❏ Eggs
❏ Gelatin desserts (sugar-free)
❏ Lentils
❏ Milk (skim or 1%; lactose-reduced milk)
❏ Oat bran (instant hot cereal)
❏ Oatmeal (instant, plain)
❏ Potatoes
❏ Puddings (no sugar added, low-fat)
❏ Salmon (canned in water)
❏ Soy milk (natural, unsweetened)
❏ Tuna (canned in water)
❏ Yogurt (low-fat, no sugar added)

Preoperative Diets

Before bariatric surgery, many doctors and dietitians recommend that you lose some weight, which may help decrease your risk. The length of time you will be on this diet varies from two weeks to three months, depending on the amount of weight you need to lose, the surgery you are going to have and the surgeon's recommendation.

Fatty liver reduction

Anyone who is obese usually has a fatty, enlarged liver. For the surgeon to get access to the stomach, part of the liver needs to be moved out of the way — part of it sits just on top of the stomach. If the liver is enlarged, it is easy to nick or injure and it could be difficult for the surgeon to get access to the stomach to perform the surgery safely. For this reason and others, many bariatric centers recommend a specialized preoperative diet designed to reduce the size of the liver.

Optifast liquid diet

The Optifast liquid diet is a specialized meal replacement plan intended for weight loss. Many surgeons recommend drinking Optifast to lose weight and drain the liver of fat prior to bariatric surgery. Optifast is a low-carbohydrate, low-fat, high-protein drink that contains vitamins and minerals. The 2-ounce (54 g) packages come in vanilla or chocolate flavor; one package is mixed with water to make an 11.5-ounce (340 mL) drink. The usual recommendation is to drink four packages per day, which provides 900 calories and 90 grams of protein, as well as 100% of vitamin and mineral needs. Optifast is lactose free. You may experience constipation while on Optifast and need to take laxatives or a fiber supplement, as recommended by your health-care professional.

The length of time this program is needed prior to surgery depends on several factors, including surgeon preference and the patient's starting BMI. Most patients can expect to be on this diet for two to four weeks before surgery.

Flavoring Optifast drinks

Some people find that Optifast shakes do not taste that great. Here are some suggestions to help make it taste better:

- Add about $\frac{1}{8}$ tsp (0.5 mL) of flavoring extracts, such as almond, banana or vanilla to each shake.
- Mix in 1 tsp (5 mL) of decaffeinated instant coffee granules.

- Mix a little sugar-free beverage powder into the vanilla shake.
- Add 1 tsp (5 mL) vanilla extract and 1 tsp (5 mL) no-sugar-added maple-flavored syrup to the vanilla shake.
- Add ice and blend the shake in the blender.
- Use very cold water to make the shakes.

Frequently Asked Questions

What else can I drink or eat while on the Optifast liquid diet?

You should keep hydrated by drinking clear, sugar-free liquids and water in addition to the Optifast drinks. If you feel you need something to chew on, you may eat no more than 2 cups (500 mL) of plain low-calorie vegetables each day. Here are some ideas:

- cauliflower
- cucumber
- spinach
- cabbage
- lettuce
- celery
- broccoli
- green peppers

Do not use any salad dressing unless it is calorie-free.

Protein-sparing modified fast

The protein-sparing modified fast (PSMF) diet is very high in lean protein, allows limited amounts of lower-carbohydrate vegetables, and is very low in fat. The high protein intake prevents the body from using its own protein stores for energy. Since very little carbohydrate is used, fat becomes the main source of energy. This quick breakdown of fat produces ketones in the body. Dehydration is a serious risk while on this diet, so you need to be sure to drink plenty of water. This diet should be followed only if medically supervised.

▶ PSMF meal plan

Breakfast	• 2-egg-white omelet • I slice whole wheat bread with $\frac{1}{2}$ tsp (2 mL) margarine • $\frac{1}{2}$ cup (125 mL) skim milk
Morning snack	• I small fruit

Lunch	• 3 oz (90 g) lean protein, such as skinless chicken breast (baked, grilled or poached) • 1 medium potato (no toppings) • 1 cup (250 mL) romaine lettuce salad with 1 tsp (5 mL) calorie-reduced dressing
Afternoon snack	• ½ cup (125 mL) Greek-style low-fat plain yogurt
Dinner	• 6 oz (180 g) lean protein such as turkey breast • ½ cup (125 mL) noodles • 1 cup (250 mL) spinach salad with 1 tsp (5 mL) calorie-reduced dressing • ½ cup (125 mL) skim milk
Evening snack	• 4 tbsp (60 mL) cottage cheese (low-fat) and 6 soda crackers

Low-calorie diet

Some surgeons and bariatric centers recommend that you follow a low-calorie, high-protein diet. For example, you may be asked to consume three ready-made high-protein, low-carbohydrate drinks and one prepared meal every day for about two weeks before your surgery.

▶ Low-calorie diet meal plan

Breakfast	• 1 cup (250 mL) high-protein, low-carbohydrate beverage
Lunch	• 1 cup (250 mL) high-protein, low-carbohydrate beverage
Afternoon snack	• 1 cup (250 mL) high-protein, low-carbohydrate beverage
Dinner	• 4 oz (125 g) lean protein, such as skinless chicken breast (baked, grilled or poached) • ½ cup (125 mL) sweet potato • 1 cup (250 mL) steamed cauliflower • 1 cup (250 mL) salad • No added fats, sauces or dressings with the food.
Throughout the day	• 5 to 6 cups (1.25 to 1.5 L) non-carbonated sugar-free liquids (water, sugar-free ice pops, sugar-free gelatin, decaffeinated tea, low-sugar fruit-flavored drinks)

Specialized liquid diet

Some centers recommend that you use ready-to-drink nutritional supplements, such as meal-replacement drinks that are high in protein and low in sugar, to replace all meals. Your surgeon or health-care team will provide you with the names of brands they recommend and tell you how many you need to drink every day and for how long. While on this diet before surgery, you must also consume non-carbonated sugar-free liquids to keep hydrated, such as water, sugar-free ice pops, sugar-free gelatin, decaffeinated tea and diet flavored drinks.

Intragastric balloon diet

The intragastric balloon procedure is used primarily to help patients who have a very high BMI lose some weight to reduce their operative risk for gastric bypass surgery. The diet usually progresses from liquids for the first three days, soft foods on days 4 to 10, and normal foods thereafter. You eat three mini meals and three snacks that are low in fat and sugar; portions are significantly smaller than usual. Be sure to drink water after eating, to rinse off the balloon. Follow the specific dietary guidelines provided by the team that inserted the intragastric balloon.

Nutritional Supplement Plan

After weight-loss surgery you will need to take vitamin and mineral supplements for the rest of your life. Additional vitamin and mineral supplements may be recommended by your doctor or dietitian, depending on your nutritional intake and laboratory (blood work) assessments. You will be advised which supplements you need to take. Take all the recommended supplements regularly as directed. It may be helpful to use a pill organizer to help you remember which vitamin and mineral supplements you need to take and when. Do not take extended-release supplements, as they may not be absorbed so well.

Recommended vitamin and mineral supplements by procedure

Gastric bypass

- complete multivitamin and mineral supplement
- calcium with vitamin D
- vitamin B_{12}
- You may also be advised to take an iron supplement.

LAGB
- complete multivitamin and mineral supplement
- You may also be advised to take a calcium and vitamin D supplement.

VSG
- complete multivitamin and mineral supplement
- vitamin B_{12}
- You may also be advised to take a calcium and vitamin D supplement.

Frequently Asked Questions

Should I take a multivitamin and mineral supplement?

Taking a multivitamin and mineral supplement every day will help you get vitamins and minerals that you may be missing or that may be malabsorbed (as is the case with a gastric bypass). The usual dosage is one to two adult multivitamin and mineral supplements every day, but this can vary based on the brand you purchase. If possible, take them with meals.

Look for a supplement that has many vitamins and minerals, especially iron, folic acid, zinc and selenium. Preferably the supplement should contain at least 18 mg iron and 400 mcg folic acid. Begin with a chewable form. Do not take children's multivitamins, as they do not have enough of the nutrients you need. If your multivitamin and mineral supplement does not contain enough iron, take an additional iron supplement. Take the multivitamin and mineral supplement separate from any calcium and iron supplements. Specialty bariatric vitamin and mineral supplements are available. Ask your doctor or dietitian for help.

Did you know?

Swallowing tips

Do not swallow whole supplements during the first six weeks after surgery. It is best to take chewable supplements or, in some cases, liquid or sublingual (dissolving) types. Some supplements can be crushed and mixed with applesauce, for example, but it might taste unpleasant. After six weeks you may be able to take supplements whole, but if the tablets are too large (more than $\frac{1}{2}$ inch/1 cm), you may need to cut them into smaller pieces first. Speak to your health-care team before beginning to swallow any medications or supplements whole.

Calcium with vitamin D

With bariatric surgery comes rapid weight loss that can decrease bone density. Taking a good calcium supplement may help to prevent this condition. With gastric bypass surgery in particular, there is the added drawback that calcium is malabsorbed. Even if you are consuming the recommended amount of calcium through food, you may still need to take a supplement every day for life.

Calcium is best absorbed in divided doses. Calcium citrate with vitamin D3 is absorbed best. Ideally the calcium supplement should include both vitamin D3 and magnesium. Vitamin D increases the amount of calcium that the body absorbs.

- Be sure to divide calcium into 500 to 600 mg doses throughout the day.
- After a gastric bypass, aim to get a total of 1,500 to 2,000 mg of elemental calcium every day.
- With a VSG or LAGB, aim to get a total of 1,500 mg elemental calcium every day, or as recommended by your health-care professional.

Vitamin B_{12}

Vitamin B_{12} is bound to protein in food. With the help of stomach acids, the B_{12} is released from the protein. It then attaches to intrinsic factor, a substance secreted by the stomach to help with the absorption of vitamin B_{12}. Deficiency in vitamin B_{12} may cause certain types of anemia and damage to nerves.

With gastric bypass surgery and VSG, there is less stomach acid and less surface area in the stomach to produce intrinsic factor, so vitamin B_{12} deficiency is quite common. Research has shown that patients who have the LAGB can also become deficient in vitamin B_{12}. Blood levels are checked to determine the appropriate level of supplementation. Vitamin B_{12} supplements are available in liquid form, as sublingual tablets or strips, as injections or as a small, round pill that can be crushed before taking.

To prevent vitamin B_{12} deficiency, all gastric bypass and VSG patients should begin vitamin B_{12} supplementation, preferably as sublingual or injections. Choose one of the following doses to start:

- 400 mcg once a day
- 1,000 mcg every other day
- 1,200 mcg every three days
- 1,000 mcg injection from your doctor every month

Iron

Iron is primarily absorbed in the first part of the small intestine, the duodenum. After gastric bypass surgery, iron deficiency is quite common. However, iron deficiency can occur with any type of weight-loss surgery. After surgery, if complications such as bleeding or ulcers arise, iron deficiency is also more likely. Women who are menstruating are at higher risk for iron deficiency.

Ensure that your multivitamin and mineral supplement contains a substantial amount of iron — at least 18 mg per tablet. If blood levels become deficient, an additional supplement may be recommended. The usual recommended starting dose is 300 mg of ferrous gluconate or fumarate once a day or up to three times a day. It is best to take iron on an empty stomach, but many people find it easier to take with food. If you do take iron with food, try to make sure the food is rich in vitamin C, such as citrus fruits, strawberries, mangos, broccoli or peppers. Vitamin C helps to increase the absorption of iron. You also need to keep your iron intake separate from calcium supplements, antacids and dairy products by at least two hours, because calcium hinders the absorption of iron.

Vitamin D

It is quite common for people who are obese to have low vitamin D levels in their blood. After weight-loss surgery, levels can also be low or depleted. Vitamin D is important for optimizing bone health and supporting a healthy immune system. Your health-care provider will direct you if you need to take a vitamin D supplement. Vitamin D is available in chewable tablets, liquid/drops or pills. The dose needed may depend on your blood levels. It is best to take vitamin D at the same time as your calcium and with a little healthy fat to help absorption.

Protein supplements

After surgery it will be difficult to take in all the protein you need through food alone. During this time your body requires extra protein for healing and to help with weight loss. You will need to drink a protein supplement every day until you can get all the protein you need from food. You may want to practice drinking protein supplements for the taste and experience. Experiment with different flavors and varieties.

Did you know?

Constipation
Iron may make you constipated. Make sure you are choosing high-fiber foods during the day and drinking plenty of water. You may need a fiber supplement or laxative to help keep you regular. Proferrin and FeraMAX are iron supplements that reduce the likelihood of constipation. Proferrin does not interact with calcium or dairy products. Speak to your health-care professional to see if these supplements are an option for you.

Frequently Asked Questions

How much protein do I need each day?
Everybody's protein needs are different, but in general you need 60 to 80 grams every day. In the initial stages after surgery, you may need more than this recommended amount. It is best to speak to your doctor or dietitian to find out how much protein you need each day.

▶ Suggested schedule for supplementation

Supplement	Dosage	Suggested schedule
Multivitamin and mineral	I to 2 tablets	breakfast and dinner
Calcium and vitamin D	500 mg three times a day	morning, afternoon and evening snack
Vitamin B_{12}	400 mcg	breakfast
Iron	as directed	as directed
Vitamin D	as directed	as directed
Protein supplements	2 to 3 drinks per day	morning, afternoon and evening snack

Use the space provided to write in other recommended vitamin and mineral supplements that you may be taking.

Eating after Weight-Loss Surgery

Immediately after your weight-loss surgery and thereafter, you will further need to change your eating habits, not only what you eat but also the quantity you eat and how you eat it. The special bariatric diet plan in this chapter has been developed by health-care professionals associated with the bariatric surgery program at Humber River Regional Hospital in Toronto.

Remember to start taking the recommended vitamin and mineral supplements. You need to take these supplements for the rest of your life. Choose liquid or chewable forms immediately after surgery, because it will be too soon to try swallowing anything whole.

Changing what you eat and how you eat is an enormous challenge, but the rewards are equally great.

Bariatric Diet Plan

This plan involves four stages that start immediately after surgery and extend through the rest of your life. The diet stages outlined here are general guidelines. Each progressive diet stage has an associated duration (length of time) that you follow until moving on to the next stage. The length of time that you are in each stage may vary, depending on your health-care team's evaluation, the type of surgery you had and your tolerance of various foods. Do not move on to the next stage until you can comfortably eat the food from the previous stage. As you progress through each stage, enjoy the taste and texture of the food items recommended. Be sure to consult the recipe section in this book for help preparing nutritious and delicious meals and snacks.

Diet stage 1: Clear fluids

Follow for 1 to 2 days after surgery
When you wake up from surgery, a nurse will assess your condition. When you are able to, you will be encouraged to start drinking water and a variety of other clear fluids in very small amounts. The usual recommendation is 1 tablespoon (15 mL) clear fluid every 15 minutes. Clear fluids are easily

---

Did you know?

Diluted juices
Diluted juices are okay to drink in diet stage 1 and while progressing to diet stage 2. But be careful not to continue with juice in the long term, because it easy to take in excessive calories from juice. After gastric bypass surgery, juice can cause you to experience dumping syndrome as well. One cup of juice contains about 6 teaspoons (30 mL) of sugar.

digested and absorbed, so they do not put too much strain on your digestive system while it is recovering from the surgery. However, clear fluids are not nutritionally complete. They should only be used temporarily before moving on to more nutritious foods and liquids.

▶ Bariatric diet stages

As you progress through each diet stage, continue with the foods from the previous stages.

Stage	Duration	Food options
Diet stage 1 Clear fluids	1 to 2 days	• Clear fluids • Non-carbonated drinks • No sugar • No caffeine
Diet stage 2 Full fluids	For 2 weeks following diet stage 1	• Blenderized soups • Strained soups • Protein-rich liquids • Low-fat milk • Protein drinks • Yogurt
Diet stage 3.1 Soft, minced and puréed protein foods	For 1 week following diet stage 2	• Soft, minced or puréed protein foods • Puréed foods from all food groups
Diet stage 3.2 Soft vegetables and fruits	For 1 week following diet stage 3.1	• Well-cooked soft vegetables • Soft or peeled ripe fruit
Diet stage 3.3 Grain products, cereals and starchy foods	For 1 week following diet stage 3.2	• Cereals, pita bread, wraps • Avoid pasta, bread and rice until you can tolerate at least 60 g protein a day.
Diet stage 4 Lifelong foods	Start after completing all phases of diet stage 3 and onward (usually start to introduce about 6 weeks or more after surgery)	• Continue to introduce a variety of acceptable foods from all food groups as tolerated

Recommended clear liquids

- water
- broth or consommé
- diluted clear fruit juice, such as apple, grape or cranberry juice
- diet fruit-flavored gelatin
- unsweetened, non-carbonated clear beverages
- unsweetened ice pops (as tolerated)
- decaffeinated coffee
- decaffeinated tea

Diet stage 2: Full fluids

Follow for 2 weeks (14 days) after diet stage 1

Full fluids include not only liquids but also some foods that are easy to swallow and generally do not require chewing. This phase of the diet is milk-based, high in protein, low in sugar and low in fat.

Frequently Asked Questions

How much should I eat in diet stage 2? How often?

Try to take in 2 tbsp (30 mL) of a full fluid every 15 minutes. If possible, consume a total of ½ to ¾ cup (125 to 175 mL) of food at every meal. Prepare to spend about an hour to an hour and a half to finish your meal. If you feel pain and/or discomfort while you are eating, stop and take a break. Try again in about 15 minutes. Take your time and eat slowly. Focus while you are eating, avoiding distractions such as television, books or computers.

What can I do to keep myself well hydrated?

Water can seem dull, but with some added flavor it can be fun. Try these strategies:
- Add a cucumber slice.
- Add an orange, lemon or lime wedge.
- Mix in low-calorie or diet flavored powders.
- Make a chilled decaffeinated herbal or fruit tea (try green tea, orange blossom tea and apple cranberry tea).

Did you know?

Diet stage 2 special needs

Aim to consume a total of 60 to 80 g of protein each day by drinking two to three high-protein supplements daily. In addition to the full fluids, try to drink 2 to 3 cups (500 to 750 mL) of water throughout the day. Keep water near you at all times to remind you to drink. All food choices should be smooth, strained, low in fat and low in sugar.

Did you know?

Blenderized soups

Including blenderized soups as part of diet stage 2 is somewhat controversial, as blenderized soups are not traditionally part of a full-fluid diet; however, blenderized soups offer more variety and increase the nutritional quality of this diet and have been safely tolerated. Many centers are now including blenderized soups as part of diet stage 2. Speak to your health-care professional for more information.

▶ Diet stage 2 food options

Be sure to also include foods that were introduced in diet stage 1.

Food group	Foods allowed	Foods to avoid
Milk and milk products	• Milk (but avoid if you are lactose intolerant) • Lactose-reduced milk • Fortified soy milk • Yogurt (smooth, no added sugar, without chunky fruit pieces) • Sugar-free pudding • Cottage cheese (mashed) • Cream soups (low-fat, strained or blenderized)	• Lactose-containing milk and milk products • Chocolate milk • Flavored soy milk • Milkshakes • Smoothies
Vegetables and fruits	• Vegetable juice (100%) • Tomato juice • Unsweetened fruit purées, such as applesauce • Blenderized soups	• Sweetened fruit purées
Grain products and cereals	• Cream of wheat • Oatmeal • Cream of rice • Steel-cut oats • Oat bran hot cereal	• Instant oatmeal (calorie-reduced and sugary varieties)
Protein supplements	• Protein drinks • Protein powder (added to food)	• Protein drinks or supplements with too much sugar or fat • Meal-replacement drinks
Fats and oils	• Small amounts of healthier fats and oils for food preparation (canola, olive and flaxseed oils, non-hydrogenated margarine, fat-free mayonnaise)	• Butter • Oils

Food group	Foods allowed	Foods to avoid
Beverages		• Juice • Coffee • Carbonated drinks • Iced tea • Lemonade • Alcoholic beverages • Smoothies • V8 Splash or Fusion • Vitamin waters
Miscellaneous	• Salt (limited amount) • Mild herbs and seasonings • Flavoring extracts	• Chile pepper • Curry powder • Coconut and coconut milk

Protein supplements

Choose a protein supplement that is made with whey protein isolate. Whey protein isolate is a readily absorbed type and contains no lactose. Otherwise, choose a whey protein concentrate supplement, which does contain some lactose. Avoid collagen-based protein supplements because they are not as nutritionally complete as whey-based formulas.

Choose a protein supplement that has 20 to 40 grams of protein and 0 to 5 grams of carbohydrate per serving. Read the Nutrition Facts label on the package to find the serving size and determine the amount of protein you will consume once the supplement is prepared.

Take, for example, the food label on page 90 for a whey isolate protein powder. This protein supplement would be appropriate for you to use because it meets the criteria given above. However, you need to be careful following the directions provided on the label. Mix the protein supplement into water or milk, not juice. If you mix it with juice, that will add sugar.

Did you know?

LAGB fills
About six weeks after LAGB surgery, the band is filled with saline solution to tighten it. This is usually repeated about every six weeks until satiety is reached. After a fill, resume diet stage 2 for two to three days, move to diet stage 3 for two to three days, then advance to the final stage. When you start to introduce soft solids after a saline fill, be careful to chew the food thoroughly to avoid blockage of the small opening in your stomach.

Diet stage 2 sample meal plans

Since your stomach pouch is now very small, it is difficult to get all the nourishment your body needs in only three meals. You will need to eat three small meals and frequent small snacks to keep nourished. Try to eat and drink mostly high-protein food choices to assist with the healing process and to maximize your nutrition intake. Be sure to sip on water throughout the day.

All of the sample menu plans assume that the protein drink is made using 1 cup (250 mL) skim milk and 1 scoop of protein powder that contains 25 grams of protein in each scoop. Therefore the approximate protein content of the prepared drink, including protein from the milk, is

- 1 cup (250 mL) = 33 g protein
- ¾ cup (175 mL) = 25 g protein
- ½ cup (125 mL) = 16.5 g protein

Menu items in bold type can be found in the recipe section of this book.

Day 1	
Early morning	• 1 serving **Almond Coffee Protein Shake** (page 330)
Breakfast	• ¼ cup (60 mL) **Fortified Cream of Wheat** (page 174) • ¼ cup (60 mL) low-fat plain yogurt
Morning snack	• ½ cup (125 mL) chocolate protein shake
Lunch	• ¼ cup (60 mL) **Low-Fat Cream of Chicken Soup** (page 195), blended • ¼ cup (60 mL) **Applesauce** (page 300)
Early afternoon snack	• ½ cup (125 mL) protein shake
Afternoon snack	• ¼ cup (60 mL) diet vanilla pudding • 2 tbsp (30 mL) **Applesauce** (page 300)
Dinner	• ¼ cup (60 mL) fat-free cottage cheese • ¼ cup (60 mL) low-fat plain yogurt • ¼ cup (60 mL) vegetable juice
Evening snack	• ¾ cup (175 mL) vanilla protein shake

Day 2	
Early morning	• I serving **Decaf Caffè Latte** (page 334) made with unsweetened soy milk
Breakfast	• ¼ cup (60 mL) hot oat bran cereal made with ¼ cup (60 mL) skim milk • ¼ cup (60 mL) low-fat plain yogurt
Morning snack	• ¼ cup (60 mL) low-fat plain yogurt • 2 tbsp (30 mL) **Applesauce** (page 300)
Lunch	• ½ cup (125 mL) fat-free cottage cheese with 2 tbsp (30 mL) unsweetened fruit sauce
Early afternoon snack	• I serving **Almond Orange Panna Cotta** (page 315)
Afternoon snack	• ½ cup (125 mL) vanilla protein shake
Dinner	• ½ cup (125 mL) **Low-Fat Cream of Cremini Mushroom Soup** (page 187), blended • ¼ cup (60 mL) tomato juice
Evening snack	• I cup (250 mL) vanilla protein shake
Day 3	
Early morning	• ½ cup (125 mL) chocolate protein shake
Breakfast	• ¼ cup (60 mL) oatmeal made with ¼ cup (60 mL) skim milk • ¼ cup (60 mL) yogurt
Morning snack	• ½ cup (125 mL) vanilla protein shake
Lunch	• ¼ cup (60 mL) **Low-Fat Cream of Asparagus Soup** (page 183), blended • ¼ cup (60 mL) **Applesauce** (page 300)
Early afternoon snack	• ½ cup (125 mL) protein shake
Afternoon snack	• I serving **Decaf Caffè Latte** (page 334)
Dinner	• ¼ cup (60 mL) fat-free cottage cheese • ¼ cup (60 mL) low-fat plain yogurt • ¼ cup (60 mL) vegetable juice
Evening snack	• I cup (250 mL) protein shake

Diet stage 3: Puréed and soft foods

Follow as directed on page 86 for stages 3.1, 3.2 and 3.3
Diet stage 3 includes more nutritious foods than the previous stages but still allows your body time to heal and learn new ways of eating, as the textures are soft. Try to include servings from all the food groups: vegetables and fruits, grain products, milk and alternatives, meat and alternatives. Choosing foods from each food group helps you get a variety of nutrients. While you are progressing through diet stage 3, puréed or blended foods are helpful for meeting your nutrition needs because they are generally easy to tolerate. Puréed or blended foods are nutritious foods that have been mashed to a smooth consistency.

▶ Foods to purée or blend for diet stage 3

Food group	Preparation
Meat, poultry and fish	Boil, roast or bake meat, poultry or fish until it separates easily from the bone or the fish flakes easily with a fork. Remove bones and skin and trim off the fat. Cut the meat or flake fish into small pieces. Add salt, pepper or herbs and seasonings to make the food taste better. **Blend.** Add a little cooking water or broth to get the right texture. Start with 1 tbsp (15 mL) water and continue to add more water as needed.
Meat alternatives	Cook dried legumes, such as beans, lentils or chickpeas, according to package directions. If using canned legumes, rinse and drain (no need to cook). If using tofu, choose a smooth tofu that is easy to blend. **Blend.** Blend the legumes with a little water or broth. Start with 1 tbsp (15 mL) water and add more water as needed.
Vegetables and fruits	Wash, peel off skins and remove seeds as necessary. Cut the vegetable or fruit into smaller pieces. Steam or boil until soft (a fork should pierce it easily). Drain and save the cooking water. **Blend.** Use some cooking water to get the right texture. Start with 1 tbsp (15 mL) water and add more water as needed. Do not add sugar, butter or margarine.

Guide to puréeing and blending food

To purée food you need a blender, a food processor or an immersion blender. The final consistency of the food should be smooth and thick enough to scoop up with a fork or spoon, similar to applesauce or baby food.

Bits and pieces

Here are some tips for managing your diet in diet stage 3:

- As you progress through diet stage 3, continue to eat food you tolerated in the previous stages.
- Use a cooking technique that keeps food moist, such as steaming, poaching or stewing. A slow cooker is ideal for preparing moist meat.
- At each meal, eat the higher-protein food first, followed by fruits and vegetables. If there is room in your stomach pouch, progress to eating the grain products.
- Avoid spicy foods, as well as very hot or very cold foods if they cause discomfort.
- Use a low-fat sauce or gravy, such as Low-Fat Tzatziki (page 301) or Low-Fat Gravy (page 240), to moisten food.
- Try only one new food at each meal so you can learn what your body will tolerate.
- Use smaller utensils to help you to take smaller bites of food.
- Be sure to chew soft solids very well — chew at least 30 times per bite.
- Choose only low-fat, low-sugar food and drinks.
- Avoid drinking and eating at the same time. Drink 30 minutes before and 30 minutes after eating.
- Feel free to enjoy soda crackers and Melba toast, as these solid foods are allowed at the beginning of stage 3. Just be sure to chew them well.
- Spoon puréed foods into ice cube trays and freeze them. Once they are frozen, store these food cubes in plastic bags or airtight containers. Be sure to date and label each batch. Depending on what food you are freezing, frozen puréed foods should generally not be stored for longer than 3 months.

▶ Diet stage 3 puréed and soft food options

Be sure to also include foods that were introduced in diet stages 1 and 2.

Food group	Foods allowed	Foods to avoid
Diet stage 3.1 (early)		
Meat and alternatives	• Minced meat, chicken or turkey • Puréed meat, chicken or turkey • Extra-lean ground beef, chicken or turkey • Lean meatballs • Meatloaf • Low-fat chili • Minced or puréed fish • Canned water-packed tuna, salmon or sardines, mashed with a fork • Thinly sliced low-fat deli meat • Poached, scrambled or hard-cooked eggs • Omelets • Egg drop soup • Well-cooked or puréed beans, lentils and other legumes • Tofu • Vegetable hot dogs • Texturized vegetable protein	• High-fat meats such as sausages, hot dogs, hamburgers, ribs, chicken wings, fried chicken or duck • Fried eggs • Oil-packed tuna, salmon or sardines
Milk and alternatives	• Low-fat ricotta cheese • Soft low-fat cheeses	• High-fat cheeses
Vegetables and fruits	• Puréed vegetables (such as beets, peas, carrots, pumpkin, squash, green beans) • Puréed fruits (such as mango and melon)	• Sweetened fruit sauces
Grain products, cereals and starchy foods	• Soda crackers (such as saltines) • Melba toast or rounds • Cornmeal • Mashed potato • Mashed sweet potato • Mashed yam	• High-fat crackers • Buttery mashed potatoes

Food group	Foods allowed	Foods to avoid
Diet stage 3.2 (mid)		
Vegetables and fruits	• Well-cooked soft vegetables (such as steamed carrots, broccoli florets, green beans) • Vegetable soups • Well-cooked soft skinless, seedless fruits (such as cooked apples, pears, peaches) • Peeled and seeded soft fruits (such as bananas, honeydew melon, watermelon, cantaloupe) • Canned water-packed fruit or fruit cups	• Gritty or very fibrous vegetables (such as corn and asparagus) • Raw vegetables and salads • Oranges and other citrus fruits • Fruits with seeds (blackberries, strawberries, raspberries), unless strained • Canned fruit packed in juice or syrup
Diet stage 3.3 (late)		
Grain products, cereals and starchy foods	• Other low-fat crackers (such as rusk, water biscuits) • Whole wheat pita bread or mini pita pockets • Whole wheat wraps (such as tortillas) • Low-sugar and high-fiber cold cereal soaked in low-fat milk • Boiled, baked or oven-roasted potatoes • Boiled, baked or oven-roasted sweet potatoes • Boiled, baked or oven-roasted yams	• Pasta, rice, noodles, bread or muffins (avoid these starches until you can tolerate at least 60 g protein a day and eat a variety of foods from diet stage 3) • Sugary or low-fiber cold cereals • French fries

▶ Herb and spice seasoning chart

Beans, tofu	Cumin, garlic, mint, oregano, parsley, thyme
Beef	Basil, cilantro, cumin, garlic, mustard, oregano, parsley, pepper, rosemary, sage, tarragon, thyme
Chicken	Allspice, basil, bay, cinnamon, dill, fennel, garlic, ginger, lemon peel, marjoram, mint, mustard, nutmeg, paprika, parsley, pepper, sage, savory, tarragon, thyme
Eggs	Basil, chervil, chives, dill, oregano, paprika, parsley, pepper, sage, tarragon, turmeric, thyme
Fish	Basil, bay, cayenne, chives, dill, garlic, ginger, lemon peel, mustard, oregano, parsley, rosemary, saffron, sage, savory, tarragon, marjoram
Fruits	Allspice, anise, cinnamon, cloves, coriander, ginger, mint
Potato	Basil, caraway, celery seed, chervil, chives, coriander, dill, marjoram, oregano, paprika, parsley, rosemary, tarragon, thyme
Soups	Basil, bay, chervil, chives, cumin, dill, fennel, garlic, marjoram, parsley, pepper, rosemary, sage, savory, thyme
Vegetables	Basil, bay, chervil, chives, cumin, dill, fennel, garlic, marjoram, parsley, pepper, rosemary, sage, savory, thyme

Did you know?

Starting over
At any stage, if you begin to experience problems such as excessive nausea, vomiting or abdominal pain, go back to diet stage 1 (clear fluids) and contact your health-care team as soon as possible.

Flavoring puréed or blended foods
You can use a variety of herbs, spices and seasonings to make blended foods palatable. Initially you may need to avoid spicy or hot seasonings, but you can try mild curry and chili powders. In the long term, most bariatric patients can tolerate a variety of herbs and spices. In the initial stages you can add the herbs and spices to your food. For example, if you are making a puréed chicken dish, add the herbs and spices before blending the food. Finely powdered spices are generally safe to add at any point. Refer to the recipe section in this book for creative and healthy puréed or blended food recipes.

Frequently Asked Questions

How much should I eat in diet stage 3?

Your daily goal is 60 to 80 grams protein and 6 to 8 cups (1.5 to 2 L) fluid, including water sipped between meals. Measure and weigh your food after it is cooked or prepared. Eat 2 to 4 tablespoons (30 to 60 mL) of food every 15 minutes and spend 60 to 90 minutes eating at each meal.

If you have had a gastric bypass or the LAGB procedure, try to consume about ½ to ¾ cup (125 to 175 mL) of food at your meal. If you have had a VSG procedure, you may be able to eat about ¾ to 1 cup (175 to 250 mL) at each meal.

Initially, be prepared to spend about an hour to an hour and a half eating a meal. In the long term you will likely become comfortable with eating your meal within half an hour. If you feel pain or discomfort while eating, stop and take a break and try again later. Take your time and eat slowly — you need to focus on your eating. Although measuring and weighing your food is important, it is best that you learn your body's own cues. Pay attention to how you are feeling with the amount you are eating.

Did you know?

Texturized vegetable protein

Also known as TVP or texturized soy protein, this food derives from defatted soy flour. TVP comes in small, dry chunks or in ground form and looks similar to dehydrated vegetables. On its own it does not have much flavor, but once it is rehydrated and seasoned, it can be used to replace all or some of the meat in dishes such as chili, hamburgers, stews and soups. It is very high in protein and low in fat and contains fiber and iron as well.

Nutritious snacks

Try to make your snack choices well balanced and nutritious by including food groups that you may have missed at mealtimes. For example, if you do not have much milk or milk products or fruit at mealtimes, snack time presents an opportunity to add in this type of nutrition. Including a source of protein helps sustain you a little longer. As well, snacks are a great time to boost your intake of fiber.

Safe snacks

Snack items in bold type can be found in the recipe section of this book.

- Low-fat cheese and high-fiber crackers
- Yogurt with fruit
- Smoked salmon on rye crispbread
- **Hard-Cooked Egg** (page 165)
- Protein shake
- High-fiber cereal and milk
- Cottage cheese and cut-up cantaloupe

- Diet pudding cup
- **Hummus** (page 304) and cut-up vegetables
- **Low-Fat Tzatziki** (page 301) with cucumber slices
- **Ricotta Cheese with Pear** (page 307) on rusk bread
- Low-fat string cheese
- Vegetable juice

Diet stage 3 sample meal plans

Here are sample meal plans to follow while progressing through each part of diet stage 3 (stages 3.1, 3.2 and 3.3). Mix and match from the three sample plans for the other days of the week. Some sample days include an early morning snack for those who prefer to start their day off with something a little lighter.

Menu items in bold type can be found in the recipe section of this book.

Diet stage 3.1 (early)	
Day 1	
Early morning	• ½ cup (125 mL) protein drink
Breakfast	• 1 **Perfect Poached Egg** (page 164) • ¼ cup (60 mL) **Applesauce** (page 300)
Morning snack	• ½ cup (125 mL) vegetable juice
Lunch	• 4 tbsp (60 mL) canned tuna, water-packed and moistened with ½ tsp (2 mL) fat-free mayonnaise • 2 pieces Melba toast
Afternoon snack	• ½ cup (125 mL) protein drink
Dinner	• 1 serving **Sweet Potato and Turkey Purée** (page 237)
Early evening snack	• 4 soda crackers with 2 tbsp (30 mL) low-fat spreadable cream cheese
Evening snack	• ¾ cup (175 mL) protein drink

Diet stage 3.1 (early)	
Day 2	
Breakfast	• ¼ cup (60 mL) **Fortified Cream of Wheat** (page 174) • ¼ cup (60 mL) low-fat yogurt
Morning snack	• ½ cup (125 mL) protein drink • 2 tbsp (30 mL) **Applesauce** (page 300) • 2 crackers
Lunch	• ½ cup (125 mL) **Tropical Chicken Purée** (page 236) • ¼ cup (60 mL) vegetable juice
Afternoon snack	• ½ cup (125 mL) protein drink
Dinner	• 3 oz (90 g) **Italian-Style Meatloaf** (page 217) • 2 tbsp (30 mL) puréed cauliflower
Early evening snack	• ½ cup (125 mL) diet pudding
Evening snack	• ¾ cup (175 mL) protein drink
Day 3	
Breakfast	• 1 serving **Stirred Scrambled Eggs** (page 166) • 2 pieces Melba toast
Morning snack	• ½ cup (125 mL) protein drink • 2 tbsp (30 mL) puréed blueberries
Lunch	• ¼ cup (60 mL) cottage cheese mixed with 2 tbsp (30 mL) puréed mango • ½ cup (125 mL) skim milk
Afternoon snack	• ½ cup (125 mL) low-fat yogurt • 2 tbsp (30 mL) mashed banana
Dinner	• 1 serving minced **Maple-Glazed Barbecue Salmon** (page 244) • ¼ cup (60 mL) **Cauliflower Mashed Potatoes** (page 294)
Early evening snack	• 1 piece low-fat string cheese • 2 pieces Melba toast
Evening snack	• ¾ cup (175 mL) protein drink

Diet stage 3.2 (mid)	
Day 1	
Early morning	• ¾ cup (175 mL) warm milk with decaffeinated coffee
Breakfast	• 1 serving **Classic Omelet** (page 167) with sautéed diced red bell peppers and mushrooms
Morning snack	• ½ cup (125 mL) low-fat yogurt
Lunch	• ¼ cup (60 mL) salmon salad • 4 Melba toast rounds • 3 soft, well-cooked baby carrots
Afternoon snack	• ½ cup (125 mL) puréed fruit salad • 1 oz (30 g) low-fat cheese
Dinner	• 1 serving **Vegetarian Chili** (page 258) • 2 to 4 tbsp (30 to 60 mL) **Herbed Mashed Potatoes** (page 295) • 1 serving **Amaretto Espresso Cups** (page 316)
Evening snack	• ¾ cup (175 mL) protein drink
Day 2	
Early morning	• ½ cup (125 mL) vegetable juice
Breakfast	• ½ cup (125 mL) steel-cut oats made with milk • 2 tbsp (30 mL) applesauce with cinnamon
Morning snack	• 4 soda crackers with 1 oz (30 g) low-fat cheese
Lunch	• ¼ cup (60 mL) egg salad • 2 Melba toast crackers • 1 well-cooked steamed broccoli floret
Afternoon snack	• ½ cup (125 mL) protein drink
Dinner	• 1 serving **Classic Chicken Stew** (page 234) • 2 tbsp (30 mL) mashed potato
Early evening snack	• ½ cup (125 mL) cut-up honeydew melon
Evening snack	• ½ cup (125 mL) protein drink

Diet stage 3.2 (mid)	
Day 3	
Early morning	• I serving **Almond Coffee Protein Shake** (page 330)
Breakfast	• I **Perfect Poached Egg** (page 164) • ½ small banana
Morning snack	• 2 tbsp (30 mL) low-fat cottage cheese • 4 soda crackers
Lunch	• I serving **Simple Sockeye Salmon Salad** (page 245) • ¼ cup (60 mL) **Steamed Green Beans** (page 288) • 2 tbsp (30 mL) mashed sweet potato
Afternoon snack	• ½ cup (125 mL) fruit cup packed in water, drained, topped with I tbsp (15 mL) plain low-fat yogurt
Dinner	• I serving **Turkey Meatloaf Muffins** (page 238) • ¼ cup (60 mL) well-cooked peas
Early evening snack	• ½ cup (125 mL) low-fat yogurt
Evening snack	• ½ cup (125 mL) protein drink
Diet stage 3.3 (late)	
Day I	
Early morning	• I serving **Decaf Caffè Latte** (page 334)
Breakfast	• ½ cup (125 mL) high-fiber cereal, soaked in ¼ cup (60 mL) skim milk
Morning snack	• I **Hard-Cooked Egg** (page 165)
Lunch	• 3 oz (90 g) **Vegetable Meatloaf** (page 218) • I small boiled potato
Afternoon snack	• 2 tbsp (30 mL) **Hummus** (page 304) • 6 well-cooked baby carrots
Dinner	• I serving **Tofu Patties** (page 267) • ¼ cup (60 mL) **Cinnamon-Glazed Carrot Coins** (page 286)
Early evening snack	• ½ cup (125 mL) yogurt
Evening snack	• ½ cup (125 mL) protein drink

Diet stage 3.3 (late)	
Day 2	
Breakfast	• ½ cup (125 mL) steel-cut oats, made with milk
Morning snack	• 1 serving **Strawberry Banana Protein Smoothie** (page 329), strained
Lunch	• 1 serving **Lentil Soup** (page 192) • ½ small wrap
Afternoon snack	• ½ cup (125 mL) pudding, mixed with ¼ chopped small banana
Dinner	• 3 oz (90 g) **Haddock in Tomato Juice** (page 243) • 4 tbsp (60 mL) well-cooked soft vegetables
Early evening snack	• 1 serving **Crustless No-Bake Pumpkin Pie** (page 313)
Evening snack	• ½ cup (125 mL) protein drink
Day 3	
Breakfast	• ½ wrap • 1 piece low-fat string cheese • ¼ cup (60 mL) fruit
Morning snack	• ½ cup (125 mL) protein drink
Lunch	• ½ cup (125 mL) **Baby Lima Bean Stew** (page 259) • 1 small pita pocket
Afternoon snack	• 1 serving **Egg and Ham Pinwheels** (page 308)
Dinner	• ½ to ¾ cup (125 to 175 mL) **Shepherd's Pie** (page 214)
Early evening snack	• 1 serving **Melon Ball Fruit Cup** (page 319), topped with 2 tbsp (30 mL) yogurt
Evening snack	• ½ cup (125 mL) protein drink

Diet stage 4: Lifelong foods

In the long term, after weight-loss surgery you can comfortably eat and enjoy a variety of foods that are low in fat and sugar and offer you good nutritional value. Most people are able to eat well-balanced nutritious meals and snacks. The lifelong diet is not much different from the way the average person should be eating — small portions, lower-fat, lower-sugar and nutritious foods.

Protein drinks

During diet stage 4, continue with the protein drinks until you are able to eat about 60 to 80 grams of protein from food every day. If you are able to eat a protein choice at breakfast and you can comfortably eat a 2- to 3-ounce (60 to 90 g) protein choice at lunch and dinner, and if you are able to consume at least two servings of milk or milk alternatives a day, you are likely getting enough protein — in which case you may be able to stop using the protein drinks. To help you add up how much protein you are getting in a day, you can refer to the chart on page 104 for the protein content of various foods. If that is too difficult for you, your dietitian or a member of your health-care team can help you decide when you no longer need protein drinks.

Food tolerance

Some of the lifelong food choices can be tricky to eat. Through trial and error you will find that you can tolerate some foods better than others. Be patient. Do not assume that if you cannot tolerate a food today you will never be able to tolerate it again. Wait a few days and try again.

Do not try the following foods until you are able to eat and tolerate a variety of the foods introduced in diet stages 1, 2 and 3, and when you can comfortably consume at least 60 grams of protein a day from food.

Raw vegetables and salads

Raw crisp vegetables can take time to introduce because it is difficult to chew them well enough. Some people can comfortably tolerate salads one month after weight-loss surgery; however, you should wait until you can comfortably eat enough protein every day before filling up on salads. When you do eat vegetables and salads, be sure to use low-fat dressings and toppings.

▶ Protein content of common foods

Food	Serving	Protein content (grams)
Canned beans	½ cup (125 mL)	8.0
Cheese, mozzarella	2 tbsp (30 mL)	7.0
Cheese, ricotta	½ cup (125 mL)	14.0
Chicken breast	2½ oz (75 g)	25.0
Chickpeas	½ cup (125 mL)	7.5
Cottage cheese	½ cup (125 mL)	14.0
Crab, steamed	3 oz (90 g)	17.0
Deli meats (low-fat ham, low-fat turkey)	1 slice, 1 oz (30 g)	5.0
Edamame (soybeans)	½ cup (125 mL)	6.0
Egg	1 large	6.0
Fish (salmon, cod, halibut, flounder)	3 oz (90 g)	21.0
Ground beef, extra-lean	2½ oz (75 g)	23.0 g
Hot dog, fat-free	1½ oz (50 g)	6.3
Lentils	½ cup (125 mL)	8.5
Milk, cow's or goat's	½ cup (125 mL)	4.0
Pork	2½ oz (75 grams)	24.0
Quinoa	½ cup (125 mL)	4.0
Shrimp	3 oz (90 g)	19.0
Soy milk, unsweetened	½ cup (125 mL)	3.5
Texturized vegetable protein, prepared	½ cup (125 mL)	24.0
Tofu	½ cup (125 mL)	10.0
Tuna, canned, water-packed	3 oz (90 g)	22.0
Yogurt	3 oz (90 g)	4.0
Yogurt, Greek-style	½ cup (125 mL)	15.0

SOURCE: USDA Nutrient Database

Fresh fruit, fruit skins and peels

Raw crisp fruit and fruit with skins and seeds are difficult to tolerate during the initial diet stages. They can comfortably be introduced after you are able to tolerate a variety of foods and textures from the previous diet stages. Most fruit skins are well tolerated except for tougher apple skins, which should be peeled; the peel can cause a lot of pain if not chewed well enough.

Grain products

Initially, leavened breads, pastas and grains can leave a heavy feeling in your stomach. In the long term, if you wish to try bread, eat toasted whole wheat bread first. Toasting the bread makes it easier to digest and tolerate. Most people can comfortably tolerate small amounts of pasta and grain products, but choose healthier alternatives such as whole wheat pasta, brown rice, quinoa or couscous.

Leftover meat

Oftentimes when leftover meat is warmed up, it tends to get overcooked and the connective tissues and meat fibers change in structure. This makes the meat tougher and more difficult to chew; you may even vomit. To add some moisture, try using leftover chicken or meat in a stew or soup. Or, when you are warming up the meat, add a low-fat broth or gravy to give it some moisture. You can also try cutting the meat into small pieces first and then sipping on a very small amount of milk, vegetable juice or water while you are chewing. If these tips do not work, you may need to give up on leftover meat for a while. Just cook what you need and try again another time.

Nut butters

Nut butters such as peanut butter, almond butter and soy nut butter are nutritious, but they should be limited in the beginning because they tend to be sticky and contain a significant amount of fat. Nut butters can be introduced gradually into your diet in small amounts.

Did you know?

Red meat

Red meat such as steak tends to be difficult to break down and tolerate. Wait three to four months before trying red meat. When you decide to have it, be sure that you choose a lean cut, limit the portion size and prepare it so that it is not dry, using a method such as stewing or braising.

▶ Foods that may be difficult to tolerate

Food group	Difficult to tolerate	Try instead
Meat and alternatives	• Red meat • Fatty cuts of meat • Whole beans with tough skins, chickpeas • Leftover meats	• Lean pork • Extra-lean ground meat • Mashed beans or chickpeas
Milk and alternatives	• Milk (lactose-containing)	• Soy milk (unsweetened) • Lactose-reduced milk • Goat's milk (fortified)
Vegetables	• Fibrous vegetables (asparagus, corn)	• Non-fibrous vegetables • Blended fibrous vegetables in soups
Fruit	• Apple skins • Dried whole fruit	• Peeled apples • Soft fresh fruit
Grain products and starchy foods	• Leavened bread (buns, baguettes, rolls, sliced bread) • Pasta • Rice • Noodles	• Wraps • Pita bread • Melba toast • Toasted whole-grain bread • Thin-sliced bread (toasted) • Rye or pumpernickel bread • Crackers • Rice noodles • Tofu noodles • Gluten-free pasta • Spelt pasta or noodles • Quinoa • Couscous • Khorasan (Kamut) • Barley • Potatoes
Beverages	• Carbonated drinks • Sugary drinks	• Non-carbonated drinks • Unsweetened or diet drinks

Food group	Difficult to tolerate	Try instead
Sugars and sweets	• Sugar • Honey • Syrup • Molasses • Brown sugar • Sugar alcohols (xylitol, mannitol, sorbitol, maltitol, isomalt, lactitol, erythritol)	• Sucralose • Aspartame • Saccharin • Cyclamate • Acesulfame potassium • No-sugar-added maple-flavored syrup
Fats and oils	• Fatty foods • Fried foods • Coconut • Avocado • Nuts • Seeds	• Baked, steamed, poached or grilled foods (see recipe section for healthy options) • Healthier fats and oils in limited amounts
Miscellaneous	• Popcorn • Candy • Chocolate • Donuts • Pastries • Cakes	• Rice crackers • Rice cakes • See recipe section for healthy options

Alcohol

Under the guidance of your doctor, an occasional drink can be enjoyed as part of your lifestyle. If you do choose to have a drink, try to select lower-calorie and non-carbonated drinks such as white wines (Zinfandel, Chablis, Chardonnay) or dry red wines. Sip the drink slowly, if possible with some food, and know your limits.

However, the general recommendation is to avoid alcohol for the first year after bariatric surgery and to limit consumption in the long term. Alcohol is absorbed into the bloodstream rapidly after gastric bypass and VSG surgery. You may find an intoxication effect after just a few sips of an alcoholic drink. Studies have shown a higher blood alcohol level in gastric bypass patients than in their counterparts after the same quantity of alcoholic drinks. The reason is simple: because of the small stomach pouch, alcohol gets absorbed into the bloodstream more quickly. Another reason for the quick intoxication effect is that when you are on a calorie-restricted diet, there is less food to hinder the absorption of alcohol.

Alcohol can irritate the lining of the digestive system as well as cause damage to the liver. During this time of rapid weight loss, the liver is already sensitive and so should not be stressed by toxins. Alcoholic drinks are empty calories that are high in sugar, and in gastric bypass surgery they can cause dumping syndrome. In the long term these extra calories may also sabotage weight-loss efforts. Nutrients in your body may be depleted, you may experience hypoglycemia (low blood sugar), and you could develop a replacement addiction. Completely avoid alcohol if you are on certain medications, or if you are experiencing complications from surgery such as vomiting or diarrhea.

Diet stage 4 sample meal plans

Here are some sample meal plans for Stage 4, lifelong foods. Take note that meal plans and portion sizes will vary based on the type of surgery you have had and your body's needs. Some people may need to eat more and some less than is outlined here. Be sure to keep hydrated with plenty of water throughout the day.

Menu items in bold type can be found in the recipe section of this book.

Day 1	
Breakfast	• 1 serving **Mexican Baked Eggs** (page 170) • ½ cup (125 mL) skim milk
Morning snack	• 1 **Mini Banana Bread Muffin** (page 309) • 3 oz (90 g) low-fat yogurt
Lunch	• 1 serving **Beef Stew with Leeks** (page 212) • 1 small fruit
Afternoon snack	• 1 serving **Green Salsa Mini Pita Pizza** (page 305)
Dinner	• 1 serving **Creamy Dijon Chicken Thighs** (page 225) • ¼ cup (60 mL) steamed vegetables • ¼ cup (60 mL) mashed potato
Early evening	• ½ cup (125 mL) skim milk
Evening snack	• 1 serving **Amaretto Espresso Cups** (page 316)

Day 2	
Early morning	• I serving **Strawberry Banana Protein Smoothie** (page 329)
Breakfast	• I serving **Apple Cinnamon Yogurt Bulgur** (page 176)
Morning snack	• ¼ cup (60 mL) low-fat cottage cheese, with 2 tbsp (30 mL) chopped strawberries
Lunch	• I serving **Spinach Soup with Oatmeal Balls** (page 189)
Afternoon snack	• 3 tbsp (45 mL) **Black Bean Dip** (page 303) • 2 pieces Melba toast • ½ cup (125 mL) skim milk
Dinner	• I serving **Swordfish Skewers** (page 247) • I serving **Khorasan Wheat with Bell Peppers** (page 280) • ¼ cup (60 mL) vegetable juice
Evening snack	• I serving **Fruit Salad with Pecans** (page 318)
Day 3	
Breakfast	• ¾ cup (175 mL) **Banana Bread Oatmeal** (page 173)
Morning snack	• I serving **Fruit Kebabs** (page 310) • I serving **Chai** (page 333)
Lunch	• I serving **Sweet Potato Chili** (page 219) • I oz (30 g) low-fat cheese
Afternoon snack	• I serving **Pearl Bocconcini with Tomato** (page 306)
Dinner	• I serving **Pad Thai with Brown Rice Noodles** (page 274) • ¼ cup (60 mL) low-fat yogurt
Evening snack	• I serving **Trail Mix Treat** (page 310) • I serving **Light Hot Chocolate** (page 336)

How to Eat

Following bariatric surgery, you will need to change the way you eat. These changes will facilitate a more successful surgery by helping to prevent problems such as pain or discomfort, vomiting, nausea, regurgitation, heartburn and/or gas.

These strategies will become part of your new lifestyle. Gone are the days of dashboard dining, eating on the run or swallowing your food before you have a chance to chew it. These tips will not only help prevent you from feeling physical side effects, they will also help prevent weight-loss failure, instilling a new, healthy attitude toward food and how you eat it.

Guidelines for how to eat

When you start to eat solid food, you must take extra care how you eat. Follow these guidelines:

Listen to your body's cues and recognize feelings of fullness

Your feelings of fullness may be different from before surgery. You may feel pressure or fullness behind the sternum (breastbone), experience a sensation that the food is stuck and/or experience heartburn from regurgitation or acid buildup. Overeating can give you pain or discomfort, make you feel nauseated and perhaps even cause you to vomit. Stop eating if you feel full or experience any of these symptoms, and contact your health-care team if this persists.

Avoid eating too much

If you eat too much you will feel sick. Over time you will be able to eat more, but at first you need to eat very small amounts of food. Use a teaspoon or small dessert fork to help you slow down. In time your stomach pouch will naturally allow you to eat larger portions. If you have had gastric bypass or LAGB surgery, try to restrict your total meal portions to $\frac{1}{2}$ to $\frac{3}{4}$ cup (125 to 175 mL) at a time. If you have had VSG surgery, try to restrict your total meal portions to $\frac{3}{4}$ to 1 cup (175 to 250 mL). In the long term you may be able to eat more, depending on your needs, but you should be careful to avoid eating too much.

Eat three meals every day

Eat three nutritious meals, spaced out during the day. Avoid skipping meals. You may not feel hunger, but this should not stop you from trying to eat. Snacks are needed in the initial months after weight-loss surgery because you are usually not able to eat enough at mealtimes. In the long term, snacks will be needed if you are not able to eat enough during mealtimes, if you wait more than three or four hours between meals or if you are very active.

Sip low-calorie non-carbonated drinks throughout the day

Liquids are necessary to stay hydrated, and water is the best choice. Drink water, skim milk and low-calorie non-carbonated beverages. Carry a water bottle at all times. Avoid high-calorie drinks such as milkshakes, soda pop, fruit juices, fruit drinks, beer, alcohol or meal substitutes. These can make you gain weight by adding calories without necessarily making you feel full. Avoid all carbonated beverages, as they can make you feel full and bloated and sometimes cause pain.

Eat well-balanced meals and nutritious foods

Make every bite count — eat high-quality, nutrient-rich food. At each meal eat the high-protein food first. After eating the high-protein food, eat the fruit or vegetable. If there is still room in your stomach pouch, eat the grain product or starch. Add foods to your diet slowly, one at a time, to test your tolerance for them.

Sit down at a table and focus while eating

Avoid distractions such as television, computers, work or other activities. Distractions can cause you to chew and swallow too quickly and to overeat, which can cause you to feel abdominal pain or discomfort. In the long term, overeating will sabotage your weight-loss efforts.

Eat and drink slowly

Set aside 30 to 60 minutes for each meal and 10 to 15 minutes for each snack. After surgery you should never gulp liquids, as this may cause you to feel pain or abdominal discomfort. Instead, sip liquids slowly. Try using a water bottle or a small glass to avoid taking large gulps. Some patients find that using a toddler's spout or sippy cup, with the flow valve removed, is helpful for drinking liquids. People tend to gulp liquids when they are dehydrated. Try to not get to the point of extreme thirst by keeping yourself hydrated throughout the day.

Did you know?

Soothing habits
Researchers have found that playing soft, slow music while eating helps people eat slowly. Smaller plates, bowls, cups and utensils encourage smaller portions.

Chew foods until they are mushy

Chewing food well grinds it into smaller pieces, making it easier for your body to handle. Initially you can cut food into small pieces — about the size of a pea — to make it easier to chew. Take very small bites, and try eating with a small teaspoon, baby spoon or dessert fork to keep bites small. Between bites, put your utensil down on the table while you are chewing. Aim to chew each bite of food 30 times.

Pay attention to taste, flavor and texture

By paying attention to the taste, flavor and texture of your food, you are becoming more mindful of not only what you are eating but also how you are eating. It provides you with an opportunity to enjoy your food. By tuning in to your body as you eat, you take control of how much you are eating and will have a better sense of when you need to stop eating.

Principles of mindful eating

- Enjoy your food.
- Appreciate the flavors and textures of food. Over time this will lead to changes in your preferences.
- Pay attention to what you are eating.
- Allow yourself to taste and savor food without feelings of guilt.
- Eat regularly, establishing a meal routine based on your schedule.
- Avoid coming to the table starving and then eating too quickly to enjoy your food. Slow down.
- Try playing some soft, slow music while eating.
- Enjoy a variety of foods from different food groups.
- Explore new tastes and flavors. Try foods from different cultures.

Be conscious of portion sizes

Monitor your portions using a weigh scale and measuring cups and spoons. Weigh and measure your food when it is ready to eat. Explain to friends and family or co-workers why you need to eat slowly, and so little, so they don't urge you to hurry up or offer you larger portions or extra servings.

Separate liquids from solid foods

Try not to drink 30 minutes before and 30 minutes after eating solid food. Drinking liquids while eating may cause nausea and dumping syndrome (for gastric bypass). It also pushes the food through the pouch faster, causing you to eat more. In the long term, for some people drinking very small amounts with meals is not a problem, but be sure to keep it to a minimum and sip slowly.

Avoid drinking straws and sports bottles

Using drinking straws or sports bottle spouts to drink liquids could cause pain or abdominal discomfort, because the sucking action can cause you to swallow air. Avoid using straws or spouted bottles to drink, and avoid any type of carbonated beverage.

Frequently Asked Questions

How do I know if I have had too much to eat or drink?
There are several clear signs of overeating:

- You may feel nausea or vomit.
- You may feel pressure or fullness behind your sternum (breastbone).
- You may feel pain in your left shoulder or in your upper back.
- You may feel pressure or discomfort in your throat.
- You may feel as if the food is stuck in your throat.

If you experience any of these symptoms, you should stop eating, even if you have not finished your meal. Try to eat again later. If this continues to happen on a regular basis, inform your health-care team.

Self-diagnosis

If after having bariatric surgery you experience problems when you are eating or drinking, you can ask yourself the following questions to help determine if you need to seek medical attention. If you continue to experience problems even though you have followed all the recommendations, seek medical attention.

If you answered no to any of these questions, work on solving those particular problems. You are following the guidelines properly if you answered yes to all of the questions. In this case there may be other reasons why you are experiencing problems, and you should seek attention from your health-care team.

▶ Self-diagnosing eating difficulties

Question	Ask yourself	Yes or No
What?	• Is this food choice part of the current diet stage I am in? • Is this food the right texture? • Is this food moist enough? • Is this food or drink low in sugar and fat?	
How?	• Am I chewing the food enough? • Am I eating slowly enough? • Am I focused on my eating? • Am I eating mindfully?	
Where?	• Am I eating at a table or a location with no distractions? • Are the TV and computer off?	
When?	• Am I eating on time? • Am I eating regular or routine meals? • Did I space out my meals and snacks appropriately? • Did I space out my drinks around my meals or snacks as recommended? • Is my stomach empty?	
Why?	• Am I eating because it is time to eat? • Am I eating because I am physically hungry?	

Frequently Asked Questions

Can I chew gum after having bariatric surgery?

Chewing gum is not recommended. The action of chewing can fill your small stomach with air, which can make you feel pain, bloating and/or abdominal discomfort. As well, with gastric bypass and LAGB surgery, if you swallow the gum by accident it may get stuck in the small, narrow opening.

Nutritional Challenges after Surgery

After weight-loss surgery, nutritional problems can arise because of the nature of the surgery. Some of these problems include malnutrition, dehydration and digestive problems such as constipation, gas and bloating, diarrhea, nausea and vomiting and lactose intolerance. Medical problems such as dumping syndrome, hypoglycemia and strictures may also occur. You need to try to prevent these problems from taking a toll on your health and well-being. However, at times they are inevitable and will need to be managed and treated by your health-care team. Don't hesitate to ask for help.

Malnutrition

Malnutrition develops when your body does not get the right amounts of nutrients to maintain healthy tissues, organs and bodily functions. It is quite common after any type of bariatric surgery to become malnourished to some degree if care is not taken to follow the recommendations provided by your health-care team.

Mild malnutrition commonly occurs after bariatric surgeries because of restricted nutritional intake and, in some cases, because of malabsorption of nutrients. There is a greater risk of becoming malnourished when post-surgical complications arise, such as strictures, leaks, infections or obstructions. In that case your health-care team may give you specific diet and supplement recommendations to prevent further malnutrition. In some cases you may need alternative methods of receiving nutrients, such as enteral or parenteral nutrition.

If you do not experience any complications or problems and you follow the recommendations provided by your health-care team, including eating a well-balanced, nutritious diet, taking all the recommended vitamin and minerals and remaining well hydrated, the likelihood of becoming malnourished is lessened.

Did you know?

Medication safety
After surgery, some medications are not safe to take and some medications may not be well absorbed. Do not make any changes to your medications without consulting a health-care professional. For example, if you take antidepressants, do not change the dose or stop taking them on your own just because you are feeling good after losing some weight. Speak to your physician or pharmacist to get more help on taking medications after weight-loss surgery.

Micronutrient deficiencies

Becoming deficient in any micronutrient is an issue primarily with gastric bypass surgery, because of the intestinal bypass. However, micronutrient deficiencies can also occur after any type of weight-loss surgery because of the decreased volume of food you are able to eat. It is imperative to eat well-balanced, nutritious meals and to take the recommended vitamin and mineral supplements every day. Routine laboratory assessments ordered by your health-care professional can detect nutrient deficiencies. For more information on nutrient deficiencies, see page 60.

▶ Common micronutrient deficiencies

After gastric bypass surgery	After LAGB	After VSG
• iron	• vitamin B_{12}	• vitamin D
• vitamin D	• iron	• vitamin B_{12}
• vitamin B_1 (thiamin)	• folate	• iron
• folate	• vitamin D	• others
• calcium	• others	
• potassium		
• vitamin B_{12}		
• zinc		
• vitamin C		
• vitamin A		
• others		

Dehydration

Dehydration can happen at any time after weight-loss surgery, especially if you do not drink enough fluids to meet your body's needs. Severe dehydration can lead to confusion, weakness and, if untreated, coma, organ failure and even death.

Dehydration is more likely to occur if you are experiencing problematic symptoms such as persistent vomiting and diarrhea. It is also quite common to develop dehydration if you have a stricture (with a gastric bypass) or if the LAGB band is too tight, resulting in poor oral intake. Exercise and excessive sweating are also risks for becoming dehydrated.

Because it is not recommended to gulp liquids after bariatric surgery, sip on fluids throughout the day to help prevent dehydration. Mild dehydration can usually be resolved at home by increasing your fluid intake, especially water, and limiting caffeinated beverages, which act as diuretics. More severe cases of dehydration will likely need medical attention and possible intravenous hydration (IV therapy).

Signs and symptoms of mild dehydration

- dry mouth or lips
- dry eyes
- dry skin
- dark, strong-smelling urine
- small amounts of urine
- headache
- fluid retention
- decreased sweating
- muscle cramps
- nausea and vomiting
- heart palpitations or elevated heart rate
- decrease in blood pressure
- flushed skin
- tiredness and irritability
- lightheadedness, dizziness
- mild confusion
- weakness

Signs and symptoms of severe dehydration

- blue lips
- blotchy skin
- confusion

- lack of energy
- cold hands or feet
- rapid breathing
- high fever
- unconsciousness

Seek medical attention immediately.

How to treat dehydration

- Sip on small amounts of clear fluids frequently:
  - ▶ water
  - ▶ diluted juice
  - ▶ low-sugar sports drink
  - ▶ diet gelatin
  - ▶ broth (diluted)
- Avoid diuretic drinks such as coffee or tea.
- Suck on ice chips.
- Rest.
- Keep cool.
- Control the symptoms causing the dehydration, such as vomiting, diarrhea or fever.
- Seek medical attention.

Frequently Asked Questions

I am struggling to get in all the water I need in the day. Are there any tips to help me keep hydrated?

After weight-loss surgery it can be difficult to get enough fluid as you learn new drinking habits and are restricted to small volumes of foods and liquids. Here are some tips to help keep you hydrated:

- Start the day by sipping on water while you are getting ready.
- Limit caffeine and alcohol because they act as diuretics and cause the body to lose water.
- For every cup of caffeinated beverage, replace it with a cup of water.
- Have a water bottle with you everywhere you go (at your desk, in the car, in your purse or bag, on your nightstand).
- Create a daily schedule to remind you to drink some water 30 minutes after every meal and snack.
- Keep a cup in the bathroom and sip on some water every time you use the toilet.
- Limit your salt intake, because salt retains fluids.
- Eat fruits, vegetables, milk and soup.

Digestive Problems

Following surgery, you may experience some common digestive problems that deserve medical attention if they persist.

Constipation

It is quite common to become constipated after weight-loss surgery. Constipation involves a decrease in the normal frequency and ease of bowel movements. You may have difficulty passing a bowel movement, straining to defecate, or have hard, dry, pebbly stools. Constipation could also mean that there is incomplete passage of stool.

Common causes of constipation after weight-loss surgery

- change in eating patterns and food intake
- inadequate fluids
- not enough fiber
- decreased physical activity
- certain pain medications
- iron supplements
- bowel obstruction (if you suspect a bowel obstruction, seek medical attention immediately)

How to improve your bowel movements

- Drink water and low-calorie fluids regularly.
- Add a fiber supplement to liquids or food.
- Eat fiber-rich foods.
- Increase your level of physical activity.
- Try a mild laxative, as directed by your health-care professional.

Gas and bloating

Gas and bloating are common, especially during the first few weeks after surgery. They could also be a sign of lactose intolerance. If gas and bloating do not improve with the suggestions provided here, speak to your health-care providers. You may want to try taking an anti-gas medication, available at your pharmacy.

How to prevent gas and bloating

- Limit liquids to 2 ounces (60 mL) at one time.
- Avoid carbonated beverages.
- Sip drinks slowly.
- Do not use a straw.
- Do not chew gum.
- Avoid sugar alcohol sweeteners.

Did you know?

Fiber facts

Women should aim to get 25 grams of dietary fiber a day and men 38 grams a day. This can be difficult to achieve after weight-loss surgery because of the restricted volumes of foods you can eat. Fiber supplements can help boost your intake. When reading food labels, aim for more than 2 grams per serving.

Diarrhea

Diarrhea may occur after bariatric surgery for several reasons. With gastric bypass surgery, the usual culprits are too much sugar or fat in the diet or lactose intolerance. If you are taking antibiotics, you may experience diarrhea as a side effect. It is important to figure out what may be causing the diarrhea, to make sure it is not a medical problem. Keep well hydrated if you do experience diarrhea. If it continues to be a problem for some time, speak to your dietitian or physician.

How to manage diarrhea

- Keep hydrated.
- Avoid foods and drinks that are high in fat or sugar.
- Try temporarily avoiding lactose (found in dairy products).
- Eat a soft, bland diet.
- Contact your health-care professional for further advice.

Nausea and vomiting

Nausea and vomiting are common during the first couple of weeks after surgery, but they can continue if you do not follow proper cooking and eating techniques. Nausea and vomiting may be a result of not chewing food well enough and/or eating too much. More specifically, nausea alone may occur if you are dehydrated or sensitive to odors.

If nausea and vomiting persist and you are following the eating guidelines carefully, this may be a sign that something is wrong, such as a stricture, acid buildup or a too-tight LAGB band. It is best to inform your physician or health-care team as soon as possible.

How to manage nausea and vomiting

- Take small bites of food and sip on fluids slowly.
- Chew your food thoroughly.
- Take your time, setting aside 30 to 45 minutes for each meal.
- Avoid drinking with meals.
- Avoid foods that are high in fat or sugar.
- If nausea and vomiting occur after eating a new food that should normally be tolerated, wait several days before trying that food again.
- Avoid cold beverages and those with caffeine or carbonation.

Lactose intolerance

Milk and dairy products contain lactose, a natural sugar molecule that is broken down into smaller molecules by the enzyme lactase. Lactose intolerance is the inability to break down this sugar. Sometimes, specifically after gastric bypass surgery, you can develop a problem with your body's ability to break down lactose. A buildup of lactose in the gut may cause any of the following symptoms:

- abdominal pain and cramping
- bloating
- gas
- diarrhea
- nausea

How to manage lactose intolerance

- Limit lactose-containing foods or drinks, choosing substitutes such as lactose-reduced milk or natural, unsweetened soy milk.
- Try heating milk to reduce its lactose content.
- Use whey protein isolate supplements, which do not contain lactose, instead of whey protein concentrates, which do contain lactose.
- Take lactase enzyme, which is available in chewable tablets or as drops, before consuming milk, other dairy products or any lactose-containing product, to help break down the lactose.

Lactose content of common dairy foods

Lactose intolerance may be temporary, and you may try to reintroduce lactose-containing foods or beverages slowly. Start with foods that contain the least amount of lactose and work your way up.

Source	Serving size	Lactose (grams)
1% milk	½ cup (125 mL)	6.7
Skim milk	½ cup (125 mL)	6.6
Goat's milk	½ cup (125 mL)	5.5
Kefir	½ cup (125 mL)	4.4
Cottage cheese, 2%	½ cup (125 mL)	3.5
Yogurt, low-fat	½ cup (125 mL)	2.5
Cream cheese, light	1 oz (30 g)	1.2
Cottage cheese, dry-curd, 0.4%	½ cup (125 mL)	1.2
Cheese (Cheddar, Gouda, blue, mozzarella, Swiss, Emmental, Parmesan)	1 oz (30 g)	<1.0

Hair loss

Some degree of hair loss is quite common between four and eight months after weight-loss surgery, usually because of rapid weight loss. Hair regrowth may begin approximately eight months after surgery. Make sure you are eating nutritious meals, getting adequate protein and taking the recommended supplements.

Some patients talk about using biotin and/or silica supplements to help prevent hair loss. There has not been enough scientific research on the usefulness of these products for bariatric patients; however, if you would like to try these supplements, be sure to inform your health-care team. Some medicated shampoos and creams have also been tried by patients, but again the research for their use after bariatric surgery is limited.

Surgical Complications

The bariatric surgery itself can present certain complications that need to be managed so that other issues do not emerge. Dumping syndrome occurs after gastric bypass surgery because of the nature of that surgery.

Dumping syndrome

Under normal circumstances, before surgery the stomach empties into the duodenum (the first part of the small intestine) at a controlled rate because of the sphincter between the two. The stomach, pancreas and liver work together to prepare food to enter the duodenum, to then mix with the digestive juices there. After gastric bypass surgery, food moves from the stomach pouch directly into the jejunum (the second part of the small intestine), which is not accustomed to handling sugar and fat molecules. In response, fluid moves from the blood to inside the intestine in an effort to dilute the contents.

Dumping syndrome symptoms

If the jejunum fills too quickly, you may feel any of the following symptoms:

- abdominal bloating
- pain
- cramping
- vomiting
- flushing of the skin
- sweating
- rapid heart rate
- lightheadedness
- diarrhea or loose stools
- explosive diarrhea
- short-lived flu-like symptoms

The symptoms usually occur 30 to 60 minutes after eating. This is referred to as early dumping syndrome, while late dumping syndrome can happen one to two hours after eating. Dumping syndrome may result in hypoglycemia, or low blood sugar.

How to prevent dumping syndrome

- Do not eat or drink anything that is high in sugar or fat.
- Read the ingredients on the food or drink label. If sugar is among the first three ingredients, do not eat or drink this product. Glucose, fructose, sucrose, cane sugar and syrups are all terms that mean sugar.

Foods and drinks to avoid in preventing dumping syndrome

- cake
- candy
- chocolate
- chocolate milk
- coconut milk
- condensed milk
- cookies
- deep-fried food
- donuts
- dried fruit
- fish and chips
- fried chicken
- fries
- frozen yogurt
- fruit juice
- gelatin desserts
- granola bars
- gravy
- honey
- hot dogs
- ice cream
- iced tea
- jam
- jellies
- ketchup
- lemonade
- meal-replacement drinks or bars
- milkshakes
- molasses
- pie
- Popsicles
- poutine
- pudding
- sausages
- sherbet
- soft drinks (regular)
- sports drinks
- sugar
- sugary cereal
- sweet pickles
- sweet rolls
- sweetened canned fruit in heavy syrup
- syrups

- Aim for less than 10 grams of sugar per serving — the lower the number, the better.
- Read the Nutrition Facts label on the food. Look for less than 5% Daily Value of fat or less than 3 grams of fat per serving.
- Avoid drinking while eating and 30 minutes before or after eating.

Hypoglycemia

Hypoglycemia (low blood sugar) may occur after gastric bypass weight-loss surgery. It is very serious. Before surgery, the pancreas was used to secreting a certain amount of insulin in response to a large amount of sugar in the diet. It is thought that after surgery the pancreas may be secreting the same amount of insulin, but there isn't enough sugar present to take it up. The result is low blood sugar, which is defined as a blood glucose reading of less than 72 mg/dL (4 mmol/L). Glucometers are devices used to check blood glucose levels and are readily available at pharmacies. A pharmacist or your physician can show you how to use a glucometer.

Hypoglycemia symptoms
- shakiness
- cold, clammy or sweaty skin
- weakness or tiredness
- pale skin
- confusion
- nervousness
- restlessness
- blurred vision
- headache
- fast heart rate
- hunger
- dizziness
- numbness of tongue, lips or mouth
- loss of consciousness/coma

How to prevent hypoglycemia
To prevent hypoglycemia, follow these simple rules:

- Eat nutritious, well-balanced meals and snacks, eat them on time and avoid skipping meals and snacks.
- Include a protein source and a carbohydrate source at each meal and snack.
- Choose whole-grain carbohydrates that are high in fiber.
- Have a nutritious snack before and after physical activity.
- Avoid alcohol.

Did you know?

Low blood sugar

Hypoglycemia may be due to a hormone called glucagon-like peptide 1 (GLP-1), which may be oversecreted. High levels may stimulate extra insulin secretion, and blood sugars can drop.

How to manage hypoglycemia

- Treat low blood sugar right away by taking 15 grams of a quick-acting sugar, such as one of the following:
  - ▸ 3 BD glucose tablets
  - ▸ 5 Dextrosol tablets
  - ▸ 6 Lifesavers (chew before swallowing)
  - ▸ 3 teaspoons (15 mL) or 3 packets table sugar dissolved in 2 ounces (60 mL) water
  - ▸ 1 tbsp (15 mL) honey
- Fifteen minutes after taking the sugar, retest your blood sugar levels, using a glucometer.
- If the level is still low, repeat the treatment and seek medical attention.
- If the level is normal, go on to have a small, healthy snack that includes protein and carbohydrate.

Strictures and acid

A stricture can occur at the gastrojejunostomy — the small opening between your stomach pouch and the small intestine — when this opening is too tight or narrow. This is exclusive to gastric bypass surgery and may result from the healing process, which can lead to scar tissue forming, or from inflammation in this area. When the opening is too tight or narrow, food cannot pass through without difficulty.

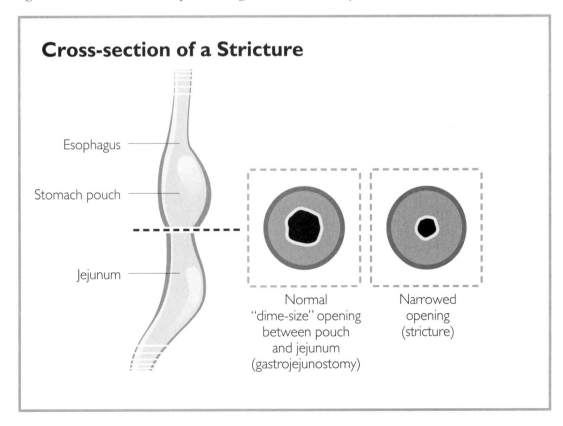

Cross-section of a Stricture

Esophagus

Stomach pouch

Jejunum

Normal "dime-size" opening between pouch and jejunum (gastrojejunostomy)

Narrowed opening (stricture)

If you are experiencing persistent vomiting or pain even when proper eating techniques are followed, this may indicate that you have a stricture.

You may also experience regurgitation of mucus or white, sticky, foam-like saliva. This reflux could indicate that you have acid buildup in the pouch. Usually a prescribed antacid medication will help. If you think you may have a stricture or an acid problem, make sure you contact your physician or surgeon.

Weight-Loss Failure

Weight-loss failure, also known as weight regain, is a possibility with any type of bariatric surgery if the patient does not comply with the bariatric diet plan and guidelines. Some patients lack adequate support, have trouble dealing with emotional eating tendencies, are not physically active or simply resort to their old eating habits and lifestyle. These patients need extra help and support in managing their new lifestyle.

Part 3

Lifestyle Changes

Challenges and Changes

Changing your lifestyle in ways that will help make your surgery successful in reducing your weight and maintaining weight loss may not be easy. It's hard to teach old dogs new tricks, but you must adopt not only the bariatric diet but also an active lifestyle if you want to ensure good health. Changing your eating habits, lifestyle and the way you think and feel about food is a process. You will need to change not only what and how you eat, but also why you eat.

There are proven techniques for making changes that last. Try not to think of change as a resolution but rather as an evolution. Remind yourself from time to time that change often takes time. And with change comes growth.

Stages of Behavioral Change

How we make changes in our lives has been studied at length, most notably in the "Stages of Change" model developed by James Prochaska and Carlo DiClemente. They identify five stages that a person must go through when changing a behavior. During each stage you need to be aware of your level of readiness. "Readiness" means simply how prepared you are to recognize what the challenge is and that you are ready to start working to change it.

Five stages of change
The five stages of change are pre-contemplation, contemplation, preparation, action and maintenance. This model is circular. People undergoing change stay at the different stages for various amounts of time. The process of change is ongoing. Having a strong support network to help you consolidate each stage of change is important. Call on family and friends or health-care professionals for support.

Stage 1: Pre-contemplation, or denial
In this stage you have not yet identified an issue or challenge. From your point of view, nothing needs to be changed, but others may have made comments or told you there may be a problem. This is news to you, and you do not agree. For example, say your physician has referred you

Stages of Change

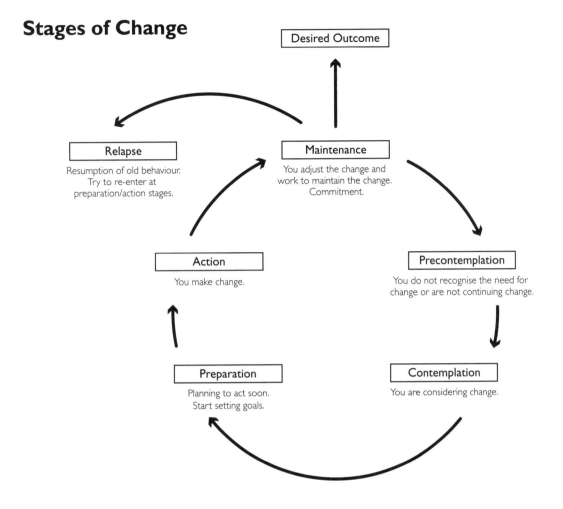

Desired Outcome

Relapse
Resumption of old behaviour.
Try to re-enter at
preparation/action stages.

Maintenance
You adjust the change and
work to maintain the change.
Commitment.

Precontemplation
You do not recognise the need for
change or are not continuing change.

Action
You make change.

Contemplation
You are considering change.

Preparation
Planning to act soon.
Start setting goals.

to a bariatric clinic for weight-loss surgery in an attempt to
resolve your type 2 diabetes. You have never thought about
this; you see no need to lose weight or resolve the diabetes.
You do not show up for any of your scheduled appointments.

Stage 2: Contemplation, or acceptance

In Stage 2 you now realize there is a problem, but you are
not ready to address it. You begin to think about what is
wrong, but you may not want to commit to making things
better. For example, you attend a general information session
at the bariatric clinic. You begin to weigh the pros and cons
of pursuing weight-loss surgery.

Stage 3: Preparation, or planning

In this stage you intend to take action. You begin making
plans to change. For example, you make preoperative
appointments and meet with the health-care team. You
begin to set goals for change, such as making healthier food
choices and taking your time to eat slowly.

Stage 4: Action

In the action stage you modify your behavior, experiences, or environment in order to overcome your problem. This is the stage where you find out what works for you and what does not. You gain access to resources to aid in your quest for change. For example, you implement the goals you've made, such as making healthier food choices by learning to read food labels. You set time aside in your busy work schedule for meals and to take your time while eating. You decide to go ahead with the weight-loss surgery.

Stage 5: Maintenance

In the maintenance stage you work on sustaining changes on a lifelong basis. You remind yourself of your successes, and you have gained skills to prevent relapse into old habits. For example, you know that you have implemented a well-structured meal routine, but during the past week you have thought about skipping lunch on a couple of occasions to catch up on work. You reconsider your work schedule and ensure that you have allotted lunch breaks.

▶ Characteristics of change

Stage	Characteristics
Pre-contemplation	• "Ignorance is bliss" • Not considering change
Contemplation	• "Sitting on the fence" • Ambivalent about change • Weighing the pros and cons of change • Not going to make change in the next month
Preparation	• "Testing the waters" • Planning to act within the next month
Action	• "Giving it a try" • Practicing new behavior for 3 to 6 months
Maintenance	• "Staying on course" • Commitment to sustained behavior • After 6 months to 5 years
Relapse	• "Falling off the wagon" • Resumption of old behavior

Relapse

Along the way, relapses are quite common and normal. Most people refer to a relapse as "falling off the wagon." Relapses are often accompanied by feelings of discouragement and failure. However, they should be viewed as a learning opportunity and a chance to make yourself stronger. When you are ready to make change again, try to resume the process at the preparation or action stages. For example, say you can't handle the pressures at work and begin to skip lunch on a regular basis. Then you pick up fast food on your way home from work because you've had such a busy and stressful day. You eat quickly because you are so hungry. During this relapse phase you have started to resume old habits. Try to get "back on the wagon" and set new goals.

Goal setting

In the preparation and action stages of change, you will set and carry out plans or goals. Setting goals will assist you and provide you with guidance as you make lifestyle changes. Spending some time now to develop SMART goals will help you in the long run. Just saying "I want to lose weight" or "I want to stop smoking" is not specific enough and does not provide you with clear direction.

"S" for Specific

You need to be specific about what you want to accomplish. Prioritize what you want to address and focus on. Then focus on what you want to do.
Example: I will begin a walking program for the month of January.

"M" for Measurable

How will you measure your progress? How will you know you have reached your goal?
Example: Every day I will write down my pedometer reading. Every Friday I will monitor my weekly progress by reviewing the daily tracking record.

"A" for Achievable

Your goal should be attainable. Keep in mind your resources and abilities. Is your goal achievable?
Example: Every Tuesday and Thursday I have craft classes, Saturdays are chore days and on Sundays I have brunch with friends, so I will be able to go for walks only on Mondays, Wednesdays and Fridays.

"R" for Realistic

Is this goal attainable in your specified time frame?
Example: Yes, because I have taken my schedule into account.

"T" for Timely

Set up a time frame. Procrastinators may struggle if they don't have a definite deadline. Having a goal date to look forward to can be quite motivating.
Example: I will review my progress on February 1 to see how January went.

Mindset for change

You will need to cultivate a mindset for change, in some cases developing new character traits such as self-acceptance and self-confidence.

- Practice self-acceptance. Take a look at yourself and love yourself as you are. Don't be hard on yourself.
- Develop self-confidence. Find ways to boost your ego. Do more of what you do well.
- Nurture yourself. Take time to care for yourself despite the demands of family and friends.
- Look forward. Focus on the present and future. Give up on past failures.
- Get in tune with your body. Listen to its cues and let your physical needs guide you.
- Be prepared to change. On your own or with the help of family and friends, assess what behaviors need to be changed. Look at things positively, not negatively.

Why We Eat

Why we eat is as important as what and how we eat. For a weight-management plan to be successful, with or without weight-loss surgery, it is crucial to build an awareness of problematic eating triggers. Think about why you eat. What situations, events or people trigger you to eat? Do these triggers cause you to have difficult feelings or emotions?

Kinds of hunger

Our society uses food to celebrate, to reward, to show love and to grieve. But we really need food to live and to grow — to be nourished physically. Learning to differentiate between the two types of hunger, head hunger and stomach hunger, will help you in your quest to avoid emotional eating.

Overeating

Debbie came to our clinic one year after gastric bypass surgery. She had found that she tended to overeat at night, especially after dinner, which is usually her down time. After a busy day at work, getting home, making dinner and cleaning up, she finally sits down around 8:30 and unwinds by watching television or surfing the Internet. Not long after she sits down she's up again, searching the kitchen for a satisfying snack. She usually has chips or cookies. Whatever the choice, she ends up sitting down again with some type of impulsive snack. We asked her, "Are you hungry at that time?" Debbie responded, "No, how could I be? I've just finished eating dinner. I think I'm just bored."

We began to strategize about the trigger that was prompting her to overeat after dinner while watching TV. The first step involved helping her develop awareness of her triggers — her emotions, current events in her life, special situations. Some of her triggers included boredom; watching TV; surfing the Internet; feeling tired; long, busy days; and wanting to reward herself. We then asked Debbie to think about ways she could nurture herself other than with food. Debbie suggested she could take a warm bubble bath and then curl up under her favorite blanket with a good book. This would help keep her distracted, away from the kitchen and any temptation to grab food. Debbie was also asked to change some of her environmental triggers. "I can stop buying and storing chips and cookies in the pantry," she volunteered. "I can keep food only in the kitchen and put it away in cupboards or the fridge, where it is not easy to see." To support her in making these changes, she said a dear friend was willing to help and was only a phone call away.

Stomach hunger

Physiological hunger, or stomach hunger, normally occurs several hours after your previous meal. The symptoms of stomach hunger include an empty feeling and rumbling in your stomach, lightheadedness, a slight headache or possibly dizziness. Stomach hunger strikes below the neck, comes on gradually and does not involve craving for a specific food.

Head hunger

Psychological hunger, also known as head hunger or emotional eating, involves cues or triggers that make you want to eat even though you are not physically hungry. Some examples of triggers include watching TV, feeling that you deserve a reward after a busy day, going on vacation, celebrating a special occasion, walking by a donut shop, and emotions such as anxiety or feeling tired. Head hunger usually strikes above the neck, suddenly and at any time, and involves craving for a specific food.

Dealing with head hunger

Most of us turn to food for emotional comfort. With any type of weight-management program, including weight-loss surgery, this habit needs to be addressed. If you eat when you are angry, stressed, bored, happy, sad or lonely, you will have to find ways to cope with those feelings or states of mind without using food. Sometimes people feel that the only thing they have control over is food. Some people turn to food to spite others. Some seek feelings of fullness because they are feeling empty spiritually or socially. Others purposely gain weight in order to be less attractive to others, which usually stems from experiences of sexual abuse. If you do not address your emotional eating tendencies, after surgery you may turn to other unhealthy coping mechanisms, which are referred to as replacement addictions. Replacement addictions may include gambling, alcoholism, shopping addiction or drug use.

Step 1: Build an awareness of triggers

- Consider situations, events, people or emotions that may trigger you to eat for the wrong reasons. Keep a list of these triggers. Continue adding to the list every time you think of a new trigger.
- Keep a food and mood journal that includes a section or column in which to record your feelings, mood and thoughts.
- For a couple of days, every time you eat take a moment to ask yourself, "Why am I eating this? Am I physically hungry? Am I having a food craving? Is this stomach or head hunger?"

Step 2: Change your environment

- Take note of daily routines and practices. Changing a lifetime of habits is not easy, but it isn't impossible. Step back and analyze your routines, obligations and responsibilities.
- Take a look at how your home and workplace are set up. For example, do you really need to keep certain foods around? Do you have a junk-food drawer at work for stressful times? Planning and organization are key components of your strategy.
- Keep fresh produce in your refrigerator accessible at eye level, not hidden away. Clean out your freezer.
- Make sure healthier foods are kept visible and easily accessible. Clean out and organize your cupboards. Keep your counter clear and clean so you won't be hindered from using it to prepare wholesome, healthy meals. Then

you will be less tempted to eat foods just because they are readily available.

- Try not to have higher-calorie fatty or sugary foods in your home, car or office or within easy reach.

Step 3: Nurture yourself

Which emotions are your triggers? Try dealing with these emotions without using food. If stress is a trigger, consider reading a book, talking to a friend or getting a massage. If a common emotional trigger is anger, perhaps you need some anger-management counseling. These strategies are sometimes referred to as positive coping mechanisms. They help you deal with difficult feelings and emotions in other ways than using food or other negative addictions such as smoking, alcohol or gambling.

Step 4: Distract yourself

- Keep yourself busy during the times that trigger eating.
- Consider distractions that move you away from food, such as taking a bath, visiting the gym, going out for a walk, gardening, going to the park or doing some laundry.
- Distract yourself with things that challenge your mind, such as crossword puzzles, craft work, scrapbooking or reading the newspaper.
- Keep handy a list of distractions that work for you, to refer to quickly when you are in need.

Step 5: Seek support

Personal and professional supports are an important component of your success and well-being. It is vital that you recognize when you need support. Having both subjective and objective perspectives on your circumstances can be beneficial. A healthy support network will undoubtedly contribute to your success.

Before having surgery, you should have both your personal and professional support network in place. Family and friends can support you at home and at social gatherings and events. Having access to a counselor, a therapist or a member of your health-care team with whom you feel comfortable will help to provide you with objective support.

Step 6: Accept the new you

Relationship changes often occur after surgery. People may be happy for you and pleased by your weight loss, but some people may have liked you better the way you were prior to surgery. It may be helpful to have "what if" conversations with loved ones before you have surgery. Open and honest

Did you know?

Benefits of support
Studies have linked post-surgery group support to long-term maintenance of weight loss. Support groups typically include a mixture of preoperative and postoperative patients. They can help you by providing information, correcting misperceptions, giving encouragement and sharing strategies for coping throughout the process.

Communication will be key to your success.

conversations with the people most important to you will help you identify existing or potential concerns or ambivalence they may have about life with you after surgery.

It may be helpful to include your loved ones in your journey through bariatric surgery. They will then have an opportunity to ask questions and perhaps address any misgivings they may have. Being included will help them feel they are not being left behind, but rather that they are part of your journey.

If you feel that you are struggling to accept the "new you," it may be time to turn to both your professional and personal supports. Life continues after surgery, and there will be stressors and upsets. Commit to a healthy lifestyle physically, mentally and socially. You are not seeking normalcy; you are seeking health.

Changing Your Eating Habits

Changing your eating habits takes time and effort. Setting SMART goals (see page 131) is a helpful way to prepare for and make the changes. Below are some suggestions to help you control your eating habits.

- Give your kitchen a makeover. Clear out unhealthy foods from your cupboards and refrigerator and make room for healthy foods only.
- Plan your meals and snacks. Planning your meals and snacks helps prevent you from eating based on cravings or impulses. Use the meal plans and recipes in this book to plan ahead. Involve your family in meal planning.
- Make a grocery list based on your weekly meal plans. Involve your family in shopping from this list as well.
- Plate your food. Use a smaller plate with a deeper center and fill only the inside part; some companies now sell divided plates that you can use. Plate your food before you sit down, and eat at a table with few or no distractions. Put away any leftover food before you eat, to help discourage you from having seconds.
- Think ahead. While preparing a meal, consider your next meal or snack. For example, if you are using red peppers for a stir-fry, slice some extra pieces and pack them away for a snack the next day.
- Avoid snack triggers. Avoid eating while watching TV, driving, using the computer, reading or doing other activities. Portion out your snack in a small bowl or cup and put the rest away.

Active Living

Anything that gets your body moving is considered activity. Not only does exercise improve your physical health, it also improves your emotional health. To help increase your activity level, set some goals for yourself. Following weight-loss surgery, your tolerance for activity should grow day by day. Just to be safe, speak to a health-care professional before beginning any type of physical activity program.

Head Start

On the first day after weight-loss surgery, someone from your health-care team (a nurse or a physiotherapist) will instruct you to breathe deeply and cough to help get rid of mucus and to prevent chest complications. As soon as you are alert and not dizzy, your blood pressure is stable and your pain is under control, you will be encouraged to start walking very slowly. You should be supervised the first time you get up from bed.

Gradually increase the length of your walk each time. You can start with a leisurely five-minute walk three times on the first day after weight-loss surgery. If you are unable to walk, the health-care team will provide you with tips on how to shift your weight in bed, to transfer from a sitting to a standing position, and vice versa.

The value of early exercise

- Prevents blood clots in the lungs and legs
- Improves overall circulation
- Prevents the development of bed sores, which can happen within two to three days
- Decreases the risk of developing heart or lung problems such as congestive heart failure or pneumonia

Deep-breathing and coughing exercises

Deep-breathing exercises after surgery encourage you to take a deep, full breath. Breathe in slowly through your nose while concentrating on expanding your diaphragm (the muscle below the ribcage). Then breathe out through your mouth and concentrate on feeling your chest sink downward and inward. When you breathe this way, the diaphragm moves farther down into the abdomen, and your lungs are then able to expand more completely within your chest cavity.

With deeper breaths, you are able to take in more oxygen and let out more carbon dioxide. This improves your healing and recovery after any type of surgery. It will also help keep your lungs clear.

In addition to deep breathing, you will be encouraged to cough, using a support or splint — a procedure referred to as supportive or splinted coughing. If you are lying down, hold a pillow over the incision sites on your abdomen and lace your fingers together over the pillow. This will help reduce some of the discomfort when you cough. You can also reduce discomfort by "splinting" your incision sites: placing one arm over your upper abdomen and the other arm lower down, as if you are hugging your belly. While supporting your abdomen, cough deeply.

To help start the cough reflex, you will need to take a few slow, deep, full breaths. Hold the third in-breath, then cough strongly. As you cough, concentrate on feeling your diaphragm force out all the air. A member of your health-care team can help you learn more about deep breathing and coughing. Consider practicing these exercises before your surgery.

Types of Physical Activity

Three forms of physical activity target three different aspects of your body: cardiovascular health, strength and flexibility. Each plays a role in helping us become physically fit — and healthier.

Cardiovascular activity

Cardiovascular activity is also known as cardio or aerobics. This type of exercise uses your large muscles for long periods of time, resulting in an increase in your heart rate. With practice your body learns to use oxygen more efficiently and your cardiovascular system (heart, lungs, circulatory system) strengthens. With this type of activity, your heart beats faster and your breathing gets harder. It includes dancing, cycling and running.

Intensity is how hard your body is working. Most people who are obese tend to have sore joints, such as knees or ankles, or even lower back pain, all of which will affect the type and intensity of physical activity they choose. As you lose weight, these types of pain may dissipate.

▶ Health effects of aerobic exercise

Intensity	Exercise types	Health effects
Light • You can comfortably sing the lyrics to a favorite song while doing the activity.	• leisure walking • bowling • fishing • golfing, using a cart • slow dancing • light housework • playing with the kids • light gardening	• relaxes you • makes you feel energized
Moderate • You can't comfortably sing the lyrics to a favorite song. • You feel slightly out of breath and tired. • You break a sweat. • Your heart rate goes up.	• walking fast • water aerobics • riding a bike (level ground) • pushing a lawnmower • golfing, walking • climbing stairs • canoeing or kayaking • carrying heavy groceries • walking up a hill	• facilitates weight loss • burns more calories than low-intensity activity
Vigorous • You feel as if you're at the point where you are pushing your boundaries. • Breathing is hard and fast. • You need to pause to take a breath while speaking. • Your heart rate becomes faster.	• jogging or running • swimming laps • riding a bike fast or on hills • playing singles tennis • playing basketball • playing hockey • rowing, canoeing or kayaking vigorously • skiing, downhill or cross-country • hiking • ice skating • roller skating • heavy yard work, chopping wood	• makes the heart work harder, making it more efficient • facilitates weight loss • burns the most calories per minute

How much aerobic exercise do I need each day?
Build up to these levels of cardiovascular exercise:

- 60 minutes of light physical activity every day, or
- 30 to 60 minutes of moderate physical activity four times a week, or
- 20 to 30 minutes of vigorous activity three to four times a week

The activity does not have to be done all at once. You can add up your activities through the day, 10 minutes at a time, to get your daily total. Take a 10-minute brisk walk during breaks at work. This will also clear your mind and can even improve your productivity. If you want to increase the intensity of your activities, slowly replace moderate-intensity ones with those that are more vigorous. One minute of high-intensity activity is about as effective as two minutes of moderate-intensity activity.

▶ Sample weekly aerobic activity log

Activity	Intensity	SUN	MON	TUES	WED
Walking	light	30 min	30 min	30 min	40 min
Running	moderate		30 min		
Dancing	moderate				
Playing hockey	vigorous	30 min			
Carrying heavy groceries	moderate				
Total (minutes)					

Strength building

Strength-building activities include exercises that require short, intense effort, such as weight-lifting, working with resistance bands, push-ups, sit-ups, heavy gardening and yoga. This type of activity strengthens your muscles and bones. Work on all the major muscle groups of your body, including your legs, hips, back, chest, abdomen, shoulders and arms. If possible, aim to do strength training at least two days a week. Exercises should include working on both the upper and lower body.

Frequently Asked Questions

Is it true that weight-lifting can help decrease the amount of excess skin I will have?

Unfortunately, when you lose a lot of weight, excess skin is a reality no matter how much you work out. But this does not negate the benefits of including strength training as part of your exercise routine to build strong muscles and bones.

THURS	FRI	SAT	Total minutes spent per week		
			Light	Moderate	Vigorous
45 min	30 min	15 min	230		
30 min				60	
	60 min			60	
					30
		15 min		15	
			230	135	30

▶ Sample strength-training program

Target area	Exercise	Routine
Upper body	• chest press • low row • pull-down • biceps curl • triceps kick-back	**Beginner** I set of 10 to 14 repetitions at least 2 times per week
Lower body	• leg extension • leg curl • leg press • calf raises	**Intermediate** 1 to 2 sets of each exercise, with 8 to 12 repetitions each, 2 to 3 times per week

Flexibility

Flexibility exercises include reaching, bending and stretching activities that keep your muscles relaxed and joints mobile. Examples include practicing yoga and doing general stretches while sitting, lying down or standing. Stretching is important before and after more energetic physical activities because it increases your flexibility and lessens the chance of injury. It also allows your muscles to loosen up and prepare for the exercises.

Gentle, slow, prolonged stretches are best. Hold each stretch for about 30 seconds, and do not bounce. Warming up with some light stretching for about five to ten minutes will help make your activities more enjoyable and prevent achiness afterward. After your activity, stretch again for about five minutes. Your muscles will be warm and supple by then and will respond well to the stretching.

How to build physical activity into your life

At home, at work or at play, including physical activity in your life is not as difficult as it may seem. Choosing activities that you can do and that you enjoy makes it that much easier.

At home
• Clean the house.
• Wash the car.
• Take the dog for a walk.
• Push the baby in the stroller.
• Dance to your favorite music.

- Build a snowman.
- Walk to the store to get groceries.
- Do stretches while watching TV.
- Ride a stationary bike while watching TV.
- Carry laundry up and down the stairs.
- Walk up and down the hall or around the room while chatting on the phone.
- Wash and dry the dishes by hand instead of using the dishwasher.
- Use a push lawnmower.
- Do your own gardening or lawn care.

At work

- Get off the bus one stop early.
- Park your car farther away.
- Go for a walk during scheduled breaks.
- Take the stairs instead of the elevator.
- Take stretch breaks during long meetings.
- Replace one of your coffee breaks with a walking break.
- Go walking with a colleague to discuss business instead of having a traditional desk meeting.
- Do some stretches while working at the computer.
- Consider organizing your company's next social gathering with activity as the focus.
- Walk to a co-worker's office to discuss an issue instead of phoning or sending an email.

At play

- Join a fun recreational activity such as skiing, bowling or ice skating.
- Learn a new sport, such as curling, soccer, basketball, tennis or bowling.
- Arrange to meet friends at your local shopping center and go mall walking.
- Play with your kids instead of just watching them — enjoy tag, hide-and-seek, throwing a Frisbee, flying a kite.
- Go ballroom dancing, folk dancing or square dancing.
- Enjoy gardening — weed, rake and prune for the fun of it.

The value of physical activity

- Optimizes the long-term success of weight-loss surgery
- Builds muscle and burns fat
- Increases overall energy levels
- Improves your ability to perform the activities of daily living
- Improves quality of life
- Keeps blood pressure under control

Coping with criticism

During a follow-up session with a group of patients who had undergone bariatric surgery, one patient, Cindy, commented that being active was a challenge for her. This was not only because of the physical discomfort she felt while trying to work out, but also because she felt embarrassed about going to the gym. She felt that people were staring at her. Once when she was walking on the treadmill, someone made a negative remark about her size, and she never went back to that gym again. Most of the other patients in the group said they felt the same way and that similar comments had been made to them.

The facilitator moved the discussion to how to deal with people who made negative comments to them while they were working out. Some of the ideas the group came up with included the following:

- Should you choose to respond, take a deep breath before speaking. Confront the person and comment that you are equally entitled to work out, no matter what your shape or size.
- Choose not to respond. Just smile — this is a good way to empower yourself. If you respond in anger, that only fuels a negative situation.
- Try to listen to music while working out. People will generally not talk to you if you can't hear them.
- If this type of behavior is consistent with one gym member, inform the manager or supervisor. Perhaps the management can post some "shape discrimination" posters or leave information materials on the front counter.

Others commented that they enjoyed doing physical activities such as going out for walks or mall walking in their community, where there was less chance of being singled out. Some people said it helped to go with someone else; your confidence is built up by having someone by your side, especially a friend or family member who will motivate and support you.

As for the physical discomfort of working out, several patients suggested that breaking up the activity into smaller, more manageable chunks really helps. Stretching is a great way to help reduce muscle soreness and discomfort. Others suggested that water aerobics at the local community center was a great way to be active without too much pain or discomfort. One patient added she did not feel comfortable wearing a swimsuit in public, so she had put together a more covered-up outfit using a water skirt and a short-sleeved water shirt.

- Improves heart health
- Improves self-esteem
- Keeps your bones strong
- Promotes joint stability, balance and posture
- Keeps muscles toned and flexible
- Improves skin elasticity
- Boosts your immune system
- Reduces stress and anxiety
- Decreases the risk of regaining weight
- Helps with weight maintenance
- Makes you feel better about yourself
- Helps you relax and sleep better
- Gives you more chances to meet new friends

Activity tips for people who are obese and or have mobility issues

- Consider consulting with a physiotherapist or personal trainer to plan exercise routines.
- Divide your exercise period into several shorter, bite-size routines so the time seems less challenging.
- If your knees or ankles hurt, use a wheelchair or scooter and try substituting seated arm and shoulder exercises such as chair aerobics, lifting weights and stretching.
- Consider water aerobics rather than walking or jogging on land.
- Try gentle yoga and tai chi movements.
- Under supervision, use an exercise ball.
- Try recreational dance classes or more formal ballroom dancing.
- Wear a pedometer to motivate you to walk more.

Exercise Schedule

During the months after surgery, you need to schedule exercise into your life to match your new lifestyle. Changing your eating habits and increasing your activities go hand in hand. The guidelines may be different for you if you have complications after surgery. After an LAGB procedure, you may be able to progress through each stage more quickly. Speak to your health-care team for advice.

Monthly plan

Every month you will gain strength and endurance — and lose weight — which will enable you to be more active.

Did you know?

Early start
People who begin some type of physical activity regimen before weight-loss surgery are twice as likely to be able to adjust to exercising after surgery.

First month

During the first month after weight-loss surgery, you may feel uncomfortable. You are still not eating much solid food and you may not have much energy. Your focus is on recovering and keeping hydrated. You need to be active, but at the same time you should not push yourself.

The first activity you should do is walking. The recommended frequency and duration are as much and as often as you can tolerate. You are encouraged to take a walk three or more times every day for at least five to ten minutes (or as much as you can tolerate). Increase the length of your walks as they become more manageable.

During the first month after weight-loss surgery you should not do any strength training, exercises with weights, heavy lifting, abdominal exercises or water aerobics.

Second and third months

After the first month you will start to feel more comfortable exercising. You are beginning to eat a greater variety of foods, so you should have more energy. With significant weight loss, you will feel ready for more activity. This is when you are encouraged to try more activities beyond just walking.

Water exercises are ideal at this time because the buoyancy of the water holds you up, helping you move more easily and making it more comfortable for your joints. Being in the water provides psychological benefits as well, including improving your mood and reducing stress and anxiety. However, do not start any swimming activities until you have been given clearance from your physician. Continue adding low- to moderate-intensity activities such as low-impact aerobics and recumbent (reclining) cycling.

Did you know?

Keeping your balance

As your body mass changes, your body's center of balance changes as well. You may be at risk of falling and injuring yourself, especially during the first six months after surgery. Avoid activities that require balance and coordination, including bike riding, lunges, squats, step-ups and yoga. Be cautious at first.

Frequently Asked Questions

When can I start lifting weights after surgery?

If all goes well and you have healed, you can start working out with weights in the third month after weight-loss surgery. Start slowly and remember to stretch before and after any type of physical activity, including weight-lifting. Be sure to speak to your health-care professional first to get clearance. Remember to avoid abdominal exercises and activities that require balance and coordination for the first six months.

Fourth to sixth months

As you continue to recover, lose more weight and gain more energy, you will be able to increase your activity accordingly. In addition to cardiovascular activities, you are now encouraged to increase your strength-training and flexibility exercises.

Sixth month and beyond

As you continue to lose weight and gain energy, you can expand the variety of your physical activity. At this time you should be able to include moderate to intense activities. Continue with strength-training exercises, increasing the weights or resistance as you get stronger.

You may now also begin abdominal exercises to improve your overall core strength. As your balance and coordination improve, you can try activities such as squats, lunges, bike riding and yoga. By this time, most people enjoy adding some light jogging when they are taking a walk.

Consider joining a walking or jogging program. Or, for that matter, consider starting a community walking or jogging program with your friends or neighbors. Physical activity is a great way to build relationships. Having friends to meet up with is a great way to get motivated, because your activity will also include catching up on each other's lives and socializing. Set an initial goal to increase your walk to 30 minutes by the end of the month. Set goals for strength training as well.

Did you know?

Preventing osteoporosis
Weight-bearing activity is a great way to prevent osteoporosis. Our bones gain strength when weight or resistance is applied to them. Performing such exercises at least three times a week can help maintain current bone mass.

▶ Long-term strength-training program

Target Area	Exercise		Routine
Upper body	• chest press • low row • pull-down • biceps curl	• triceps kick-back • shoulder press	**Beginner** I set of 10 to 15 repetitions at least twice per week
Lower body	• leg extension • leg curl • leg press	• wall squat • lunge • calf raise	**Intermediate** I to 2 sets of each exercise, with 8 to 12 repetitions each, 2 to 3 times per week
Torso (core)	• abdominal crunch • abdominal rotation	• lower back extension	

▶ Review of activity progression after weight-loss surgery

When	What	Avoid
In the hospital	• Deep breathing • Supportive or splinted coughing • Sit in a chair or on the side of the bed. • Stand. • Lie down and turn from side to side. • Transfer from sitting to standing, with assistance if needed. • Calf pumping (while lying down, point your toes forward and back again; keep repeating) • Walk for 5 minutes 3 times a day, increasing duration and frequency daily, as tolerated (ideally under supervision).	• Abdominal exercises • Heavy lifting, pushing or pulling
First month	• Continue deep breathing and supportive or splinted coughing if needed. • Walk 3 or more times every day for at least 5 to 10 minutes, or as much as you can tolerate. Increase the length of each walk as tolerated. • Easy stairs • Light household chores • Light activities of daily living, including getting dressed and undressed and showering • Driving short distances (if no longer taking prescription pain medication and alert)	• Water exercises • Abdominal exercises • Moderate- to vigorous-intensity exercises • Strength/resistance training (lifting weights) • Any activity that requires balance or coordination • Heavy lifting, pushing or pulling, such as vacuuming or carrying heavy groceries

When	What	Avoid
Second and third months	• Water exercises • Frequent walks of longer duration and more intensity • Low- to moderate-intensity activities	• Abdominal exercises • Vigorous-intensity exercises • Strength/resistance training (lifting weights) • Any activity that requires balance or coordination • Heavy lifting, pushing or pulling, such as vacuuming or carrying heavy groceries
Fourth and fifth months	• Water exercises • Cardiovascular or endurance activities of moderate intensity • Strength training • Flexibility exercises (stretching)	• Any activity that requires balance or coordination • Abdominal exercises • Vigorous-intensity exercises
Six months and beyond	• Increase the variety of physical activity. • Include moderate- to vigorous-intensity activities such as jogging. • Continue with strength training, increasing the weight or resistance. • Abdominal exercises • Balance and coordination exercises	

CASE HISTORY

Feeling energized

One year after weight-loss surgery, Andrew came to our clinic for a follow-up visit. When we asked what he is doing for physical activity, Andrew's face lit up. He had just started coaching his daughter's soccer team. "Getting out on the field and doing drills with my daughter and the team is a wonderful and fulfilling feeling," he commented. "You get so much more satisfaction than just sitting on the bench watching." Andrew has become more active in other areas of his life as well. At work he is taking walk breaks, he works out at a gym twice a week, he plays squash with his friends every Monday night, and on Friday nights he and his wife enjoy a water aerobics class together.

Tips for safe activity

- To prevent or minimize muscle aches, begin with light activities and progress gradually to moderate- and vigorous-intensity activities.
- Wear comfortable shoes that provide support and good cushioning.
- Wear comfortable and appropriate clothing that suits the activity and the weather.
- Use safety gear as appropriate, such as a helmet for cycling, knee, elbow and wrist protectors for inline skating and protective goggles for playing squash.
- Before engaging in any type of physical activity, speak to your physician.

Frequently Asked Questions

When can I start swimming after my weight-loss surgery? Can I go in a hot tub?

It is generally recommended that you wait about one month after surgery to go swimming or do water exercises. Be sure that your incision sites are healed before going into a public swimming pool, a lake or the ocean. Hot tubs are fine to use after the first month, as long as they are clean and properly disinfected. Be careful to not stay in too long, as there is a risk of dizziness, dehydration and changes in blood pressure.

Activity logs

Keeping track of your physical activities and their intensity level can be rewarding in itself. Depending on your level of tolerance, set SMART goals (see page 131) for yourself and enjoy your successes.

Sample long-term activity goals

Aerobic
- 60 minutes of light-intensity physical activity every day (420 minutes per week), or
- 30 to 60 minutes of moderate physical activities 4 times a week (120 to 160 minutes per week), or
- 20 to 30 minutes of vigorous activity 3 to 4 times a week (60 to 120 minutes per week)

Strength
- Muscle and bone strengthening activities 2 to 3 times a week

Flexibility
- Flexibility activities 4 to 7 times a week

Lifelong Success

If you follow the bariatric nutrition guide and enjoy an active lifestyle, lifelong success is not out of your reach. The challenge ahead lies in maintaining your weight and your new lifestyle. If your weight loss is truly coupled with lifestyle change and not just another diet, your chances of continued success are far greater than you may ever have imagined. Continue to choose healthier foods, being mindful of your eating habits, and continue physical activities and setting realistic goals. You are the key to your lifelong success.

Follow-up Care

Regular follow-up with your health-care team is essential. Follow-up visits will include physical examinations, weight monitoring, assessment of mental well-being and routine laboratory assessments to screen for nutrient deficiencies.

Come well prepared. To get the most out of each appointment, keep a journal in which you write down observations and questions. Remember to ask the questions — your health-care team is there to support you. Once you have been discharged from the bariatric clinic, continue to receive follow-up medical care from your physician.

Support Groups

Support groups, whether professional or personal, are an important part of lifelong success. Many patients have formed bariatric support groups in their communities. If your local community does not have one, consider starting your own support group with other people who have had bariatric surgery or are thinking about the surgery. Support groups provide a great venue for sharing stories and experiences and picking up tips.

Check online for support groups in your area, or ask a member of your health-care team to help you. Some bariatric clinics have professionally run support groups that may be an option for you.

Social Dining

Attending parties and social functions can be initially challenging, especially since food is usually the focus of social gatherings. If you have to attend a special function while you are at a particular diet stage, you may need to bring your own food or eat before you attend. In the long term you can enjoy eating out and attending parties and social functions. Just be careful not to overeat, to choose healthier foods and beverages, and to take your time eating and drinking.

Tips for dining out, parties and social functions

- Use a small plate or ask to have your meal put on a smaller plate.
- Share your meal with someone else.
- If possible, order a half-portion or appetizer size.
- Pack some of your meal to go.
- Eat slowly, pacing yourself.
- Avoid anything high in fat or sugar.
- Avoid anything breaded, battered or fried, such as calamari, chicken wings or egg rolls.
- Ask the server not to bring a bread basket.
- Avoid creamy sauces and dressings.
- Ask for dressings and sauces on the side, and use them sparingly, if at all.
- Ask the server or host how the food was prepared.
- Talk more – you'll eat less.
- Walk around and mingle.

Top 5 Tips for Lifelong Success

Copy this list and post it on your refrigerator door. You can succeed in losing weight and maintaining weight loss after bariatric surgery. Congratulations!

1. Follow the bariatric diet program for mindful eating.
2. Practice the principles of active living.
3. Change what you eat, how you eat and why you eat.
4. Take the required vitamin and minerals for life to prevent deficiencies.
5. Cooperate with your health-care team and join or create a support group.

▶ Healthier eating options for dining out

Avoid	Choose instead
Breakfast and lunch	
• fried eggs and bacon • croissants • egg sandwiches • buttered bagels and/or toast • French toast • muffins and pastries • hash browns or fried potatoes	• poached or boiled egg without sauce • scrambled egg • rye bread, unbuttered • cottage cheese and fruit • low-fat yogurt with fruit • diet jam • light cream cheese
Appetizers and snacks	
• chicken wings • egg rolls or fried spring rolls • cheese bread • cheesy dipping sauces • onion rings • fried calamari	• bruschetta • raw vegetables, without dip • mussels in tomato sauce • cold or fresh spring rolls
Soups and salads	
• cream soups • French onion soup • Caesar salad	• vegetable soup • mixed green salad (no bacon bits, dressing on the side)
Asian	
• fried rice • chicken balls • fried chicken • ribs • sushi rolls with creamy sauces or tempura • tempura • plum or teriyaki sauce	• lemon chicken (not fried) • grilled tofu • steamed or grilled fish • steamed vegetables • steamed rice • sushi rolls without creamy sauces or tempura • sashimi • light soy sauce

Avoid	Choose instead
Greek	
• breaded and fried shrimp • fried calamari • saganaki (flaming cheese)	• grilled chicken • only one of pita, rice or potatoes • tzatziki (small amounts)
Italian	
• lasagna • pasta with cream or meat sauce • thick-crust pizza with meat and/or cheese	• Italian wedding soup • pasta with tomato sauce (small portion) • steamed vegetables • grilled or poached fish • grilled chicken • mussels in tomato sauce • thin-crust whole wheat pizza with vegetables
Mexican	
• nachos • tacos • quesadillas or enchiladas	• chicken fajita (toppings on the side; focus on chicken and vegetables) • chili with beans
Fast food	
• hamburger • fried fish or chicken burger • hot dog • onion rings • fries • poutine	• grilled chicken burger • grilled chicken wrap • salad (check nutritional information) • baked potato
Traditional	
• ribs • chicken pot pie • chicken fingers • fish and chips	• roast chicken (white meat, no skin) • baked potato • steamed vegetables

Part 4

Nutritious and Enjoyable Recipes

Introduction to the Recipes

Congratulations! You are embarking on a journey to prepare healthy, nutritious food for yourself, your family and your loved ones. These recipes are intended not only for those who are considering or have had weight-loss surgery, but for anyone who wants to eat healthier without compromising taste and quality.

The Development and Testing of the Recipes

All of these recipes were developed and tested by Sue Ekserci, a registered dietitian experienced in counseling people who have had or are candidates for weight-loss surgery. She is the mother of two young children and has several good friends who have had weight-loss surgery. The taste testers included people of all ages and cultures: Sue's friends and family, her colleagues (experienced registered dietitians and social workers) and, most importantly, people who have had weight-loss surgery.

Using the Recipes

Read each recipe all the way through before starting to make it. Make sure you have all the ingredients and equipment on hand before beginning.

Tips and variations

Each recipe includes kitchen tips, weight-loss surgery tips and/or variations. The kitchen tips provide interesting facts and helpful ideas to assist you in preparing the recipe. The weight-loss surgery tips give you important information about tolerance of the recipe and helpful details about nutrition. The variations give you options if you do not have an ingredient on hand or prefer a different ingredient. They allow you to keep things interesting. Don't stop at just these variations! Once you've tried the recipes, let your creative side shine and come up with some variations of your own.

You will notice that each recipe mentions a serving size, or recommended portion — these are just guides so that we could provide nutrient information specific to that serving size. Most of the recipes can be doubled or halved, depending on how many people you are making the recipe for. In some cases, leftovers can be stored in the refrigerator or freezer, which will save you lots of time when it comes to future meals. Be sure to read the kitchen tips for storage advice.

Diet stages

You will notice a Diet Stage tag located near the top of each recipe in the sidebar. This tag will tell you whether the recipe is appropriate for you, based on what diet stage you are in.

Nutrient information

Each recipe provides detailed nutrition information, including the number of calories; the grams of fat, carbohydrate, fiber, sugar and protein; and the milligrams of sodium, calcium and iron in each serving. Nutrient values have been rounded to one decimal place, with the exception of those for calories, sodium and calcium, which have been rounded to the nearest whole number.

About the nutrient analysis

Computer-assisted nutrient analysis of the recipes was prepared by Kimberly Zammit, HBSc (the project supervisor was Len Piché, PhD, RD, Division of Food & Nutritional Sciences, Brescia University College, London, ON), using Food Processor® SQL, version 10.5, ESHA Research Inc., Salem, OR (this software contains the entire Canadian Nutrient File, 2007b). The nutrient database was the Canadian Nutrient File, version 2007b, supplemented when necessary with documented data from reliable sources.

The analysis was based on:

- imperial weights and measures (except for foods typically packaged and used in metric quantities);
- the larger number of servings (the smaller portion) when there was a range;
- the smaller ingredient quantity when there was a range;
- the first ingredient listed when there was a choice of ingredients.

Unless otherwise stated, recipes were analyzed using canola oil, non-hydrogenated margarine, skim (0%) milk and 0% yogurt with no added sugar. When protein powder was used (flavored or unflavored), it was assumed that whey protein isolate was used. Each scoop (28 g) of the protein powder provides 100 calories, 23 grams protein, 2 grams carbohydrate, 0 grams sugar and 0 grams fat. Calculations involving meat and poultry use lean portions without skin and with visible fat trimmed. A pinch of salt and salt to taste was calculated as $\frac{1}{8}$ tsp (0.5 mL). All recipes were analyzed prior to cooking. Optional ingredients and garnishes, and ingredients that are not quantified, were not included in the calculations.

Equipping Your Kitchen

The list below includes essential kitchen items that will help you prepare and enjoy tasty and nutritious food after weight-loss surgery. There's no need to run out and buy everything at once. If you need to, borrow from a friend or neighbor, buy the items as you need them or use alternatives and make do with what you have on hand.

Essential kitchen items

- Bamboo skewers: 6-inch (15 cm) and 12-inch (30 cm)
- Box grater
- Casserole dishes: 8-cup (2 L) and 6-cup (1.5 L)
- Chef's knife: 10-inch (25 cm)
- Cutting boards
- Fine-mesh sieve
- Foil
- Food processor, blender and/or immersion (hand) blender
- Food storage bags
- Freezer-safe containers with lids
- Glass baking dish: 11- by 7-inch (28 by 18 cm)

- Glass loaf pan: 9- by 5-inch (23 by 13 cm)
- Glass pie plate: 9-inch (23 cm)
- Ice cube tray
- Kitchen scale
- Kitchen timer
- Measuring cups: dry and liquid
- Measuring spoons
- Melon baller
- Metal baking pans: 13- by 9-inch (33 by 23 cm) and 8-inch (20 cm) square
- Mixing bowls (various sizes)
- Nonstick muffin pans: 12-cup regular-size and mini
- Nonstick rimmed baking sheets

- Nonstick skillets: small, medium and large
- Paper baking cups
- Parchment paper
- Paring knife
- Plastic wrap
- Popsicle sticks
- Ramekins: $\frac{1}{2}$ cup (125 mL) and $\frac{3}{4}$ cup (175 mL)
- Saucepans with lids: small, medium and large
- Silicone baking cups (mini)
- Silicone spatula
- Steamer
- Strainer or colander
- Vegetable peeler
- Whisk
- Wooden spoons

Common Ingredients

Before you head off to the grocery store, flip through this book and decide which recipes you want to try over the coming days, then make a list of the ingredients you'll need to prepare them. Below are listed some commonly used items that you should try to keep on hand for quick decisions and last-minute meal preparation.

Meat and meat alternatives

- Chicken breasts, boneless skinless
- Chickpeas, canned and/or dried
- Eggs
- Ground beef, extra-lean
- Ground turkey or chicken, extra-lean
- Lentils, dried (red, green, brown)
- Mixed beans, canned
- Peanut butter, all-natural
- Salmon, canned
- Tuna, canned (water-packed)

Milk, milk products and milk alternatives

- Cheddar cheese, light
- Milk, skim or 1%
- Spreadable light Swiss cheese, such as Laughing Cow (La vache qui rit)
- Yogurt, low-fat (plain, Greek-style, flavored)

Vegetables and fruits

- Apples
- Applesauce, unsweetened
- Bananas
- Bell peppers (red, yellow, green)
- Blueberries
- Carrots
- Celery
- Cucumbers
- Garlic
- Green onions
- Lemons
- Lettuce (iceberg, romaine, mixed spring greens)
- Limes
- Mixed vegetables, frozen
- Mushrooms (button, cremini, portobello)
- Onions (white, red, yellow, Spanish)
- Pears
- Potatoes
- Spinach, fresh and frozen
- Strawberries
- Sweet potatoes
- Tomatoes, fresh (any variety)
- Tomatoes, canned (diced and crushed)

Grain products

- Couscous (medium-grain, pearl)
- Crackers, whole wheat
- Cream of wheat cereal
- Dry bread crumbs, whole wheat (seasoned or unseasoned)
- Flour, all-purpose and whole wheat
- Flour tortillas, whole wheat (small)
- Long-grain brown rice
- Melba toast or rounds
- Oats, steel-cut and quick-cooking rolled
- Pitas, whole wheat (regular and mini pockets)
- Quinoa

Fats and oils

- Canola oil
- Light nonstick cooking spray
- Mayonnaise, low-fat
- Margarine, non-hydrogenated
- Olive oil

Herbs, spices and seasonings

- Basil, dried
- Black pepper
- Cinnamon, ground
- Cumin, ground
- Garlic powder
- Ginger, ground
- Herbes de Provence
- Italian herb seasoning
- Nutmeg, ground
- Oregano, dried
- Paprika
- Parsley, fresh
- Rosemary, dried
- Salt

Beverages

- Coffee, decaffeinated (brewed or instant)
- Sugar-free fruit drinks, such as Crystal Light or No-Sugar-Added Kool-Aid
- Tea, decaffeinated

Miscellaneous items

- Artificial sweetener (granulated sucralose, such as Splenda)
- Baking powder
- Baking soda
- Bouillon cubes or powder (chicken, vegetable, beef), reduced-sodium
- Chicken stock, low-fat, reduced-sodium
- Dijon mustard
- Gelatin, no-sugar-added
- Maple-flavored syrup, no-sugar-added, such as E.D. Smith
- Soy sauce, reduced-sodium
- Tomato juice, reduced
- Sodium
- Tomato paste
- Tomato sauce
- Vegetable stock, low-fat, reduced-sodium
- Vanilla extract
- Vinegar, balsamic and white

Breakfasts

You have heard time and time again that breakfast is the most important meal of the day. Breakfast provides you with the energy you need to start your day and is a great time to get in fiber, protein and many important nutrients. These simple breakfast recipes will help you take your breakfast from plain, boring and ordinary to extraordinary. In a crunch for time at lunch or supper? Try these recipes any time of day. The Mexican Baked Eggs and the Eggs en Cocotte are crowd pleasers and are a wonderful choice if you're hosting a brunch. The Cranberry Spelt Muffins are also a great choice for a snack.

Here is a two-week menu plan for diet stage 4 to get your day started off right with a nutritious breakfast.

WEEK	1	2
SUNDAY	Stirred Scrambled Eggs (page 166) and Decaf Caffè Latte (page 334)	Veggie Scrambled Eggs (page 166) and yogurt
MONDAY	Maple Walnut Steel-Cut Oats (page 171) and Chai (page 333)	Banana Bread Oatmeal (page 173) and Light Hot Chocolate (page 336)
TUESDAY	Berry Fruit Cream of Wheat (page 175)	Berry Yogurt Granola (page 177) and Skinny High-Protein Cappuccino (page 335)
WEDNESDAY	Hard-Cooked Eggs (page 165) and fruit	Easy Eggs (page 164) and yogurt
THURSDAY	Apple Cinnamon Yogurt Bulgur (page 176)	Fortified Cream of Wheat (page 174) and fruit
FRIDAY	Peanut Butter and Banana Roll-Up (page 177) and milk	Hot Oat Bran Cereal with Prunes (page 172) and milk
SATURDAY	Eggs en Cocotte (page 169) and Melba rounds for dipping	Mexican Baked Eggs (page 170) and pitas for dipping

Easy Eggs

Makes 1 serving

Diet Stages 3 to 4

Nutrients
PER SERVING

Calories	63
Fat	4.4 g
Sodium	62 mg
Carbohydrate	0.3 g
Fiber	0 g
Sugar	0.3 g
Protein	5.5 g
Calcium	23 mg
Iron	0.8 mg

- **Small silicone baking cup or ¾ cup (175 mL) ramekin**

I	egg	I
	Salt and freshly ground black pepper (optional)	

1. In baking cup, stir egg lightly with a fork until blended.

2. Microwave on High for 30 seconds. Let cool for 2 minutes. If desired, season to taste with salt and pepper.

Variation

Stir 1 tbsp (15 mL) shredded light Cheddar cheese into the egg before cooking.

Perfect Poached Egg

Makes 1 serving

Diet Stages 3 to 4

4 cups	water	I L
½ tsp	salt	2 mL
½ tsp	white vinegar	2 mL
I	egg	I
	Freshly ground black pepper	

Nutrients
PER SERVING

Calories	64
Fat	4.4 g
Sodium	62 mg
Carbohydrate	0.5 g
Fiber	0.1 g
Sugar	0.3 g
Protein	5.6 g
Calcium	24 mg
Iron	0.8 mg

1. In a medium saucepan, bring water to a boil over high heat. Add salt and vinegar. Reduce heat to a simmer.

2. Crack egg into a small dish, then slide it into the simmering water. Using a slotted spoon, gather the bits of egg white together, making a nice clump. Increase heat to medium and cook for 2 to 3 minutes or until yolk is just beginning to harden. Using a slotted spoon, remove egg from water. Season to taste with pepper.

Variation

If you prefer the yolk cooked through, cook the egg for 4 to 5 minutes.

Hard-Cooked Eggs

**Makes 1 to
2 servings**

Diet Stages 3 to 4

These are among the easiest foods to prepare. Cook extra and keep them in the fridge to have as a snack, to make an egg salad or to add to your favorite salad.

Kitchen Tips

To make peeling the hard-cooked egg easier, roll it back and forth on a hard surface, applying light pressure. Peel the cracked shell under cold running water, starting at the large end.

For an elegant look, cut the peeled egg in half lengthwise and sprinkle with a pinch of paprika or ground turmeric.

Store unpeeled hard-cooked eggs in a container in the refrigerator for up to 1 week.

Nutrients PER SERVING	
Calories	63
Fat	4.4 g
Sodium	62 mg
Carbohydrate	0.3 g
Fiber	0 g
Sugar	0.3 g
Protein	5.5 g
Calcium	23 mg
Iron	0.8 mg

2	eggs	2

Cold water

Salt and freshly ground black pepper (optional)

1. Place eggs in a saucepan with a tight-fitting lid and add enough cold water to cover. Bring to a boil over high heat. Turn off heat, cover and let stand for 15 minutes.

2. Drain off hot water and place eggs under cold running water. Crack the bottoms of the eggs and immerse in cold water for 2 minutes. (The cold water helps the shell separate from the egg.) Drain, then peel off shells. Season to taste with salt and pepper (if using).

Variation

For soft-cooked eggs, let stand for 3 to 4 minutes in step 1. To peel a soft-cooked egg, cool it briefly under cold running water. Place the egg, small end down, in an egg cup. Using a spoon or knife, crack the top of the large end and carefully peel off the top part of the shell.

Stirred Scrambled Eggs

2	eggs, separated	2
$\frac{1}{4}$ tsp	margarine	1 mL
$\frac{1}{8}$ tsp	salt (or to taste)	0.5 mL
	Freshly ground black pepper	

1. In a small bowl, lightly beat egg yolks, just enough to break them.
2. In a small saucepan, melt margarine over medium heat. Add egg whites, stirring continuously with a wooden spoon. Once whites start to get cloudy, with visible strands, add beaten egg yolks. Continue stirring until egg is cooked but still moist. Season with up to $\frac{1}{8}$ tsp (0.5 mL) salt and pepper to taste.

Nutrients
PER SERVING

Calories	67
Fat	4.8 g
Sodium	66 mg
Carbohydrate	0.3 g
Fiber	0 g
Sugar	0.3 g
Protein	5.5 g
Calcium	23 mg
Iron	0.8 mg

Veggie Scrambled Eggs

$\frac{1}{4}$ tsp	margarine	1 mL
1 tbsp	grated zucchini	15 mL
1 tbsp	grated carrot	15 mL
1 tbsp	finely chopped onion	15 mL
2	eggs	2
1 tbsp	low-fat cottage cheese	15 mL
$\frac{1}{8}$ tsp	salt (or to taste)	0.5 mL
	Freshly ground black pepper	

1. In a nonstick skillet, melt margarine over medium-high heat. Sauté zucchini, carrot and onion for 1 to 2 minutes or until starting to soften.
2. In a small bowl, lightly beat eggs. Stir in cottage cheese. Add to skillet and reduce heat to medium. Cook, stirring with a wooden spoon or silicone spatula, until egg is cooked but still moist. Season with up to $\frac{1}{8}$ tsp (0.5 mL) salt and pepper to taste.

Nutrients
PER SERVING

Calories	75
Fat	4.8 g
Sodium	97 mg
Carbohydrate	1.5 g
Fiber	0.2 g
Sugar	1.0 g
Protein	6.5 g
Calcium	30 mg
Iron	0.9 mg

Classic Omelet

Diet Stages 3 to 4

Don't be intimidated by the thought of making an omelet — it's just as simple as making scrambled eggs.

Kitchen Tips

To test whether the skillet is hot enough, add a drop of water; if it hisses, the skillet is ready.

If you prefer, you can use light nonstick cooking spray instead of margarine.

2	eggs	2
2 tbsp	skim milk	30 mL
1/8 tsp	salt (or to taste)	0.5 mL
	Freshly ground black pepper	
1/2 tsp	margarine	2 mL

1. In a medium bowl, lightly beat eggs until pale yellow. Whisk in milk and season with up to 1/8 tsp (0.5 mL) salt and pepper to taste.

2. Heat a small nonstick skillet over medium-low heat. Melt margarine, swirling to coat. Pour in egg mixture, without stirring. Cook for 1 to 2 minutes or until starting to set. Gently push one edge of the egg into the center of the pan while tilting the pan to allow the still liquid egg to flow underneath. Repeat with the other edges until no liquid remains.

3. Slide omelet onto a plate, then return to the pan, flipped over. Cook for 1 minute or until no liquid remains. Using a spatula, lift one edge of the omelet and fold it across and over, so that the edges line up. Cook for 1 minute. Transfer to a plate and cut in half if you are sharing.

Variation

Before folding the omelet in step 3, you can add your choice of fillings. Some ideas include sautéed diced onion and/or mushrooms, shredded light Cheddar cheese, chopped tomatoes, fresh parsley, diced ham and salsa. The possibilities are endless.

Nutrients
PER SERVING

Calories	75
Fat	5.1 g
Sodium	75 mg
Carbohydrate	1.1 g
Fiber	0 g
Sugar	1.1 g
Protein	6.1 g
Calcium	42 mg
Iron	0.8 mg

Deviled Eggs

*Deviled eggs are excellent
at breakfast or as a simple
healthy snack.*

Kitchen Tips

Deviled eggs are great to
make ahead of time. Store
them in an airtight container
in the refrigerator for up
to 24 hours. Sprinkle with
paprika just before serving.

For a moister egg yolk
mixture, add a little water or
skim milk.

If you don't own a piping
bag, you can improvise one.
Spoon the egg mixture into
a plastic food storage bag
and push it into the bottom
corner, making a cone shape.
Using sharp scissors, snip
off the corner. Squeeze the
mixture into each egg white.

4	hard-cooked eggs (see page 165)	4
1 tsp	finely chopped fresh chives	5 mL
1 tbsp	low-fat mayonnaise	15 mL
1 tsp	Dijon mustard	5 mL
1/4 tsp	ground paprika	1 mL

1. Cut eggs in half lengthwise. Scoop the yolks into a
   bowl and mash with a fork. Stir in chives, mayonnaise
   and mustard.

2. Using a small spoon or a piping bag, fill egg whites with
   yolk mixture. Sprinkle with paprika.

Variation

Replace the low-fat mayonnaise with spreadable
light cream cheese or low-fat plain yogurt.
Flavored light cream cheeses, such as herb and
garlic, smoked salmon and chives, work well.

Nutrients
PER SERVING

Calories	74
Fat	5.4 g
Sodium	107 mg
Carbohydrate	1.0 g
Fiber	0.1 g
Sugar	0.4 g
Protein	5.6 g
Calcium	24 mg
Iron	0.8 mg

Eggs en Cocotte

Makes 1 serving

Diet Stages 3 to 4

Cocotte *is the French word for "ramekins" — the little dishes these eggs are cooked in.*

Kitchen Tip

For a runny yolk, bake for 6 to 7 minutes and serve with Melba toast or crisp pitas for dipping.

- **Preheat oven to 375°F (190°C)**
- **¹/₂ cup (125 mL) ramekin, lightly sprayed with light nonstick cooking spray**
- **Small baking dish**

¹/₂ oz	sliced smoked salmon	15 g
1	egg	1
1 tbsp	spreadable light Swiss cheese (such as Laughing Cow/La vache qui rit)	15 mL
	Boiling water	
	Freshly ground black pepper	
	Chopped fresh chives	

1. Place smoked salmon in prepared ramekin. Break egg on top of salmon. Place cheese on top.

2. Set the ramekin in a baking dish. Add boiling water to the baking dish until it reaches halfway up the sides of the ramekin.

3. Bake in preheated oven for 10 to 14 minutes or until egg is set. Season to taste with pepper. Garnish with chives.

Variations

Any little surprise can be added to the bottom of the ramekin in place of the smoked salmon. Try puréed spinach or cooked spinach leaves, diced ham, cooked beans or sautéed mushrooms.

Use light ricotta cheese in place of the Swiss.

Nutrients
PER SERVING

Calories	106
Fat	6.4 g
Sodium	359 mg
Carbohydrate	1.2 g
Fiber	0.1 g
Sugar	1.0 g
Protein	10.0 g
Calcium	67 mg
Iron	1.0 mg

Mexican Baked Eggs

Mid Diet Stage 3 to Diet Stage 4

Here's a simple way to make eggs packed with flavor. The sour cream provides a smooth texture, and the salsa adds zing. Enjoy these eggs with crisp pitas.

Kitchen Tips

For a runny yolk, bake for 6 to 7 minutes and serve with Melba toast or crisp pitas for dipping.

This recipe also makes a tasty, low-budget, quick dinner option.

- **Preheat oven to 375°F (190°C)**
- **½ cup (125 mL) ramekin, lightly sprayed with light nonstick cooking spray**
- **Small baking dish**

1 tsp	reduced-fat (light) sour cream	5 mL
3	fresh chives, finely chopped	3
1 tbsp	shredded light Cheddar cheese	15 mL
1	egg	1
	Freshly ground black pepper (optional)	
	Boiling water	
1 tbsp	mild salsa	15 mL
1 tsp	chopped fresh cilantro	5 mL

1. Place sour cream in ramekin, then add chives and cheese. Crack egg on top. Season with pepper (if using).

2. Set the ramekin in a baking dish. Add boiling water to the baking dish until it reaches halfway up the sides of the ramekin.

3. Bake in preheated oven for 10 to 14 minutes or until egg is set. Garnish with salsa and cilantro.

Nutrients
PER SERVING

Calories	87
Fat	5.3 g
Sodium	173 mg
Carbohydrate	2.3 g
Fiber	0 g
Sugar	1.2 g
Protein	7.6 g
Calcium	63 mg
Iron	0.8 mg

Maple Walnut Steel-Cut Oats

Steel-cut oats are also known as Irish oats. They have a lower glycemic index than instant oats, which makes them a healthier alternative.

Kitchen Tip

To speed up the cooking process, soak the oats in the 2 cups (500 mL) water overnight in the refrigerator. In the morning, bring to a boil as directed, then decrease the simmering time to 9 to 12 minutes or until oats are tender and thickened.

Weight-Loss Surgery Tip

To serve this in diet stages 2 or 3, omit the walnuts. Add the nuts once you are able to tolerate their texture.

Nutrients PER SERVING	
Calories	126
Fat	5.8 g
Sodium	8 mg
Carbohydrate	16.6 g
Fiber	2.5 g
Sugar	0.2 g
Protein	3.6 g
Calcium	17 mg
Iron	0.2 mg

1/2 cup	steel-cut oats	125 mL
2 cups	water	500 mL
1/4 cup	chopped walnuts	60 mL
1 tbsp	no-sugar-added maple-flavored syrup	15 mL

1. In a medium saucepan, combine oats and water. Bring to a boil over high heat. Reduce heat and boil gently, stirring, for 2 to 3 minutes or until oats start to thicken. Reduce heat to low, cover and simmer, stirring occasionally, for about 30 minutes or until oats are tender and thickened.

2. Remove from heat and stir in walnuts and syrup.

Variations

Use any chopped nuts, such as almonds, pecans or Brazil nuts, instead of walnuts.

For extra protein and nutrition, use skim milk instead of water to cook the oats.

Top with a dollop of low-fat yogurt or a splash of skim milk for added protein.

Top with fresh fruit, such as seasonal berries, for added fiber.

Hot Oat Bran Cereal with Prunes

2	pitted prunes, finely chopped	2
½ cup	skim milk	125 mL
⅛ tsp	ground cinnamon	0.5 mL
2 tbsp	oat bran cereal	30 mL

Makes 1 serving

Diet Stage 4

Oat bran cereal is packed with fiber and vitamin B_1 — key nutrients needed after weight-loss surgery.

Weight-Loss Surgery Tips

Be sure to chop the prunes finely and chew them well.

To serve this in diet stages 2 or 3, either omit the prunes or use 2 tbsp (30 mL) puréed baby prunes instead. Progress to using finely chopped prunes once you are able to tolerate their texture.

1. In a small saucepan, combine prunes, milk and cinnamon. Bring to a gentle boil over medium-high heat. Gradually stir in oat bran cereal; reduce heat to medium and boil gently, stirring frequently, for about 2 minutes or until cereal thickens.

Variations

Use any type of dried fruit, such as apricots or raisins, in place of the prunes.

For extra protein, add 1 scoop unflavored protein powder to the cooked cereal.

To make this recipe lactose-free, use water instead of milk and add unflavored whey protein isolate. Or prepare it with lactose-reduced skim milk or unsweetened soy milk.

Nutrients
PER SERVING

Calories	102
Fat	0.5 g
Sodium	73 mg
Carbohydrate	20.7 g
Fiber	2.0 g
Sugar	7.2 g
Protein	5.3 g
Calcium	176 mg
Iron	2.3 mg

Banana Bread Oatmeal

The banana increases the fiber content and enhances the flavor of traditional oatmeal, giving it a little extra natural sweetness.

Kitchen Tip

Store leftovers in a covered microwave-safe bowl in the refrigerator for up to 3 days. To reheat, add a few spoonfuls of milk to thin the oatmeal, then microwave, uncovered, on High for 2 to 3 minutes or until warmed through. Let stand for a few minutes before serving.

Weight-Loss Surgery Tip

To serve this in diet stages 2 or 3, omit the walnuts. Add the nuts once you are able to tolerate their texture.

1 1/2 cups	skim milk	375 mL
1/4 tsp	ground cinnamon	1 mL
1/8 tsp	ground nutmeg	0.5 mL
1/8 tsp	salt	0.5 mL
1 cup	quick-cooking rolled oats	250 mL
1/2	banana, mashed	1/2
2 tbsp	chopped walnuts	30 mL
	Sucralose artificial sweetener, such as Splenda (optional)	

1. In a small saucepan, combine milk, cinnamon, nutmeg and salt. Bring to a gentle boil over medium-high heat. Stir in oats and return to a boil. Reduce heat and simmer, stirring occasionally, for about 1 minute or until desired texture is achieved. Remove from heat and stir in banana, walnuts and sweetener to taste (if using).

Variations

For extra protein, add 1 scoop unflavored protein powder to the cooked oatmeal.

To make this recipe lactose-free, use water instead of milk and add unflavored whey protein isolate. Or prepare it with lactose-reduced skim milk or unsweetened soy milk.

If you want to use old-fashioned (large-flake) rolled oats instead of quick-cooking oats, increase the simmering time to about 5 minutes.

Nutrients
PER SERVING

Calories	153
Fat	4.0 g
Sodium	98 mg
Carbohydrate	23.2 g
Fiber	3.1 g
Sugar	8.2 g
Protein	6.8 g
Calcium	136 mg
Iron	1.6 mg

Fortified Cream of Wheat

Makes 2 servings

Diet Stages 2 to 4

Protein powder turns a basic cereal into a nutrient-packed high-protein breakfast.

Kitchen Tip

Store leftovers in a covered microwave-safe bowl in the refrigerator for up to 3 days. To reheat, add a few spoonfuls of milk to thin the cereal, then microwave, uncovered, on High for 2 to 3 minutes or until warmed through. Let stand for a few minutes before serving.

Weight-Loss Surgery Tip

When you are able to tolerate fruit, top with chopped fresh fruit, a sprinkle of ground cinnamon and a drizzle of no-sugar-added maple-flavored syrup.

1¼ cups	skim milk	300 mL
⅛ tsp	salt (optional)	0.5 mL
3 tbsp	cream of wheat cereal	45 mL
1	scoop unflavored protein powder	1

1. In a small saucepan, combine milk and salt (if using). Bring almost to a boil over medium-high heat. Slowly add cream of wheat, stirring constantly, and bring to boil. Reduce heat and simmer, stirring frequently, for 3 minutes or until cereal thickens. Stir in protein powder.

Variations

For a sweeter cereal, stir in artificial sweetener to taste.

To make this recipe lactose-free, use water instead of milk and add unflavored whey protein isolate. Or prepare it with lactose-reduced skim milk or unsweetened soy milk.

Nutrients
PER SERVING

Calories	162
Fat	0.3 g
Sodium	279 mg
Carbohydrate	21.0 g
Fiber	0.6 g
Sugar	7.8 g
Protein	18.3 g
Calcium	218 mg
Iron	4.8 mg

Berry Fruit Cream of Wheat

Fresh blueberries and a touch of strawberry spread give traditional cream of wheat a sweeter taste.

Kitchen Tip

Store leftovers in a covered microwave-safe bowl in the refrigerator for up to 3 days. To reheat, add a few spoonfuls of milk to thin the cereal, then microwave, uncovered, on High for 2 to 3 minutes or until warmed through. Let stand for a few minutes before serving.

Weight-Loss Surgery Tips

For diet stage 2, use seedless fruit spread and omit the blueberries.

For diet stage 4, top the cooked cereal with 1 tbsp (15 mL) chopped walnuts.

1 ¼ cups	skim milk	300 mL
⅛ tsp	salt	0.5 mL
3 tbsp	cream of wheat cereal	45 mL
3 tbsp	blueberries	45 mL
1 tbsp	no-sugar-added strawberry spread	15 mL
	Ground cinnamon (optional)	

1. In a small saucepan, combine milk and salt. Bring almost to a boil over medium-high heat. Slowly add cream of wheat, stirring constantly, and bring to a boil. Reduce heat and simmer, stirring frequently, for 3 minutes or until cereal thickens. Stir in blueberries, strawberry spread and cinnamon (if using).

Variations

For extra protein, add 1 scoop unflavored protein powder to the cooked cereal.

To make this recipe lactose-free, use water instead of milk and add unflavored whey protein isolate. Or prepare it with lactose-reduced skim milk or unsweetened soy milk.

Nutrients
PER SERVING

Calories	121
Fat	0.4 g
Sodium	279 mg
Carbohydrate	22.8 g
Fiber	0.9 g
Sugar	9.2 g
Protein	6.9 g
Calcium	215 mg
Iron	4.9 mg

Cornmeal Porridge

Nutrients PER SERVING	
Calories	69
Fat	0.4 g
Sodium	54 mg
Carbohydrate	11.9 g
Fiber	0.6 g
Sugar	6.3 g
Protein	4.8 g
Calcium	154 mg
Iron	0.3 mg

1 cup	skim milk	250 mL
2 tbsp	fine cornmeal	30 mL
	Salt (optional)	

1. Pour milk into a small saucepan and whisk in cornmeal. Season to taste with salt (if using). Bring to a boil over medium-high heat, whisking frequently to prevent lumps. Reduce heat and simmer, stirring frequently, for 15 to 20 minutes or until cornmeal starts to thicken.

Variation

To make this recipe lactose-free, use water instead of milk and add unflavored whey protein isolate. Or prepare it with lactose-reduced skim milk or unsweetened soy milk.

Apple Cinnamon Yogurt Bulgur

Nutrients PER SERVING	
Calories	159
Fat	1.5 g
Sodium	79 mg
Carbohydrate	29.4 g
Fiber	2.8 g
Sugar	14.2 g
Protein	7.5 g
Calcium	198 mg
Iron	0.6 mg

1/4 cup	finely ground bulgur (bulgur #1)	60 mL
3/4 cup	low-fat plain yogurt	175 mL
1/4 cup	skim milk	60 mL
1	apple, peeled and grated	1
	Ground cinnamon	
	Artificial sweetener (optional)	

1. In a small bowl, combine bulgur, yogurt and milk; let stand for 10 minutes. Stir in apple, cinnamon and sweetener to taste (if using).

Variations

Use grated pear or chopped fresh berries instead of apple.

Use no-sugar-added maple-flavored syrup instead of artificial sweetener.

Berry Yogurt Granola

Nutrients PER SERVING	
Calories	107
Fat	2.2 g
Sodium	57 mg
Carbohydrate	17.2 g
Fiber	0.4 g
Sugar	7.5 g
Protein	4.4 g
Calcium	105 mg
Iron	0.1 mg

2 tbsp	mixed berries (such as raspberries, blueberries and sliced strawberries)	30 mL
1/4 cup	low-fat plain yogurt	60 mL
2 tbsp	reduced-sugar granola	30 mL
I tsp	no-added-sugar maple-flavored syrup	5 mL

1. Place berries in a small serving bowl. Layer yogurt, granola and syrup on top.

Peanut Butter and Banana Roll-Up

Nutrients PER SERVING	
Calories	165
Fat	5.7 g
Sodium	86 mg
Carbohydrate	24.3 g
Fiber	2.8 g
Sugar	7.2 g
Protein	4.3 g
Calcium	3 mg
Iron	0.9 mg

I tbsp	all-natural peanut butter	15 mL
I	small whole wheat flour tortilla	I
I	small banana	I

1. Spread peanut butter evenly over tortilla. Lay banana on peanut butter and gently straighten out the curve of the banana. Roll tortilla up tightly and slice into 6 small rounds.

Variation

Use any nut butter, such as almond butter or soy nut butter, in place of the peanut butter.

Cranberry Spelt Muffins

Makes 12 muffins

Serving size: 1 muffin

Diet Stage 4

Spelt is an ancient grain with a mellow, nutty flavor that's perfect for muffins.

Kitchen Tip

Make sure to use granulated sucralose artificial sweetener that measures like sugar, not the packets.

Weight-Loss Surgery Tip

Muffins are usually not well tolerated initially, but in the long term most people can comfortably tolerate a healthy version that is high in fiber and low in sugar and fat.

- **Preheat oven to 400°F (200°C)**
- **12-cup muffin pan, lightly sprayed with light nonstick cooking spray**

1½ cups	whole wheat flour	375 mL
¾ cup	spelt flour	175 mL
2 tbsp	wheat germ	30 mL
1 tbsp	baking powder	15 mL
½ tsp	ground cinnamon	2 mL
⅛ tsp	salt	0.5 mL
½ cup	granulated sucralose artificial sweetener, such as Splenda	125 mL
1 tbsp	grated orange zest	15 mL
1	egg	1
¾ cup	low-fat plain yogurt	175 mL
½ cup	skim milk	125 mL
½ cup	unsweetened applesauce	125 mL
½ cup	low-calorie orange juice	125 mL
½ cup	dried cranberries (preferably unsweetened)	125 mL

1. In a medium bowl, whisk together whole wheat flour, spelt flour, wheat germ, baking powder, cinnamon and salt.

2. In a large bowl, whisk together sweetener, orange zest, egg, yogurt, milk, applesauce and orange juice until well blended. Whisk in flour mixture until just blended. Fold in cranberries.

3. Divide batter equally among prepared muffin cups. Bake in preheated oven for 25 minutes or until a tester inserted in the center comes out clean. Let cool in pan on a wire rack for 10 minutes, then transfer to the rack to cool completely.

Variations

Replace the spelt flour with ground millet flour, which is also rich in protein.

Substitute fresh blueberries for the dried cranberries.

Nutrients
PER SERVING

Calories	108
Fat	1.0 g
Sodium	183 mg
Carbohydrate	22.0 g
Fiber	2.6 g
Sugar	8.5 g
Protein	4.0 g
Calcium	73 mg
Iron	0.8 mg

Soups

Soups provide a nutritious meal option, especially when you have difficulty eating solid foods after weight-loss surgery. These recipes are delicious and easy to make, yet provide good-quality nutrition. Another benefit of soups is that they can easily be frozen for a quick meal on a day when you are too busy to cook.

The serving sizes for these soups are based on their nutritional quality. If the soup provides a good amount of protein and a variety of nutrients, it can be considered a main course, and the serving size is ¾ cup (175 mL). If the soup is lower in protein and other nutrients, the serving size is ½ cup (125 mL) so you can enjoy a protein-rich food along with it or added to it. Depending on the surgery you had, your tolerance and which diet stage you are in, you may need to the adjust the serving size.

Adding Protein to Soups

Here are some easy ways to add more protein to soups in diet stages 3 and 4, to help you get the nutrition you need.

Egg Sauce

In a bowl, beat 2 eggs well with a fork or wire whisk. Beat in the juice of 1 lemon. Gradually whisk egg mixture into the simmering soup and simmer, stirring, for 1 to 2 minutes or until egg mixture is light and fluffy. This works well with clear soups, such as Vegetable Stock or Spinach Soup with Oatmeal Balls.

Cheesy Egg Sauce

In a bowl, beat 2 eggs well with a fork or wire whisk. Whisk in 2 tbsp (30 mL) grated or shredded light cheese (any variety will do, but Parmesan works especially well). If desired, whisk in 1 tsp (5 mL) finely chopped fresh parsley. Gradually whisk egg mixture into the simmering soup and simmer, stirring, for 1 to 2 minutes or until egg mixture is light and fluffy. This works well with clear soups, such as Vegetable Stock or Spinach Soup with Oatmeal Balls.

Chicken or Turkey

After preparing your soup, toss in some leftover cooked chicken or turkey. Shredded or chopped pieces work well. Warm through and serve. Tastes great in Potato and Leek Soup or Oven-Roasted Tomato Soup.

Mini Meatballs

Add leftover cooked mini meatballs to simmering soup and warm through. Tastes great in Vegetable Stock, Lentil Soup or Oven-Roasted Tomato Soup.

Seafood or Fish

After preparing your soup, toss in leftover cooked shrimp or precooked cocktail shrimp and simmer until heated through. Or add thawed frozen seafood mix or chunks of fish and simmer for about 5 minutes or until seafood is firm and opaque or fish flakes easily with a fork. Try adding chunks of salmon to the Potato and Leek Soup or shrimp to the Oven-Roasted Tomato Soup.

Tofu

Add chopped firm or extra-firm tofu to simmering soup and warm through. The tofu pieces will absorb flavor from the soup. Try adding it to the Oven-Roasted Tomato Soup, Hearty Minestrone, Pearl Couscous Chickpea Soup or Low-Fat Cream of Asparagus Soup. Or add silken or soft tofu to any soup that will be puréed.

Legumes

A handful of canned or cooked dried beans, lentils or other legumes goes a long way when you are in a hurry to prepare a quick soup. If using canned legumes, drain and rinse them before adding them to soup. Toss them into the soup of your choice, then warm through. For example, add navy or kidney beans to Oven-Roasted Tomato Soup or Vegetable Stock.

Yogurt

Spoon a dollop of low-fat Greek-style plain yogurt into soup just before serving. Yogurt tastes great in Oven-Roasted Tomato Soup, Green Lentil Soup with Swiss Chard, Spinach Soup with Oatmeal Balls or Carrot and Red Lentil Soup. (Yogurt can be added to soups during diet stage 2.)

Light Cheese

Sprinkle some finely grated or shredded light cheese into soup just before serving.

Protein Powder

Stir unflavored protein powder into soup just before serving. (Protein powder can be added to soups during diet stage 2.)

Vegetable Stock

This homemade low-fat vegetable stock can be used in any recipe that calls for vegetable stock or broth. Make extra to freeze, and thaw it when you're ready to make soup.

Kitchen Tip

Vegetable stock freezes well. Let cool completely, pour individual portions into airtight containers and store in the freezer for up to 4 months. Be sure to leave some room for expansion.

2 tsp	olive oil	10 mL
2	carrots, chopped	2
2	stalks celery, chopped	2
1	large onion, chopped	1
3	cloves garlic, minced	3
6	sprigs fresh parsley	6
4	sprigs fresh thyme	4
2	bay leaves	2
6 cups	water	1.5 L
⅛ tsp	salt (or to taste)	0.5 mL
	Freshly ground black pepper	

1. In a pot, heat oil over medium heat. Sauté carrots, celery and onion for 6 to 7 minutes or until tender. Add garlic and sauté for 1 minute (being careful not to burn garlic).

2. Add parsley, thyme, bay leaves and water. Bring to a boil over high heat. Reduce heat and simmer for about 30 minutes or until vegetables are very soft. Remove from heat and let cool for 10 minutes. Strain through a fine-mesh sieve, discarding solids. Season with up to ⅛ tsp (0.5 mL) salt and pepper to taste.

Variations

Instead of straining the stock, use a slotted spoon to remove the bay leaves and herb sprigs. Enjoy as is, or use a blender or food processor to purée it and enjoy during diet stages 2 to 4.

Substitute 1 sliced leek (white and light green parts only) for the onion.

Nutrients
PER SERVING

Calories	28
Fat	1.2 g
Sodium	66 mg
Carbohydrate	4.0 g
Fiber	1.1 g
Sugar	1.3 g
Protein	0.6 g
Calcium	25 mg
Iron	0.3 mg

Chicken Stock

*This chicken stock is better
than store-bought and is
easy to make. You can use
it in any recipe that calls
for chicken stock or broth.
Make extra to freeze, and
thaw it when you're ready to
make soup.*

Kitchen Tip

This stock freezes well.
Store in individual portions
in airtight containers in the
freezer for up to 3 months.
Be sure to leave some room
for expansion.

1 lb	skinless bone-in chicken breasts, fat trimmed	500 g
3	cloves garlic, sliced	3
2	carrots, chopped	2
2	stalks celery, chopped	2
1	large onion, chopped	1
6	sprigs fresh parsley	6
4	sprigs fresh thyme	4
2	bay leaves	2
8 cups	cold water	2 L
⅛ tsp	salt (or to taste)	0.5 mL
	Freshly ground black pepper	

1. In a large pot, combine chicken, garlic, carrots, celery, onion, parsley, thyme, bay leaves and cold water. Bring to a boil over high heat. Reduce heat to low, cover and simmer for 1 hour. Remove from heat and let cool for 10 minutes. Season with up to ⅛ tsp (0.5 mL) salt and pepper to taste.

2. Remove cooked chicken. (If you are in diet stage 3 to 4, save it to use in another recipe or shred and add to soup). Strain stock through a fine-mesh sieve into a large bowl, discarding solids. Cover and refrigerate overnight. The next day, use a spoon to remove any hardened fat that has risen to the top of the stock.

Nutrients PER SERVING	
Calories	11
Fat	0.1 g
Sodium	40 mg
Carbohydrate	2.6 g
Fiber	0.7 g
Sugar	0.9 g
Protein	0.4 g
Calcium	13 mg
Iron	0.2 mg

Low-Fat Cream of Asparagus Soup

Asparagus is packed with nutrients, including vitamin A, vitamin C and iron, and this low-fat creamy soup incorporates all that goodness.

Kitchen Tips

When buying asparagus, choose firm, bright green or pale ivory stalks with tight tips.

Asparagus breaks naturally where the spear becomes tough. Hold the top of the asparagus with one hand and the bottom with the other and break off the tough end.

Sprinkle soup with a little grated light Parmesan cheese.

Nutrients
PER SERVING

Calories	80
Fat	2.6 g
Sodium	101 mg
Carbohydrate	11.2 g
Fiber	2.4 g
Sugar	4.9 g
Protein	4.1 g
Calcium	102 mg
Iron	1.6 mg

- **Food processor, blender or immersion blender**

1 tsp	olive oil	5 mL
1 lb	asparagus, cut into 2-inch (5 cm) pieces	500 g
1	small onion, chopped	1
1	stalk celery, chopped	1
1	small potato, peeled and chopped	1
2 cups	Vegetable Stock (see recipe, page 181) or reduced-sodium vegetable broth	500 mL
1 cup	skim milk	250 mL
½ cup	reduced-fat (light) sour cream	125 mL

1. In a pot, heat oil over medium heat. Sauté asparagus, onion, celery and potato for 10 to 15 minutes or until tender. Add stock and bring to a boil. Reduce heat and simmer for 20 minutes or until vegetables are soft. Remove from heat and let cool for 10 minutes.

2. Working in batches, transfer soup to food processor (or use immersion blender in pot) and purée until smooth. Return soup to pot (if necessary) and stir in milk and sour cream; heat over medium-low heat, stirring constantly, until warmed through (do not let boil).

Variation

Use Chicken Stock (see recipe, page 182) or reduced-sodium low-fat chicken broth in place of the vegetable stock.

Best-Ever Broccoli Cheddar Soup

This is a classic soup, made lower in fat. The flavor combination of broccoli and Cheddar cheese is yummy.

Kitchen Tip

You can use 2 cups (500 mL) leftover chopped cooked broccoli or thawed frozen broccoli if you wish, but reduce the stock to 3 1/2 cups (875 mL) and the cooking time by 15 to 20 minutes.

• **Food processor, blender or immersion blender**

4 cups	Vegetable Stock (see recipe, page 181) or reduced-sodium vegetable broth	1 L
2 cups	coarsely chopped broccoli (about 1 small head)	500 mL
1	small onion, chopped	1
1	clove garlic, minced	1
1/3 cup	finely shredded light Cheddar cheese	75 mL
1/8 tsp	salt (or to taste)	0.5 mL
	Freshly ground black pepper	

1. In a pot, bring stock to a boil over high heat. Add broccoli, onion and garlic; reduce heat and simmer for 25 to 30 minutes or until broccoli is very tender. Remove from heat and let cool for 10 minutes.

2. Working in batches, transfer soup to food processor (or use immersion blender in pot) and purée until smooth. Return soup to pot, if necessary. Stir in cheese and heat over medium-low heat, stirring constantly, until melted. Season with up to 1/8 tsp (0.5 mL) salt and pepper to taste.

Nutrients
PER SERVING

Calories	48
Fat	2.1 g
Sodium	136 mg
Carbohydrate	6.1 g
Fiber	1.8 g
Sugar	2.0 g
Protein	2.5 g
Calcium	69 mg
Iron	0.5 mg

Carrot and Red Lentil Soup

Packed full of fiber, protein and antioxidants, this smooth soup makes a great meal served with a couple of slices of Melba rounds. It tastes wonderful hot or cold.

Kitchen Tip

This soup can be frozen in an airtight container for up to 4 months. Be sure to leave some room for expansion.

Weight-Loss Surgery Tip

For extra protein, top each serving with 1 tbsp (15 mL) Greek-style low-fat plain yogurt.

- **Food processor, blender or immersion blender**

1 tbsp	olive oil	15 mL
8 oz	carrots, chopped	250 g
1	small onion, chopped	1
½	red bell pepper, chopped	½
1	clove garlic, minced	1
1 ½ tsp	grated gingerroot	7 mL
3 cups	Chicken Stock (see recipe, page 182) or reduced-sodium low-fat chicken broth	750 mL
½ cup	dried red lentils, rinsed	125 mL
1 tsp	freshly squeezed lemon juice	5 mL
⅛ tsp	salt (or to taste)	0.5 mL

1. In a pot, heat oil over medium heat. Sauté carrots, onion and red pepper for 3 minutes. Add garlic and ginger; sauté for 2 minutes.

2. Add stock and lentils; bring to a boil. Reduce heat and simmer, stirring occasionally, for 15 to 20 minutes or until lentils are soft. Remove from heat. Add lemon juice. Season with up to ⅛ tsp (0.5 mL) salt. Let stand for 10 minutes.

3. Working in batches, transfer soup to food processor (or use immersion blender in pot) and purée until smooth. Return soup to pot (if necessary) and heat over medium-low heat, stirring constantly, until warmed through.

Nutrients
PER SERVING

Calories	88
Fat	2.2 g
Sodium	90 mg
Carbohydrate	14.0 g
Fiber	3.6 g
Sugar	3.3 g
Protein	4.1 g
Calcium	29 mg
Iron	1.0 mg

Variations

For a vegetarian soup, use Vegetable Stock (see recipe, page 181) or reduced-sodium vegetable broth instead of chicken stock.

If you're in diet stage 4, you can top this soup with a dollop of parsley cream for an extra-special treat. To make parsley cream, combine ½ cup (125 mL) finely chopped fresh parsley, 1 finely chopped green onion, ¾ cup (175 mL) reduced-fat (light) sour cream and a pinch of cayenne pepper.

Cool Cucumber and Yogurt Soup

This cool soup is refreshing on a hot summer day. For more protein, use Greek-style low-fat plain yogurt and use skim milk instead of water.

Weight-Loss Surgery Tip

Once you're in diet stage 4, you can cut the cucumber into matchsticks, then simply combine it with the salt, yogurt and cold water in a large bowl, rather than puréeing them. Garnish with 1 tbsp (15 mL) finely chopped fresh mint.

- **Food processor or blender**

1	large cucumber, peeled	1
⅛ tsp	salt	0.5 mL
4 cups	low-fat plain yogurt	1 L
1 cup	cold water	250 mL
6	ice cubes	6

1. Cut cucumber lengthwise and remove the seeds. Cut into chunks.
2. In food processor, combine cucumber, salt, yogurt and cold water; purée until smooth. Transfer to a large bowl, cover and refrigerate for 1 to 2 hours or until chilled.
3. Place 1 ice cube in each serving bowl. Divide cucumber mixture evenly among bowls.

Variation

For extra flavor, add 1 minced clove garlic with the cucumber and salt.

Nutrients
PER SERVING

Calories	105
Fat	2.1 g
Sodium	155 mg
Carbohydrate	11.6 g
Fiber	0.3 g
Sugar	11.3 g
Protein	7.6 g
Calcium	275 mg
Iron	0.1 mg

Low-Fat Cream of Cremini Mushroom Soup

Cremini mushrooms are immature portobello mushrooms, and they offer a fuller flavor than everyday white mushrooms.

Weight-Loss Surgery Tip

If you blend the soup or strain it through a fine-mesh sieve, discarding the solids, you can eat it during diet stage 2.

1 tsp	olive oil	5 mL
1½ cups	sliced cremini mushrooms	375 mL
2	cloves garlic, minced	2
¾ cup	Vegetable Stock (see recipe, page 181) or reduced-sodium vegetable broth	175 mL
¾ cup	skim milk	175 mL
1 tbsp	cornstarch	15 mL
2 tbsp	cold water	30 mL
⅛ tsp	salt (or to taste)	0.5 mL
	Freshly ground black pepper	

1. In a pot, heat oil over medium heat. Sauté mushrooms for 2 minutes. Add garlic and stock; bring to a boil. Add milk, reduce heat and simmer, stirring occasionally, for 10 minutes (do not let boil).

2. In a small bowl, dissolve cornstarch in cold water. Stir into soup, increase heat to medium-high and bring to a boil; boil, stirring frequently, for 1 minute. Season with up to ⅛ tsp (0.5 mL) salt and pepper to taste.

Nutrients
PER SERVING

Calories	53
Fat	1.8 g
Sodium	119 mg
Carbohydrate	7.1 g
Fiber	0.8 g
Sugar	3.3 g
Protein	2.7 g
Calcium	71 mg
Iron	0.3 mg

Potato and Leek Soup

Potatoes and leeks are perfectly matched flavors. Make this large batch of soup and freeze extras to use as a base for your own creative recipes!

Kitchen Tip

This soup freezes well. Store in individual portions in airtight containers in the freezer for up to 4 months. Be sure to leave some room for expansion.

Weight-Loss Surgery Tip

Just before eating, swirl 1 tbsp (15 mL) Greek-style low-fat plain yogurt or 1 scoop unflavored protein powder into each bowl for added protein.

Nutrients
PER SERVING

Calories	70
Fat	2.3 g
Sodium	72 mg
Carbohydrate	9.8 g
Fiber	1.7 g
Sugar	1.9 g
Protein	1.5 g
Calcium	23 mg
Iron	0.7 mg

- **Food processor, blender or immersion blender**

2 tbsp	olive oil	30 mL
1	small onion, chopped	1
1 cup	thinly sliced leeks (white and light green parts only)	250 mL
2	medium potatoes, peeled and chopped	2
2	bay leaves	2
2	sprigs fresh thyme	2
4 cups	Chicken Stock (see recipe, page 182) or reduced-sodium low-fat chicken broth	1 L
2 tsp	freshly squeezed lemon juice	10 mL
¼ tsp	salt (or to taste)	1 mL
	Freshly ground black pepper	

1. In a large pot, heat oil over medium-high heat. Sauté onion and leeks for about 3 minutes or until softened.

2. Stir in potatoes, bay leaves, thyme and stock; bring to a boil. Reduce heat and simmer for about 20 minutes or until potatoes are very soft. Remove from heat and let cool for 10 minutes. Discard bay leaves and thyme.

3. Working in batches, transfer soup to food processor (or use immersion blender in pot) and purée until smooth. Return soup to pot (if necessary) and stir in lemon juice. Season with up to ¼ tsp (1 mL) salt and pepper to taste. Heat over medium-low heat until warmed through.

Variations

Add ½ cup (125 mL) chopped carrot and/or celery with the leeks.

For diet stage 4, add 1 cup (250 mL) corn with the lemon juice.

For mid diet stage 3 to diet stage 4, toss in 1 cup (250 mL) sautéed mushrooms with the lemon juice.

Garnish with finely chopped fresh cilantro or chives.

Spinach Soup with Oatmeal Balls

Makes 8 servings

Serving size: ½ cup (125 mL)

Late Diet Stage 3 to Diet Stage 4

This soup sounds silly but tastes delicious. Give it a try — you will love it!

Kitchen Tips

If you cannot find finely ground bulgur, use a coffee grinder to grind coarser-textured bulgur.

When making the oatmeal balls, wet your hands with a little warm water to prevent the mixture from sticking to them.

This soup can be stored in airtight containers in the freezer for up to 4 months. Be sure to leave some room for expansion.

Nutrients
PER SERVING

Calories	121
Fat	2.6 g
Sodium	325 mg
Carbohydrate	15.2 g
Fiber	3.8 g
Sugar	1.4 g
Protein	10.7 g
Calcium	41 mg
Iron	1.8 mg

Oatmeal Balls

¾ cup	quick-cooking rolled oats	175 mL
¼ cup	finely ground bulgur (bulgur #1)	60 mL
½ tsp	salt	2 mL
¼ cup	water	60 mL

Soup

3 cups	Chicken Stock (see recipe, page 182) or reduced-sodium low-fat chicken broth	750 mL
½ tsp	olive oil	2 mL
¼	small onion, finely chopped	¼
8 oz	fresh baby spinach or frozen spinach, thawed and drained	250 g
½ cup	chopped tomato	125 mL
⅛ tsp	salt (or to taste)	0.5 mL
	Freshly ground black pepper	

1. *Oatmeal Balls:* In a bowl, knead together oats, bulgur, salt and water. Shape into balls about the size of a cherry. Set aside.

2. *Soup:* In a large pot, bring stock to a boil over high heat. Add oatmeal balls, reduce heat and simmer for 5 minutes.

3. Meanwhile, in a small nonstick skillet, heat oil over medium-high heat. Sauté onion for 2 to 4 minutes or until golden brown. Add to the stock, along with spinach and tomato. Simmer for 5 to 8 minutes or until spinach is soft. Season with up to ⅛ tsp (0.5 mL) salt and pepper to taste.

Variations

For a vegetarian soup, use Vegetable Stock (see recipe, page 181) or reduced-sodium vegetable broth instead of chicken stock.

Make an egg sauce to add protein to this soup (see page 179).

Oven-Roasted Tomato Soup

Roasting the tomatoes in the oven gives this soup a rustic, authentic taste.

Kitchen Tips

This soup is intended to be thick; if you prefer a thinner consistency, add more chicken stock.

If you tolerate pasta, this soup can do double duty as a pasta sauce.

Weight-Loss Surgery Tip

To add some protein, stir in 1 scoop unflavored protein powder into each bowl. Or top each bowl with a dollop of low-fat Greek style plain yogurt.

Nutrients
PER SERVING

Calories	29
Fat	0.9 g
Sodium	52 mg
Carbohydrate	4.9 g
Fiber	0.9 g
Sugar	2.5 g
Protein	0.8 g
Calcium	15 mg
Iron	0.4 mg

- **Preheat oven to 450°F (230°C)**
- **8-cup (2 L) casserole dish**
- **Food processor or blender**

1 lb	tomatoes (about 3 medium)	500 g
¼ cup	chopped onion	60 mL
1 tbsp	Italian herb seasoning	15 mL
1 tsp	olive oil	5 mL
1	clove garlic, minced	1
1 cup	Chicken Stock (see recipe, page 182) or reduced-sodium low-fat chicken broth	250 mL
2 tbsp	tomato paste	30 mL
⅛ tsp	salt (or to taste)	0.5 mL
	Freshly ground black pepper	

1. In casserole dish, toss tomatoes with onion, Italian seasoning and oil. Roast in preheated oven for 20 minutes or until tomatoes start to brown and the skin begins to shrivel. Let cool for 10 minutes.

2. Transfer tomato mixture to food processor and purée until smooth. Pour into a large pot and stir in garlic, stock and tomato paste. Bring to a simmer over medium heat; reduce heat and simmer for 5 minutes. Season with up to ⅛ tsp (0.5 mL) salt and pepper to taste.

Variations

For a vegetarian soup, use Vegetable Stock (see recipe, page 181) or reduced-sodium vegetable broth instead of chicken stock.

Stir in 3 tbsp (45 mL) reduced-fat (light) sour cream just before serving.

Hearty Minestrone

*This hodgepodge of
nutritious vegetables
requires very little
measuring. I love to make
this soup when I want to
clean out my fridge.*

Kitchen Tips

If you prefer a thinner soup,
add extra chicken stock.

One 19-oz (540 mL)
can of navy beans yields
about 2 cups (500 mL). If
you use 2 smaller cans or
1 larger can, measure 2 cups
(500 mL), then refrigerate
any extras in an airtight
container for up to 3 days or
freeze for up to 3 months.

Nutrients
PER SERVING

Calories	150
Fat	4.0 g
Sodium	362 mg
Carbohydrate	23.3 g
Fiber	5.5 g
Sugar	3.4 g
Protein	6.3 g
Calcium	58 mg
Iron	1.7 mg

2 tbsp	olive oil	30 mL
1	stalk celery, chopped	1
1	carrot, chopped	1
1	small onion, chopped	1
1	small red bell pepper, finely chopped	1
2 cups	Chicken Stock (see recipe, page 182) or reduced-sodium low-fat chicken broth	500 mL
1 cup	chopped Savoy cabbage	250 mL
2	cloves garlic, minced	2
2	plum (Roma) tomatoes, chopped	2
1	small potato, peeled and diced	1
1	small zucchini, peeled and chopped	1
1	bay leaf	1
2 cups	drained rinsed canned navy beans	500 mL
⅛ tsp	salt (or to taste)	0.5 mL
	Freshly ground black pepper	
	Chopped fresh parsley	

1. In a large pot, heat oil over medium heat. Sauté celery, carrot and onion for 6 minutes. Add red pepper and sauté for 2 minutes.

2. Stir in stock and bring to a boil. Stir in cabbage, garlic, tomatoes, potato, zucchini and bay leaf. Reduce heat to low, cover and simmer for 12 to 15 minutes or until potato is tender but not falling apart.

3. Add beans and simmer for about 2 minutes or until warmed through. Discard bay leaf. Season with up to ⅛ tsp (0.5 mL) salt and pepper to taste. Serve garnished with parsley.

Variation

For a vegetarian soup, use Vegetable Stock (see recipe, page 181) or reduced-sodium vegetable broth instead of chicken stock.

Lentil Soup

*This quick and easy soup
offers many nutritional
benefits, and thanks to the
soft texture of the vegetables
and lentils, it's a great
transition to solid foods.*

Weight-Loss Surgery Tips

Vary the cooking time
according to the texture
you want to achieve. For
example, cook the soup
longer for softer-textured
vegetables and lentils.

If you purée this soup, you
can eat it during diet stage 2.

1 tsp	olive oil	5 mL
3	stalks celery, chopped	3
2	carrots, chopped	2
2	cloves garlic, minced	2
1	onion, chopped	1
4 cups	Vegetable Stock (see recipe, page 181) or reduced-sodium vegetable broth	1 L
¾ cup	water	175 mL
¾ cup	dried brown lentils, rinsed	175 mL
¼ tsp	salt (or to taste)	1 mL
	Freshly ground black pepper	

1. In a large pot, heat oil over medium heat. Sauté celery, carrots, garlic and onion for 10 minutes.

2. Stir in stock and water; bring to a boil over medium-high heat. Stir in lentils and return to a boil. Reduce heat and simmer for about 30 minutes or until lentils and vegetables are tender. Season with up to ¼ tsp (1 mL) salt and pepper to taste.

Nutrients
PER SERVING

Calories	116
Fat	1.9 g
Sodium	169 mg
Carbohydrate	20.0 g
Fiber	4.6 g
Sugar	3.8 g
Protein	6.5 g
Calcium	43 mg
Iron	2.1 mg

Green Lentil Soup with Swiss Chard

This soup is full of garlic flavor — and full of fiber and iron from the green lentils and Swiss chard.

Kitchen Tips

Adjust the amount of garlic to your liking.

This soup freezes well. Store in individual portions in airtight containers in the freezer for up to 4 months. Be sure to leave some room for expansion.

Weight-Loss Surgery Tip

If you purée this soup, you can eat it during diet stage 2.

Nutrients
PER SERVING

Calories	70
Fat	1.0 g
Sodium	138 mg
Carbohydrate	12.6 g
Fiber	3 g
Sugar	1.7 g
Protein	3.9 g
Calcium	44 mg
Iron	1.7 mg

½ cup	dried green lentils, rinsed	125 mL
5¼ cups	water, divided	1.3 L
12 oz	Swiss chard, chopped	375 g
2 tbsp	freshly squeezed lemon juice	30 mL
1 tsp	olive oil	5 mL
1	large onion, finely chopped	1
4	cloves garlic, minced	4
1 tsp	dried mint	5 mL
1 tsp	ground cumin	5 mL
2 tbsp	all-purpose flour	30 mL
⅛ tsp	salt (or to taste)	0.5 mL
	Freshly ground black pepper	

1. In a large pot, combine lentils and 5 cups (1.25 L) of the water. Bring to a boil over medium heat. Reduce heat and simmer for 15 minutes. Stir in Swiss chard and lemon juice; simmer for 15 minutes.

2. Meanwhile, in a nonstick skillet, heat oil over medium-high heat. Sauté onion for 4 minutes or until golden brown. Add to soup, along with garlic, mint and cumin.

3. In a small bowl, whisk together flour and the remaining water until smooth. Add to soup and simmer, stirring often, for 5 minutes or until thickened. Season with up to ⅛ tsp (0.5 mL) salt and pepper to taste.

Variation

Use chopped spinach instead of Swiss chard.

Pearl Couscous Chickpea Soup

Pearl couscous, also known as Israeli or Middle Eastern couscous, is pearl-sized and made of semolina wheat. It cooks like pasta, and can be found in the rice aisle of most grocery stores or at a specialty market.

Kitchen Tips

This soup freezes well. Store in individual portions in airtight containers in the freezer for up to 3 months. Be sure to leave some room for expansion.

This recipe can easily be divided in half if you want to make a smaller batch.

Nutrients
PER SERVING

Calories	84
Fat	1.6 g
Sodium	283 mg
Carbohydrate	14.1 g
Fiber	3.1 g
Sugar	2.9 g
Protein	3.7 g
Calcium	44 mg
Iron	1.1 mg

1½ cups	water	375 mL
	Salt	
¼ cup	pearl couscous	60 mL
¼ cup	finely chopped onion	60 mL
¼ cup	diced celery	60 mL
¼ cup	diced carrot	60 mL
¼ cup	finely chopped red or yellow bell pepper	60 mL
3 cups	Vegetable Stock (see recipe, page 181) or reduced-sodium vegetable broth	750 mL
2 cups	drained rinsed canned chickpeas	500 mL
1 cup	chopped baby spinach	250 mL
¾ tsp	ground cumin	3 mL
⅛ tsp	ground cinnamon (optional)	0.5 mL
	Freshly ground black pepper	

1. In a small saucepan, bring water and ¼ tsp (1 mL) salt to a boil over high heat. Add couscous, reduce heat and simmer for 25 to 30 minutes or until tender. Drain and set aside.

2. Meanwhile, in a medium pot, combine onion, celery, carrot, red pepper and stock. Bring to a boil over high heat. Reduce heat and simmer for about 10 minutes or until vegetables are tender. Stir in reserved couscous, chickpeas, spinach, cumin and cinnamon (if using); simmer for 2 to 3 minutes or until spinach is wilted. Season with up to ⅛ tsp (0.5 mL) salt and pepper to taste.

Variation

Substitute any type of legumes, such as navy beans or black-eyed peas, for the chickpeas.

Low-Fat Cream of Chicken Soup

Makes 5 servings

Serving size: ¾ cup (175 mL)

Mid Diet Stage 3 to Diet Stage 4

This soup tastes creamy without a drop of cream added. It's a much healthier version of traditional or canned cream soups.

Weight-Loss Surgery Tip

If you purée this soup, you can eat it during diet stage 2.

1 tsp	olive oil	5 mL
½ cup	chopped onion	125 mL
½ cup	sliced carrots	125 mL
½ cup	sliced mushrooms	125 mL
¼ tsp	dried basil	1 mL
1 cup	cubed cooked chicken breast	250 mL
1 cup	Chicken Stock (see recipe, page 182) or reduced-sodium low-fat chicken broth	250 mL
1¾ cups	skim milk	425 mL
2 tbsp	cornstarch	30 mL
3 tbsp	cold water	45 mL
¼ tsp	salt (or to taste)	1 mL
	Freshly ground black pepper	

1. In a large saucepan, heat oil over medium heat. Sauté onion and carrots for 4 to 5 minutes or until tender. Add mushrooms and basil; sauté for 5 minutes. Stir in chicken, stock and milk; bring to a simmer (do not let boil).

2. In a small bowl, whisk cornstarch with cold water. Add to soup and cook, stirring, for 1 minute. Reduce heat and simmer for 5 minutes. Season with up to ¼ tsp (1 mL) salt and pepper to taste.

Variation

Add ½ cup (125 mL) thawed frozen peas with the chicken.

Nutrients
PER SERVING

Calories	93
Fat	2.0 g
Sodium	211 mg
Carbohydrate	11.6 g
Fiber	1.2 g
Sugar	6.2 g
Protein	7.7 g
Calcium	125 mg
Iron	0.3 mg

No-Noodle Chicken Soup

This twist on traditional chicken soup omits the noodles and scoops some seasoned mashed potatoes on top.

Kitchen Tip

Use leftover grilled or baked chicken to make this quick and easy soup. If you don't have any cooked chicken handy, simply poach a 6-oz (175 g) boneless skinless chicken breast in water until no longer pink inside. Drain off the water, shred the meat and add it to the soup.

Weight-Loss Surgery Tip

If you purée this soup, you can eat it during diet stage 2.

Nutrients
PER SERVING

Calories	99
Fat	2.9 g
Sodium	266 mg
Carbohydrate	9.2 g
Fiber	2.1 g
Sugar	2.2 g
Protein	9.8 g
Calcium	30 mg
Iron	0.5 mg

1 tsp	olive oil	5 mL
1	carrot, sliced	1
1	stalk celery, finely diced	1
1	onion, finely chopped	1
1	clove garlic, minced	1
2½ cups	Chicken Stock (see recipe, page 182) or reduced-sodium low-fat chicken broth	625 mL
1	green onion, thinly sliced	1
1 cup	shredded cooked chicken breast	250 mL
1 tsp	dried parsley	5 mL
½ tsp	dried thyme	2 mL
¼ tsp	salt (or to taste)	1 mL
	Freshly ground black pepper (optional)	
½ cup	leftover mashed potatoes	125 mL
1	fresh chive, finely chopped (optional)	1

1. In a medium saucepan, heat oil over medium heat. Sauté carrot, celery and onion for 10 minutes or until onion is lightly browned.

2. Stir in garlic and stock; bring to a boil. Add green onion, chicken, parsley and thyme; reduce heat and simmer for 10 minutes or until soup is flavorful. Season with up to ¼ tsp (1 mL) salt and pepper to taste (if using)

3. Pour into individual bowls and spoon mashed potatoes on top, dividing equally. Garnish potatoes with chives (if using).

Variation

Instead of chicken, use chopped extra-firm tofu or cooked beef, pork or turkey — any type of protein, really.

Classic Canadian Ham and Pea Soup

This low-fat soup is a great way to use leftover ham, and it's quite inexpensive to make.

Kitchen Tips

This soup is quite thick. For a thinner consistency, stir in some Vegetable Stock (see recipe, page 181) or reduced-sodium vegetable broth.

Store this soup in airtight containers in the freezer for up to 3 months. Be sure to leave some room for expansion.

- **Food processor, blender or immersion blender**

I	small onion, chopped	I
I cup	dried green split peas, rinsed	250 mL
1/2 cup	chopped carrots	125 mL
1/2 cup	chopped celery	125 mL
1/2 tsp	dried savory	2 mL
1/4 tsp	ground cloves	Pinch
3 cups	water	750 mL
1/2 tsp	liquid smoke	2 mL
I	bay leaf	I
3/4 cup	diced cooked ham	175 mL
1/8 tsp	salt (or to taste)	0.5 mL
	Freshly ground black pepper	

1. In a large pot, combine onion, peas, carrots, celery, savory, cloves, water and liquid smoke. Bring to a boil over medium-high heat. Reduce heat and simmer for about 20 minutes or until vegetables are soft. Remove from heat and let cool for 10 minutes. Discard bay leaf.

2. Working in batches, transfer soup to food processor (or use immersion blender in pot) and purée until smooth. Return soup to pot (if necessary) and stir in ham. Season with up to 1/8 tsp (0.5 mL) salt and pepper to taste. Bring to a simmer over medium-low heat and simmer for 2 to 4 minutes or until ham is warmed through.

Nutrients
PER SERVING

Calories	117
Fat	1.0 g
Sodium	165 mg
Carbohydrate	17.9 g
Fiber	0.5 g
Sugar	1.7 g
Protein	9.4 g
Calcium	13 mg
Iron	1.1 mg

New England Clam Chowder

Clams provide protein, iron and zinc, making this simple chowder a healthy option for the whole family. It tastes even better the next day!

Kitchen Tips

While any variety of potato will work in this recipe, Yukon golds are preferred, as they provide a moist and succulent texture.

This soup can be frozen in airtight containers for up to 4 months. Be sure to leave some room for expansion.

1 tsp	canola oil	5 mL
½ cup	chopped onion	125 mL
½ cup	chopped celery	125 mL
2	cans (each 3 oz/85 g) chopped clams, with liquid	2
1	clove garlic, minced	1
1	small potato, peeled and diced	1
2	sprigs fresh thyme	2
1	bay leaf	1
1	bottle (8 oz/236 mL) clam juice	1
2 tbsp	all-purpose flour	30 mL
¾ cup	skim milk	175 mL
	Freshly ground black pepper	

1. In a large pot, heat oil over medium-high heat. Sauté onion and celery for 2 minutes.

2. Drain liquid from clams through a fine-mesh sieve into a small bowl. Set clams aside.

3. Add clam liquid, garlic, potato, thyme, bay leaf, and clam juice to the onion mixture; bring to a boil. Reduce heat and simmer for about 15 minutes or until potato is tender. Discard thyme and bay leaf.

4. In a small bowl, whisk together flour and milk until smooth. Add to soup and simmer, stirring frequently, for about 5 minutes or until thickened. Add clams and simmer for 2 minutes or until clams are warmed through. Season to taste with pepper.

Nutrients
PER SERVING

Calories	150
Fat	2.7 g
Sodium	471 mg
Carbohydrate	22.5 g
Fiber	1.5 g
Sugar	5.7 g
Protein	10.0 g
Calcium	130 mg
Iron	11.3 mg

Salads

Some salads may initially be difficult to tolerate after weight-loss surgery, but in the long term most patients can comfortably digest a variety of healthy salads. Salads make an easy and quick lunch or supper choice, or a terrific accompaniment to a well-balanced meal.

Adding Protein to Salads

Here are some easy ways to add more protein to salads, to help you get the nutrition you need.

Light Cheese

Shredded, grated or sliced, a little bit of cheese adds protein and a lot of flavor to your salad. Try Cheddar, goat cheese, Parmesan or Havarti — just be sure to choose low-fat or light versions.

Hard-Cooked or Poached Eggs

Slice or chop a hard-cooked egg into your favorite salad. Or lay a chilled poached egg on top of a bed of salad greens.

Chicken, Turkey, Pork or Beef

Toss in some leftover chopped or shredded cooked meat, such as chicken, turkey, pork or beef. Sliced low-fat deli meat works well. Or throw in some canned flaked chicken. If you tolerate red meat, thinly sliced beef tastes great in Asian-style salads.

Seafood or Fish

Add leftover cooked shrimp, precooked cocktail shrimp, canned tuna (flavored or plain) or salmon or any type of cooked fish.

Tofu

Grilled firm or extra-firm tofu works wonders in a salad, taking on some of the flavor of the dressing.

Legumes

A handful of canned or cooked dried beans, lentils or other legumes goes a long way. Drain and rinse canned beans and store them in an airtight container in the refrigerator for up to 3 days. For a quick meal, toss the beans into the salad of your choice.

Nuts and Seeds

If you can tolerate the texture of nuts and seeds, add some to your salad for extra crunch and protein. Remember, though, that they also add fat, and be careful to not use too much.

Yogurt

Make your dressing using regular or Greek-style low-fat plain yogurt.

Unflavored Protein Powder

Mix some unflavored protein powder into your favorite low-fat and/or low-calorie dressing.

Classic Coleslaw

Nutrients
PER SERVING

Calories	48
Fat	2.9 g
Sodium	155 mg
Carbohydrate	5.4 g
Fiber	1.1 g
Sugar	2.5 g
Protein	0.8 g
Calcium	27 mg
Iron	0.2 mg

¼ cup	low-fat mayonnaise	60 mL
2 tbsp	reduced-fat (light) sour cream	30 mL
2 tsp	cider vinegar	10 mL
½ tsp	Dijon mustard	2 mL
	Artificial sweetener equivalent to ½ tsp (2 mL) granulated sugar	
2 cups	shredded cabbage	500 mL
¼ cup	grated carrot	60 mL

1. In a large bowl, whisk together mayonnaise, sour cream, vinegar, mustard and sweetener. Add cabbage and carrots; toss to coat. Refrigerate for at least 1 hour, until chilled, or overnight.

Egg Salad

Nutrients
PER SERVING

Calories	78
Fat	5.1 g
Sodium	264 mg
Carbohydrate	2.7 g
Fiber	0.8 g
Sugar	0.8 g
Protein	5.9 g
Calcium	38 mg
Iron	1.0 mg

2 tsp	low-fat mayonnaise	10 mL
½ tsp	Dijon mustard	2 mL
⅛ tsp	paprika	0.5 mL
2	hard-cooked eggs, peeled and chopped (see recipe, page 165)	2
1	stalk celery, diced	1
1	green onion, sliced	1
⅛ tsp	salt (or to taste)	0.5 mL
	Freshly ground black pepper	

1. In a small bowl, combine mayonnaise, mustard and paprika. Stir in eggs, celery and green onion. Season with up to ⅛ tsp (0.5 mL) salt and pepper to taste. Serve immediately.

Fattouch Salad

Diet Stage 4

This Lebanese-style salad is made with a variety of fresh vegetables and crispy pita bread.

Kitchen Tip

Sumac is a dark purple spice that provides a tangy, lemony flavor. It is commonly used in Greek, Sicilian and Middle Eastern dishes. Look for ground sumac in the spice aisle of your grocery store or at a Middle Eastern market. There is no good substitute for the unique flavor sumac provides; if you really must substitute, use paprika for color and add a little extra lemon juice for tang.

Nutrients
PER SERVING

Calories	101
Fat	7.4 g
Sodium	330 mg
Carbohydrate	7.8 g
Fiber	2.0 g
Sugar	2.5 g
Protein	1.5 g
Calcium	31 mg
Iron	0.9 mg

- Preheat broiler
- Rimmed baking sheet

Crispy Pita Bread

1	9-inch (23 cm) whole wheat pita, cut into bite-size pieces	1
1 tbsp	olive oil	15 mL

Dressing

1	clove garlic, minced	1
1/4 cup	finely chopped onion	60 mL
1 tsp	salt	5 mL
1/2 tsp	freshly ground black pepper	2 mL
1/4 tsp	ground sumac	1 mL
1/4 cup	freshly squeezed lemon juice	60 mL
3 tbsp	olive oil	45 mL

Salad

12	radishes, sliced (about 1 cup/250 mL)	12
2	green onions, sliced	2
1	head romaine lettuce, (about 6 cups/1.5 L) chopped	1
1	small green bell pepper, chopped	1
1	tomato, chopped	1
1	small cucumber, peeled, seeded and chopped	1
1	stalk celery, chopped	1
1/2 cup	chopped fresh parsley	125 mL

1. *Pita Bread:* Place pita pieces on baking sheet and drizzle with oil. Broil for about 2 minutes, turning halfway through, until crisp and light golden brown on both sides. Let cool to room temperature.

2. *Dressing:* In a small bowl, whisk together garlic, onion, salt, pepper, sumac, lemon juice and oil.

3. *Salad:* In a large bowl, combine radishes, green onions, romaine, green pepper, tomato, celery and parsley. Add pita pieces. Pour dressing over salad and toss gently to coat. Serve immediately.

Lemon Poppy Seed Salad

Makes 7 servings

Diet Stage 4

Without a doubt, this salad is alluring. The dressing also makes a great dip for vegetables such as cucumbers, snow peas, baby carrots and celery sticks.

Weight-Loss Surgery Tip

Top with grilled chicken breast or broiled salmon to make this salad a complete meal.

Dressing

1 tsp	minced onion	5 mL
1 tsp	poppy seeds	5 mL
1 tsp	granulated sucralose artificial sweetener, such as Splenda	5 mL
1/4 tsp	salt	1 mL
2 tbsp	low-fat plain yogurt	30 mL
1 tbsp	freshly squeezed lemon juice	15 mL
1 tsp	canola oil	5 mL

Salad

3 cups	torn heart of romaine lettuce (about 1 heart)	750 mL
1/4 cup	blueberries	60 mL
2 tbsp	whole wheat croutons	30 mL
2 tbsp	chopped almonds	30 mL

1. *Dressing:* In a small bowl, whisk together onion, poppy seeds, sweetener, salt, yogurt, lemon juice and oil.

2. *Salad:* In a large bowl, combine romaine, blueberries, croutons and almonds. Drizzle dressing over salad and toss to coat. Serve immediately.

Nutrients
PER SERVING

Calories	35
Fat	2.3 g
Sodium	75 mg
Carbohydrate	3.0 g
Fiber	0.7 g
Sugar	1.4 g
Protein	1.2 g
Calcium	29 mg
Iron	0.4 mg

Spring Greens Chicken and Avocado Salad

Makes 4 servings

Diet Stage 4

Chicken adds protein and iron to this delicious salad. The creamy avocado contributes healthy fat, and the strawberries provide vitamin C to boost the absorption of iron.

Dressing

2 tsp	balsamic vinegar	10 mL
2 tsp	olive oil	10 mL
½ tsp	Dijon mustard	2 mL
½ tsp	no-added-sugar strawberry jam	2 mL
1 tbsp	finely chopped red onion	15 mL
¼ tsp	salt	1 mL
	Freshly ground black pepper	

Salad

½	avocado, chopped	½
1 cup	chopped grilled chicken breast	250 mL
2 cups	mixed spring greens	500 mL
½ cup	quartered strawberries	125 mL

1. *Dressing:* In a small bowl, whisk together vinegar, oil, mustard and jam. Whisk in onion, salt and pepper to taste.

2. *Salad:* In a large bowl, combine avocado, chicken, spring greens and strawberries. Pour dressing over salad and toss to coat. Serve immediately.

Variations

For a vegetarian version, use grilled tofu in place of chicken.

Replace the strawberries with any type of berry you have on hand, such as blueberries, blackberries or raspberries.

Nutrients
PER SERVING

Calories	130
Fat	8.0 g
Sodium	203 mg
Carbohydrate	6.0 g
Fiber	3.1 g
Sugar	1.9 g
Protein	9.9 g
Calcium	23 mg
Iron	0.6 mg

Chicken Caesar Salad

Makes 5 servings

Diet Stage 4

Who says you have to give up eating Caesar salad? This recipe is low in fat and high in protein, and is perfect for a light, nutritious lunch.

- **Preheat broiler**
- **Rimmed baking sheet**

Chicken

¼ tsp	ground cumin	I mL
¼ tsp	garlic powder	I mL
I tsp	Worcestershire sauce	5 mL
6 oz	boneless skinless chicken breast, cut into 1-inch (2.5 cm) wide strips	175 g

Caesar Dressing

I	anchovy fillet, rinsed and patted dry, mashed with a fork	I
½ tsp	garlic powder	2 mL
I tsp	freshly squeezed lemon juice	5 mL
¾ tsp	olive oil	3 mL
½ tsp	Dijon mustard	2 mL
I tbsp	grated light Parmesan cheese	15 mL
2 tbsp	low-fat plain yogurt	30 mL
⅛ tsp	salt (or to taste)	0.5 mL
	Freshly ground black pepper	

Salad

3 cups	torn heart of romaine lettuce (about I heart)	750 mL
¼ cup	whole wheat croutons	60 mL

1. *Chicken:* In a medium bowl, combine cumin, garlic powder and Worcestershire sauce. Add chicken and toss to coat. Spread out on baking sheet and broil for 5 minutes per side or until chicken is no longer pink inside. Let cool slightly.

2. *Dressing:* In a small bowl, quickly whisk together anchovy, garlic powder, lemon juice, oil and mustard to form a paste. Whisk in Parmesan and yogurt. Season with up to ⅛ tsp (0.5 mL) salt and pepper to taste.

3. *Salad:* In a large bowl, combine chicken, lettuce and croutons. Pour dressing over salad and toss to coat. Serve immediately.

Nutrients
PER SERVING

Calories	83
Fat	3.0 g
Sodium	170 mg
Carbohydrate	3.8 g
Fiber	0.9 g
Sugar	1.2 g
Protein	10.3 g
Calcium	41 mg
Iron	0.5 mg

Tuna Apple Salad

Serve a portion of this tuna salad wrapped in a leaf of Boston lettuce. Or use it as a filling for a whole wheat tortilla wrap or to make a mini pita sandwich.

Weight-Loss Surgery Tip

If you want to try eating tuna salad early in diet stage 3, omit the celery and apple.

2 tbsp	low-fat plain yogurt	30 mL
2 tsp	low-fat mayonnaise	10 mL
1 tsp	freshly squeezed lemon juice	5 mL
1	can (6 oz/170 g) water-packed flaked tuna, drained	1
½	small apple, peeled, cored and grated	½
2 tbsp	diced celery	30 mL
1 tsp	chopped fresh tarragon	5 mL
⅛ tsp	salt (or to taste)	0.5 mL
	Freshly ground black pepper	

1. In a small bowl, combine yogurt, mayonnaise and lemon juice. Stir in tuna, apple, celery and tarragon. Season with up to ⅛ tsp (0.5 mL) salt and pepper to taste. Serve immediately.

Variations

Substitute ¼ cup (60 mL) chopped green onion or grated carrots for the apple.

Replace the tuna with canned flaked chicken or ¾ cup (175 mL) diced cooked chicken.

Substitute ¼ cup (60 mL) chopped onion for the apple and 1 can (6½ oz/185 g) salmon, drained, for the tuna.

Nutrients
PER SERVING

Calories	138
Fat	1.7 g
Sodium	464 mg
Carbohydrate	6.9 g
Fiber	0.9 g
Sugar	4.8 g
Protein	22.8 g
Calcium	49 mg
Iron	1.5 mg

Asian Crab Salad

Makes 2 servings

Late Diet Stage 3 to Diet Stage 4

The combined flavors of crab, soy sauce and rice vinegar give this salad Asian flare. Enjoy it on its own or serve it on top of thin rice crackers.

Kitchen Tips

To julienne the red pepper, slice it into very thin strips that resemble matchsticks.

For a cheaper alternative to crabmeat, use ¾ cup (175 mL) shredded imitation crab.

This recipe is delicious served over rice, if you're able to tolerate it.

If you tolerate sesame seeds, sprinkle some in just before serving.

1	small cucumber, peeled, seeded and grated	1
¼	red bell pepper, halved and julienned (see tip, at left)	¼
½ tsp	salt	2 mL
1	can (6 oz/170 g) white crabmeat, drained	1
1 tsp	granulated sucralose artificial sweetener, such as Splenda	5 mL
1½ tsp	rice vinegar	7 mL
1 tsp	reduced-sodium soy sauce	5 mL

1. In a medium bowl, combine cucumber and red pepper. Sprinkle with salt and let stand for 15 minutes. Transfer to a fine-mesh sieve and rinse under cold running water; drain. Return to bowl and stir in crabmeat.

2. In a small bowl, whisk together sweetener, vinegar and soy sauce. Pour over salad and stir with a fork until combined. Serve immediately.

Nutrients
PER SERVING

Calories	96
Fat	1.2 g
Sodium	692 mg
Carbohydrate	3.0 g
Fiber	0.8 g
Sugar	1.6 g
Protein	18.7 g
Calcium	72 mg
Iron	0.6 mg

Italian Salad Dressing

*Better than store-bought
dressing, this vinaigrette
tastes great drizzled over
any of your favorite salads.
For a simple, classic
Italian salad, enjoy it over
mixed greens and sliced
cucumber, tomato and
onion. Add grilled calamari
or light bocconcini cheese
for protein.*

Kitchen Tip

Store extra dressing in
an airtight container in
the refrigerator for up to
1 week. Let it come to room
temperature before use.

¼ tsp	dried oregano	1 mL
¼ tsp	dried basil	1 mL
¼ tsp	onion powder	1 mL
¼ tsp	garlic powder	1 mL
3 tbsp	olive oil	45 mL
1½ tbsp	red wine vinegar	22 mL
1 tsp	freshly squeezed lemon juice	5 mL
⅛ tsp	salt (or to taste)	0.5 mL
	Freshly ground black pepper	

1. In a small bowl, whisk together oregano, basil, onion powder, garlic powder, oil, vinegar and lemon juice. Season with up to ⅛ tsp (0.5 mL) salt and pepper to taste.

Nutrients
PER SERVING

Calories	77
Fat	8.4 g
Sodium	47 mg
Carbohydrate	0.3 g
Fiber	0.1 g
Sugar	0.1 g
Protein	0 g
Calcium	3 mg
Iron	0.1 mg

Simple Balsamic Vinaigrette

This dressing is effortless to prepare, but adds tons of flavor to any salad. It also makes a great marinade for chicken.

Kitchen Tip

You can double this recipe and store any extra in an airtight container in the refrigerator for up to 1 week. Let it to come to room temperature before use.

2 tsp	balsamic vinegar	10 mL
1 tsp	Dijon mustard	5 mL
3 tbsp	olive oil	45 mL
⅛ tsp	salt (or to taste)	0.5 mL
	Freshly ground black pepper	

1. In a small bowl, whisk together vinegar and mustard. Slowly whisk in oil. Season with up to ⅛ tsp (0.5 mL) salt and pepper to taste.

Nutrients
PER SERVING

Calories	97
Fat	10.5 g
Sodium	76 mg
Carbohydrate	0.5 g
Fiber	0 g
Sugar	0.4 g
Protein	0 g
Calcium	1 mg
Iron	0 mg

Herbes de Provence Salad Dressing

This savory dressing takes full advantage of herbes de Provence, a wonderful blend of dried herbs that includes basil, fennel, lavender, marjoram, rosemary, sage, savory and thyme.

Kitchen Tip

You can double this recipe and store any extra in an airtight container in the refrigerator for up to 1 week. Let it to come to room temperature before use.

2 tsp	red wine vinegar	10 mL
½ tsp	Dijon mustard	2 mL
3 tbsp	olive oil	45 mL
1 tsp	herbes de Provence	5 mL
⅛ tsp	salt (or to taste)	0.5 mL
	Freshly ground black pepper	

1. In a small bowl, whisk together vinegar and mustard. Slowly whisk in oil. Season with herbes de Provence, up to ⅛ tsp (0.5 mL) salt and pepper to taste.

Nutrients
PER SERVING

Calories	96
Fat	10.6 g
Sodium	66 mg
Carbohydrate	0.2 g
Fiber	0.1 g
Sugar	0 g
Protein	0 g
Calcium	4 mg
Iron	0.1 mg

Raspberry Yogurt Salad Dressing

The yogurt gives this dressing a creamy texture, while the raspberry jam provides sweetness, making it a delicious option for a summertime salad.

Kitchen Tip

You can double this recipe and store any extra in an airtight container in the refrigerator for up to 1 week. Let it to come to room temperature before use.

1 tbsp	no-sugar-added raspberry jam	15 mL
1 tbsp	low-fat plain yogurt	15 mL
1 tbsp	cider vinegar	15 mL
2 tsp	olive oil	10 mL
⅛ tsp	salt (or to taste)	0.5 mL
	Freshly ground black pepper	

1. In a small bowl, whisk together raspberry jam, yogurt, vinegar and oil. Season with up to ⅛ tsp (0.5 mL) salt and pepper to taste.

Nutrients
PER SERVING

Calories	27
Fat	2.4 g
Sodium	62 mg
Carbohydrate	1.6 g
Fiber	0 g
Sugar	0.3 g
Protein	0.2 g
Calcium	7 mg
Iron	0 mg

Meat and Poultry

Handling Raw Meat and Poultry

- Wash your hands thoroughly with warm water and soap before and after handling raw meat and poultry.
- Disinfect and clean surface areas, utensils and cutting boards thoroughly.
- Keep raw meat and poultry separate from other ingredients to avoid cross-contamination.
- Keep raw meat and poultry sealed in the refrigerator until you're ready to cook them.
- Thaw frozen meat and poultry in the refrigerator or defrost it in the microwave. Do not thaw meat or poultry at room temperature.

Cooking Meat and Poultry

- Ensure that all meat and poultry is cooked thoroughly according to safe internal temperature guidelines.

- Always use a clean meat thermometer to check the internal temperature. Insert the thermometer directly into the thickest part of the meat.

Storing Meat and Poultry

- Raw meat and poultry can be stored in airtight packaging in the refrigerator for up to 2 days or in the freezer for up to 3 months.
- Leftover cooked meat and poultry can be stored in an airtight container in the refrigerator for up to 3 days or in the freezer for up to 3 months.

For more detailed food safety guidelines, including temperature charts, visit FoodSafety.gov at www.foodsafety.gov or the Canadian Partnership for Consumer Food Safety Education at www.canfightbac.org.

Beef Stew with Leeks

This stew is warm, hearty and full of flavor. Serve it with Herbed Mashed Potatoes (page 295).

Kitchen Tip

Although this stew tastes great as is, experiment by adding more seasoning, such as dried oregano, thyme, basil, sage and/or rosemary, with the tomato.

Weight-Loss Surgery Tip

Beef is usually not well tolerated after surgery; however, stewing tenderizes the meat, and the sauce keeps it moist. Try a little when you feel ready. The first time you try beef, cut the tender meat into pea-size pieces and be sure to chew each bite very well.

Nutrients PER SERVING	
Calories	266
Fat	12.0 g
Sodium	190 mg
Carbohydrate	11.5 g
Fiber	2.2 g
Sugar	4.4 g
Protein	28.0 g
Calcium	43 mg
Iron	4.4 mg

1 tbsp	canola oil	15 mL
1 lb	stewing beef, cut into chunks	500 g
2	leeks (white and light green parts only), chopped	2
1	large onion, thinly sliced	1
¼ tsp	salt (or to taste), divided	1 mL
1	tomato, diced	1
1	can (5½ oz/156 mL) tomato paste	1
3 cups	water	750 mL
	Freshly ground black pepper	

1. In a large pot, heat oil over medium-high heat. Cook beef, stirring, for about 5 minutes or until browned on all sides. Stir in leeks and onion; cook, stirring, for 2 minutes, scraping up any brown bits from bottom of pan.

2. Stir in ⅛ tsp (0.5 mL) of the salt, tomato, tomato paste and water; reduce heat and simmer, stirring occasionally for 1½ hours or until beef is fork-tender. Season with up to ⅛ tsp (0.5 mL) salt and pepper to taste.

Variations

Substitute stewing veal for the beef.

Eggplant with Ground Beef

Mid Diet Stage 3 to
Diet Stage 4

This recipe, which is similar to lasagna, uses eggplant as the "noodles" and meat sauce as a high-protein, hearty filling.

Kitchen Tip

This recipe freezes well. Let the baked dish cool, then transfer individual portions to airtight containers and freeze for up to 3 months.

- **Preheat oven to 350°F (180°C)**
- **13- by 9-inch (33 by 23 cm) glass baking dish, lightly sprayed with light nonstick cooking spray**

2	large eggplants	2
1 tbsp	salt	15 mL
1 lb	extra-lean ground beef	500 g
1	onion, finely chopped	1
1 cup	Tomato Basil Sauce (see recipe, page 272) or store-bought tomato pasta sauce	250 mL
½ cup	finely chopped tomatoes	125 mL
1 tsp	ground cinnamon	5 mL
	Freshly ground black pepper	

1. Cut off stems and cut eggplants lengthwise into ¼-inch (0.5 cm) thick slices. Sprinkle each slice with salt and place in a large bowl. Let stand for 1 hour. Dry eggplant with a paper towel.

2. In a large nonstick skillet, cook beef over medium-high heat, breaking it up with the back of a wooden spoon, for about 8 minutes or until no longer pink. Add onion, tomato sauce, tomatoes, cinnamon and pepper to taste; reduce heat and simmer, stirring often, for 10 minutes.

3. Arrange one-third of the eggplant slices in prepared baking dish, trimming eggplant to fit as necessary. Spread half the meat sauce over top. Repeat layers. Arrange the remaining eggplant on top.

4. Cover and bake in preheated oven for 30 minutes or until eggplant is tender and sauce is bubbling. Uncover and broil for 2 minutes or until lightly browned.

Variation

Sprinkle ½ cup (125 mL) shredded part-skim mozzarella cheese over the top layer just before broiling.

Nutrients
PER SERVING

Calories	117
Fat	2.7 g
Sodium	968 mg
Carbohydrate	12.0 g
Fiber	5.7 g
Sugar	4.4 g
Protein	13.1 g
Calcium	30 mg
Iron	1.6 mg

Shepherd's Pie

Makes 8 servings

Late Diet Stage 3 to
Diet Stage 4

*Traditionally, shepherd's
pie is made from lamb, but
this recipe uses extra-lean
ground beef to help reduce
the fat content. When beef
is used, some call this all-in-
one dish cottage pie.*

Kitchen Tips

Use leftover mashed
potatoes as the top layer
to cut down on preparation
time.

You can also mix the thawed
frozen mixed vegetables
right into the meat layer
instead of having them as a
separate layer.

Leftover shepherd's pie
can be stored in an airtight
container in the refrigerator
for up to 3 days.

Nutrients
PER SERVING

Calories	142
Fat	5.6 g
Sodium	255 mg
Carbohydrate	10.0 g
Fiber	1.6 g
Sugar	2.3 g
Protein	12.5 g
Calcium	32 mg
Iron	1.4 mg

- **Preheat oven to 400°F (200°C)**
- **8-inch (20 cm) square glass baking dish,
  lightly sprayed with light cooking spray**

Top Layer

1 cup	chopped peeled potato	250 mL
1 cup	chopped butternut squash	250 mL
1/4 cup	skim milk	60 mL
1 tbsp	margarine	15 mL
1/4 tsp	salt (or to taste)	1 mL
	Freshly ground black pepper (optional)	
1 tbsp	dry whole wheat bread crumbs	15 mL

Bottom Layer

1 tbsp	olive oil	15 mL
1	green onion, finely chopped	1
1/3 cup	finely chopped carrots	75 mL
1/3 cup	finely chopped celery	75 mL
1/3 cup	chopped green bell pepper	75 mL
1	chicken bouillon cube	1
1 lb	extra-lean ground beef	500 g
1	small tomato, finely chopped	1
1 tsp	cornstarch	5 mL
1/4 tsp	ground paprika	1 mL
	Freshly ground black pepper	
1 tsp	reduced-sodium soy sauce	5 mL

Middle Layer

2 cups	thawed frozen mixed vegetables	500 mL

1. *Top Layer:* In a large pot, combine potato and squash.
Add enough water to cover. Bring to a boil over high
heat. Reduce heat and simmer for about 20 minutes
or until tender.

Kitchen Tips

Prepare this recipe through step 4 the night before. Cover and refrigerate. When you are ready to make dinner the next day, proceed with step 5, increasing the baking time by about 15 minutes.

You can also make individual mini shepherd's pies in small ramekins. Place the ramekins on a baking sheet and bake for 20 minutes or until bubbling.

Weight-Loss Surgery Tip

This recipe provides an option that is moist and easy to tolerate if you are having difficulty eating meat.

2. *Bottom Layer:* Meanwhile, in a large nonstick skillet, heat oil over medium heat. Sauté green onion, carrots, celery and green pepper for 2 minutes. Stir in bouillon cube and sauté for about 2 minutes or until vegetables are softened. Add beef and cook, breaking it up with the back of a wooden spoon, for about 8 minutes or until no longer pink. Add tomato, cornstarch, paprika, pepper to taste and soy sauce; cook, stirring, for 3 minutes. Spread mixture evenly in bottom of prepared baking pan.

3. *Middle Layer:* Top meat layer with mixed vegetables. Set aside.

4. Drain and mash potato and squash. Stir in milk and margarine. If desired, season with up to $1/4$ tsp (1 mL) salt and pepper to taste. Spread over middle layer and sprinkle with bread crumbs.

5. Bake in preheated oven for 30 minutes or until bubbling. If desired, broil for the last few minutes to brown the top layer.

Variations

Use plain mashed potato, mashed squash or cornmeal porridge for the top layer.

Substitute any type of extra-lean ground meat, such as chicken or turkey. You can also use lean ground lamb or a mixture of lamb and beef.

Armenian-Style Hamburgers

These hamburgers are an old favorite in my family and are sure to become one in yours, too. Serve with steamed rice or vegetables.

Kitchen Tip

These burgers are also excellent on the barbecue. Prepare patties, cover and refrigerate for 1 to 2 hours to help them set. Spray the grill with light nonstick cooking spray and preheat to medium-high. Grill, turning once, for 4 to 5 minutes per side or until no longer pink inside.

Weight-Loss Surgery Tip

This recipe provides a choice that is moist enough to introduce during diet stage 3.

Nutrients
PER SERVING

Calories	122
Fat	3.1 g
Sodium	112 mg
Carbohydrate	7.7 g
Fiber	1.2 g
Sugar	1.9 g
Protein	15.9 g
Calcium	11 mg
Iron	1.6 mg

- **Preheat broiler**
- **Large, heavy baking sheet, lined with foil**

1 lb	extra-lean ground beef	500 g
1	large onion, finely chopped	1
1/4 cup	finely ground bulgur (bulgur #1)	60 mL
3 tbsp	finely chopped green bell pepper	45 mL
2 tbsp	finely chopped fresh parsley	30 mL
3/4 cup	reduced-sodium tomato juice	175 mL
1/8 tsp	salt	0.5 mL

1. In a large bowl, combine beef, onion, bulgur, green pepper, parsley, tomato juice and salt. Knead with your hands until well combined. Let stand for 10 minutes.

2. Using about 1/4 cup (60 mL) per patty, shape beef mixture into 18 mini patties, about 3/4 inch (2 cm) thick. Place in a single layer on prepared baking sheet.

3. Broil for 5 to 6 minutes, turning once, until no longer pink inside.

Variations

Replace 4 oz (125 g) of the ground beef with lean ground lamb.

Substitute dry whole wheat bread crumbs for the bulgur.

Italian-Style Meatloaf

Mmm ... mozzarella, tomato sauce and rosemary give this amazing meatloaf Italian flare.

Kitchen Tips

Freezing mozzarella for about 30 minutes makes it easier to shred. Shred extra and store it in an airtight container in the refrigerator for up to 3 weeks.

Prepare this recipe through step 1 the night before. Cover and refrigerate. When you are ready to make dinner the next day, proceed with step 2 and increase the baking time by about 15 minutes.

You can also use this meat mixture to make meatballs or mini burgers.

Nutrients
PER SERVING

Calories	110
Fat	3.1 g
Sodium	175 mg
Carbohydrate	6.8 g
Fiber	1.2 g
Sugar	0.2 g
Protein	13.4 g
Calcium	56 mg
Iron	1.7 mg

- **Preheat oven to 350°F (180°C)**
- **9- by 5-inch (23 by 13 cm) glass loaf dish, sprayed with light cooking spray**

1 lb	extra-lean ground beef	500 g
1/4 cup	shredded part-skim mozzarella cheese	60 mL
1/4 cup	dry whole wheat bread crumbs	60 mL
2 tbsp	Italian herb seasoning	30 mL
1 tbsp	dried rosemary	15 mL
	Freshly ground black pepper (optional)	
1	egg	1
1/3 cup	Tomato Basil Sauce (see recipe, page 272) or store-bought tomato pasta sauce	75 mL

1. In a large bowl, combine beef, mozzarella, bread crumbs, Italian seasoning, rosemary, pepper to taste (if using), egg and tomato sauce. Knead with your hands until well combined.

2. Spoon into prepared loaf pan, patting down to form an even loaf. Bake in preheated oven for 1 to $1\frac{1}{2}$ hours or until a meat thermometer inserted in the center of the meatloaf registers 160°F (71°C). Broil for 2 to 3 minutes or until top is browned.

Variation

Substitute any type of extra-lean ground meat, such as chicken or turkey.

Vegetable Meatloaf

Makes 8 servings

Diet Stages 3 to 4

The grated vegetables in this meatloaf are a healthy way to add moisture to the meat while also adding nutrition and fiber.

Kitchen Tips

Instead of grating the vegetables, you can finely chop them, if you wish.

Prepare this recipe through step 1 the night before. Cover and refrigerate. When you are ready to make dinner the next day, proceed with step 2 and increase the baking time by about 15 minutes.

If necessary, drain off any excess liquid before broiling.

Weight-Loss Surgery Tip

This is an excellent recipe to try during diet stage 3, when you're introducing solids.

Nutrients
PER SERVING

Calories	96
Fat	3.0 g
Sodium	164 mg
Carbohydrate	4.6 g
Fiber	1.0 g
Sugar	0.8 g
Protein	12.6 g
Calcium	36 mg
Iron	1.6 mg

- **Preheat oven to 350°F (180°C)**
- **9- by 5-inch (23 by 13 cm) glass loaf dish, sprayed with light cooking spray**

1 lb	extra-lean ground beef	500 g
1/3 cup	grated zucchini, with skin	75 mL
1/3 cup	grated peeled carrots	75 mL
1/4 cup	dry whole wheat bread crumbs	60 mL
1 tbsp	dried oregano	15 mL
1 tsp	garlic powder	5 mL
1/4 tsp	salt	1 mL
1/8 tsp	freshly ground black pepper	0.5 mL
1	egg	1
1/4 cup	skim milk	60 mL

1. In a large bowl, combine beef, zucchini, carrots, bread crumbs, oregano, garlic powder, salt, pepper, egg and milk. Knead with your hands until well combined.

2. Spoon into prepared loaf pan, patting down to form an even loaf. Bake in preheated oven for 1 to $1\frac{1}{2}$ hours or until a meat thermometer inserted in the center of the meatloaf registers 160°F (71°C). Broil for 2 to 3 minutes or until top is browned.

Variation

Substitute any vegetables you have on hand, such as onions or bell peppers, for the zucchini and carrots.

Sweet Potato Chili

Thanks to the sweet potato and red pepper, this hearty chili is super-nutritious.

Kitchen Tips

One 19-oz (540 mL) can of kidney beans yields about 2 cups (500 mL).

This chili freezes well. Transfer individual portions to airtight containers and freeze for up to 3 months.

Try making this chili in a slow cooker. First brown the beef in a skillet, then add all ingredients to the slow cooker. Cover and cook on Low for 4 hours or on High for 6 hours.

1 lb	extra-lean ground beef	500 g
1 cup	chopped onion	250 mL
1 cup	chopped red bell pepper	250 mL
2 tsp	chili powder	10 mL
1 tsp	ground cumin	5 mL
2 cups	chopped peeled sweet potato	500 mL
1 cup	chopped tomato	250 mL
2 cups	reduced-sodium beef broth	500 mL
1	can (5 1/2 oz/156 mL) tomato paste	1
2 cups	drained rinsed canned kidney beans	500 mL
1/4 tsp	salt (or to taste)	1 mL
	Freshly ground black pepper	

1. In a large pot, cook beef over medium-high heat, breaking it up with the back of a wooden spoon, for about 8 minutes or until no longer pink. Add onion, red pepper, chili powder and cumin; cook, stirring often, for 4 minutes or until vegetables are softened.

2. Stir in sweet potato, tomato, broth and tomato paste; bring to a boil. Reduce heat and simmer, stirring occasionally, for 25 minutes or until sweet potato is tender. Stir in beans and cook for about 5 minutes or until warmed through. Season with up to 1/4 tsp (1 mL) salt and pepper to taste.

Variations

Substitute extra-lean ground turkey or chicken for the beef.

Use Chicken Stock (see recipe, page 182) or reduced-sodium low-fat chicken broth in place of the beef broth.

For a more traditional chili, substitute 1 1/2 cups (375 mL) corn kernels for the sweet potato.

If you can tolerate a bit of spice, add 1 canned chipotle pepper, chopped, and 2 tbsp (30 mL) adobo sauce.

Nutrients
PER SERVING

Calories	206
Fat	3.2 g
Sodium	147 mg
Carbohydrate	25.2 g
Fiber	7.9 g
Sugar	7.3 g
Protein	19.1 g
Calcium	19 mg
Iron	1.9 mg

Baked Brown Sugar Ham

Baked ham is a festive favorite for special occasions, but why wait? Enjoy it any day of the week — the preparation couldn't be easier.

Kitchen Tip

Chop leftover ham and add it to scrambled eggs or omelets, or use it to make Classic Canadian Ham and Pea Soup (page 197).

- **Preheat oven to 325°F (160°C)**
- **Roasting pan with rack**

¼ cup	brown sugar substitute (such as Splenda Brown Sugar Blend)	60 mL
1 tsp	dry mustard	5 mL
⅛ tsp	ground cloves	0.5 mL
3 tbsp	unsweetened applesauce	45 mL
2 lbs	smoked ham	1 kg

1. In a bowl, combine brown sugar substitute, mustard, cloves and applesauce. Rub all over ham. Place ham on rack on roasting pan.

2. Bake in preheated oven for 40 to 60 minutes or until a meat thermometer inserted in the thickest part of the ham registers 155°F (68°C). Transfer ham to a cutting board, cover loosely with foil and let rest for 10 minutes before slicing.

Nutrients
PER SERVING

Calories	113
Fat	2.2 g
Sodium	817 mg
Carbohydrate	7.7 g
Fiber	0.1 g
Sugar	1.0 g
Protein	16.3 g
Calcium	6 mg
Iron	0.4 mg

Pork and Apple Roast

The classic combination of pork and apple makes this roast an ideal dinner choice for an autumn meal.

Kitchen Tip

To clean leeks, after slicing them, place them in a strainer and rinse under cold running water.

- **Preheat oven to 350°F (180°C)**
- **6-cup (1.5 L) shallow glass baking dish**

2 tsp	olive oil, divided	10 mL
8 oz	pork tenderloin	250 g
	Salt and freshly ground black pepper	
1	leek (white and light green parts only), finely sliced	1
1	small carrot, finely chopped	1
1½ tsp	all-purpose flour	7 mL
1 cup	Vegetable Stock (see recipe, page 181) or reduced-sodium vegetable broth	250 mL
1 tsp	dried thyme	5 mL
1 tsp	dried rosemary	5 mL
1 tsp	Dijon mustard	5 mL
1	small apple, peeled and sliced	1

1. In a large nonstick skillet, heat 1 tsp (5 mL) oil over medium-high heat. Cook pork, turning often, for about 5 minutes or until browned on all sides. Transfer to baking dish and season with up to ⅛ tsp (0.5 mL) salt and pepper to taste. Set aside.

2. Add the remaining oil to the skillet and heat over medium-high heat. Sauté leeks and carrots for about 3 minutes or until leeks are softened. Sprinkle with flour and cook, stirring constantly, for 1 minute. Gradually whisk in stock, thyme, rosemary and mustard. Cook, stirring often, for 2 minutes. Season with up to ⅛ tsp (0.5 mL) salt.

3. Arrange some apple slices on top of pork and add the rest to the baking dish. Pour sauce over apples.

4. Bake in preheated oven for 35 to 45 minutes or until a meat thermometer inserted in the thickest part of the pork registers 155°F (68°C) and just a hint of pink remains inside. Transfer pork to a cutting board, cover loosely with foil and let rest for 10 minutes.

5. Thinly slice pork and serve with apples and sauce spooned over top.

Nutrients
PER SERVING

Calories	231
Fat	12.2 g
Sodium	291 mg
Carbohydrate	11.8 g
Fiber	2.2 g
Sugar	6.1 g
Protein	18.4 g
Calcium	43 mg
Iron	1.9 mg

Orange Ginger Pork Tenderloin

Makes 4 to 6 servings

Diet Stages 3 to 4

The orange marmalade adds sweetness to this roast, while ginger provides a touch of zest. Serve with Oven-Baked Sweet Potatoes (page 293).

- **Preheat oven to 350°F (180°C)**
- **8-cup (2 L) shallow glass baking dish**

2 tsp	canola oil	10 mL
1 lb	pork tenderloin	500 g
1/8 tsp	salt (or to taste)	0.5 mL
	Freshly ground black pepper	
1/3 cup	no-sugar-added orange marmalade	75 mL
2 tsp	cider vinegar	10 mL
1/2 tsp	dry mustard	2 mL
1/4 tsp	ground ginger	1 mL

1. In a large nonstick skillet, heat oil over medium-high heat. Cook pork, turning often, for 5 minutes or until browned on all sides. Transfer to baking dish and season with up to 1/8 tsp (0.5 mL) salt and pepper to taste. Set aside.

2. In a small pot, combine marmalade, vinegar, mustard and ginger. Cook over medium heat, stirring occasionally, for about 3 minutes or until slightly reduced. Pour glaze over pork.

3. Bake in preheated oven for 40 to 50 minutes, basting with drippings halfway through, until a meat thermometer inserted in the thickest part of the pork registers 155°F (68°C) and just a hint of pink remains inside. Transfer pork to a cutting board, cover loosely with foil and let rest for 10 minutes before slicing.

Variation

Substitute no-sugar-added orange jam for the marmalade.

Nutrients
PER SERVING

Calories	119
Fat	3.2 g
Sodium	89 mg
Carbohydrate	5.4 g
Fiber	0 g
Sugar	4.5 g
Protein	15.9 g
Calcium	4 mg
Iron	0.8 mg

Grilled Pork Kebabs

The onion and white wine help to tenderize the pork, making it moist and flavorful. Serve with whole wheat pita bread and Low-Fat Tzatziki (page 301).

Kitchen Tip
You can also use the broiler to cook these kebabs. Place them on a broiler pan and broil about 6 inches (15 cm) from the heat for about 12 minutes, turning halfway through, until browned and just a hint of pink remains inside.

- **Six 6-inch (15 cm) wooden skewers**

2	cloves garlic, minced	2
1	large onion, thinly sliced	1
2 tsp	dried oregano	10 mL
1/4 cup	dry white wine	60 mL
2 tbsp	olive oil	30 mL
1 lb	pork tenderloin, cut into 1 1/4-inch (3 cm) cubes	500 g
1/8 tsp	salt (or to taste)	0.5 mL
	Freshly ground black pepper	
	Juice of 1/2 lemon	

1. In a large bowl, combine garlic, onion, oregano, wine and oil. Add pork and toss to coat. Cover and refrigerate for at least 2 hours or overnight.

2. Soak skewers in water for 30 minutes. Preheat barbecue grill to medium-high.

3. Remove pork from marinade, discarding marinade. Thread pork cubes onto skewers, dividing equally. Grill, covered, for 10 minutes, turning occasionally, until browned on all sides and just a hint of pink remains inside.

4. Transfer kebabs to a serving platter and season with up to 1/8 tsp (0.5 mL) salt and pepper to taste. Squeeze lemon juice over meat.

Variation
If you tolerate beef, substitute boneless beef, such as sirloin, for the pork and add some steak seasoning to the marinade.

Nutrients	
PER SERVING	
Calories	147
Fat	6.4 g
Sodium	90 mg
Carbohydrate	3.7 g
Fiber	0.7 g
Sugar	1.3 g
Protein	16.3 g
Calcium	22 mg
Iron	1.1 mg

Lemon Pepper Chicken

This old favorite is easy to make with readily available ingredients.

Kitchen Tip

Cook only the amount of marinated chicken you will serve. Freeze the rest in the marinade in an airtight container for up to 6 months. Thaw overnight in the refrigerator before cooking.

* **11- by 7-inch (28 by 18 cm) glass baking dish, lined with foil**

1	clove garlic, minced	1
½	small onion, minced	½
2 tsp	freshly ground black pepper	10 mL
1 tbsp	grated lemon zest	15 mL
¼ cup	freshly squeezed lemon juice	60 mL
1 tbsp	olive oil	15 mL
8	chicken drumsticks, skin removed and fat trimmed	8
⅛ tsp	salt (or to taste)	0.5 mL

1. In a medium bowl, combine garlic, onion, pepper, lemon zest, lemon juice and oil. Add chicken and turn to coat. Cover and refrigerate for at least 2 hours or overnight.
2. Preheat oven to 375°F (190°C). Remove chicken from marinade, discarding marinade. Arrange drumsticks in a single layer in prepared baking dish.
3. Bake for 35 minutes or until juices run clear when chicken is pierced and a meat thermometer inserted in the thickest part of a drumstick registers 165°F (74°C). Season with up to ⅛ tsp (0.5 mL) salt.

Nutrients
PER SERVING

Calories	96
Fat	3.9 g
Sodium	91 mg
Carbohydrate	1.5 g
Fiber	0.2 g
Sugar	0.4 g
Protein	12.9 g
Calcium	11 mg
Iron	0.7 mg

Creamy Dijon Chicken Thighs

These chicken thighs are moist and tasty, with just a hint of flavor from the Dijon mustard to give them an extra kick.

Kitchen Tips

Instead of baking these thighs, you can grill them on the barbecue over medium-high heat for about 5 minutes per side or until juices run clear when thighs are pierced.

Use any cut of chicken, such as breasts or legs. Be sure to remove the skin and any visible fat before marinating, and adjust the cooking time as necessary.

- **11- by 7-inch (28 by 18 cm) glass baking dish, lightly sprayed with light nonstick cooking spray**

1	clove garlic, minced	1
1/3 cup	Chicken Stock (see recipe, page 182) or reduced-sodium low-fat chicken broth	75 mL
3 tbsp	low-fat plain yogurt	45 mL
1 tbsp	Dijon mustard	15 mL
6	boneless skinless chicken thighs (about 1 lb/500 g total), trimmed of fat	6

1. In a medium bowl, combine garlic, stock, yogurt and mustard. Add chicken and turn to coat. Cover and refrigerate for at least 1 hour or overnight.

2. Preheat oven to 400°F (200°C). Remove chicken from marinade, discarding marinade. Arrange chicken in a single layer in prepared baking dish.

3. Cover and bake for 20 minutes. Uncover and bake for 15 minutes or until juices run clear when thighs are pierced.

Nutrients
PER SERVING

Calories	88
Fat	2.8 g
Sodium	98 mg
Carbohydrate	0.9 g
Fiber	0.1 g
Sugar	0.6 g
Protein	14.0 g
Calcium	21 mg
Iron	0.7 mg

Chicken with Cranberry Raspberry Sauce

Makes 4 servings

Diet Stage 4

Here's an easy recipe when you're in a rush to make a quick meal. While the chicken is baking, prepare a simple, healthy side dish, such as Steamed Green Beans (page 288) or Boiled Mini Potatoes (page 296).

- **Preheat oven to 400°F (200°C)**
- **8-cup (2 L) shallow glass baking dish**

1 tsp	olive oil	5 mL
2	boneless skinless chicken breasts (about 12 oz/375 g total), trimmed of fat	2
1/8 tsp	salt (or to taste) Freshly ground black pepper	0.5 mL
1/4 cup	finely chopped onion	60 mL
1 tbsp	balsamic vinegar	15 mL
1/3 cup	Chicken Stock (see recipe, page 182) or reduced-sodium low-fat chicken broth	75 mL
2 tbsp	chopped fresh or thawed frozen cranberries	30 mL
2 tbsp	mashed raspberries	30 mL

1. In a nonstick skillet, heat oil over medium-high heat. Cook chicken for about 3 minutes per side or until browned on both sides. Transfer to baking dish and season with up to 1/8 tsp (0.5 mL) salt and pepper to taste. Set aside.

2. Add onion to the skillet and sauté over medium-high heat for 1 minute. Add vinegar and scrape up any brown bits from bottom of pan. Stir in stock, cranberries and raspberries; cook for 1 minute. Pour over chicken.

3. Cover and bake in preheated oven for 25 minutes or until chicken is no longer pink inside and a meat thermometer inserted in the thickest part of a breast registers 165°F (74°C). Let stand for 5 minutes before serving.

Variations

Substitute 12 oz (375 g) turkey cutlets for the chicken and decrease the baking time to about 15 minutes or until turkey is cooked through.

Replace the raspberries with mashed blackberries.

Nutrients
PER SERVING

Calories	97
Fat	2.6 g
Sodium	108 mg
Carbohydrate	3.4 g
Fiber	0.5 g
Sugar	1.6 g
Protein	14.0 g
Calcium	14 mg
Iron	0.5 mg

Greek-Style Chicken

This chicken recipe is easy to make, yet inviting enough to serve to guests.

Kitchen Tips

This chicken is also excellent grilled on the barbecue. Simply thread the cubed chicken onto soaked wooden skewers and grill over medium heat, turning often, for 10 to 12 minutes or until browned on all sides and no longer pink inside.

Freeze the chicken in the marinade in an airtight container for up to 6 months. Thaw overnight in the refrigerator before cooking.

Weight-Loss Surgery Tip

This is an excellent choice when you're introducing solids into your diet.

Nutrients
PER SERVING

Calories	139
Fat	4.7 g
Sodium	96 mg
Carbohydrate	1.0 g
Fiber	0.2 g
Sugar	0.2 g
Protein	22.0 g
Calcium	15 mg
Iron	0.8 mg

- **11- by 7-inch (28 by 18 cm) glass baking dish, lightly sprayed with light nonstick cooking spray**

2	cloves garlic, minced	2
1 tsp	dried oregano	5 mL
1/4 tsp	paprika	1 mL
2 tbsp	freshly squeezed lemon juice	30 mL
1 tbsp	olive oil	15 mL
1 lb	boneless skinless chicken breasts, cut into 1-inch (2.5 cm) cubes	500 g
1/8 tsp	salt (or to taste)	0.5 mL
	Freshly ground black pepper	

1. In a medium bowl, combine garlic, oregano, paprika, lemon juice and oil. Add chicken and toss to coat. Cover and refrigerate for at least 1 hour or overnight.

2. Preheat oven to 375°F (190°C). Remove chicken from marinade, discarding marinade. Arrange chicken in a single layer in prepared baking dish.

3. Cover and bake for 15 minutes. Uncover and bake for about 10 minutes or until chicken is no longer pink inside. Season with up to $1/8$ tsp (0.5 mL) salt and pepper to taste.

Chicken with Cherry Tomatoes

This moist and succulent chicken dish looks fabulous served alongside steamed green beans.

Weight-Loss Surgery Tip

This chicken is moist enough to try when you're introducing solids in diet stage 3. But avoid eating the cherry tomatoes during this stage, as the skin and seeds may be troublesome.

2 tbsp	all-purpose flour	30 mL
	Salt and freshly ground black pepper	
1 lb	boneless skinless chicken breasts (about 3 small breasts), trimmed of fat and cut in half	500 g
1 tbsp	olive oil	15 mL
5	cloves garlic, minced	5
¾ cup	Chicken Stock (see recipe, page 182) or reduced-sodium low-fat chicken broth	175 mL
2 tbsp	freshly squeezed lemon juice	30 mL
1 tsp	dried oregano	5 mL
⅛ tsp	ground cinnamon (optional)	0.5 mL
2½ cups	cherry tomatoes, halved	625 mL
1½ tsp	cornstarch	7 mL
1 tbsp	cold water	15 mL

1. On a plate, combine flour, ⅛ tsp (0.5 mL) salt and ⅛ tsp (0.5 mL) pepper. Dredge chicken in seasoned flour, shaking off excess. Discard any excess flour.

2. In a large nonstick skillet, heat oil over medium heat. Cook chicken for 5 minutes per side or until golden brown on both sides and no longer pink inside. Using tongs, transfer chicken to a plate.

3. Add garlic to the skillet and sauté for 30 seconds. Stir in stock, lemon juice, oregano and cinnamon (if using); cook, stirring occasionally, for 2 minutes. Add tomatoes and cook, stirring occasionally, for 4 minutes.

4. In a small bowl, whisk together cornstarch and water. Add to skillet and cook, stirring, for 1 minute. Return chicken and any accumulated juices to the pan and cook for 1 minute or until chicken is warmed through. Season with up to ¼ tsp (1 mL) salt and pepper to taste.

Nutrients
PER SERVING

Calories	167
Fat	4.8 g
Sodium	104 mg
Carbohydrate	7.1 g
Fiber	1.2 g
Sugar	2.0 g
Protein	23.0 g
Calcium	27 mg
Iron	1.1 mg

Cilantro Chicken Fajitas

*Make tonight fajita night!
For a complete meal, serve
this delectable chicken
mixture wrapped in a small
whole wheat flour tortilla
or over brown rice. Top
with diced tomatoes, salsa,
low-fat sour cream and/
or shredded low-fat cheese.
Or, for a different twist,
top with Peanut Dipping
Sauce (page 233).*

Kitchen Tip

If you don't have time to
marinate the chicken, you
can cook it right away, but
the marinating time allows
the flavors to combine and
tenderizes the chicken.

Weight-Loss Surgery Tip

Omit the chili powder if you
cannot tolerate spice.

Nutrients PER SERVING	
Calories	130
Fat	4.4 g
Sodium	219 mg
Carbohydrate	4.8 g
Fiber	1.3 g
Sugar	1.9 g
Protein	17.6 g
Calcium	22 mg
Iron	1.1 mg

1 cup	finely chopped fresh cilantro	250 mL
1 tbsp	chili powder (optional)	15 mL
1 tsp	ground cumin	5 mL
2 tbsp	reduced-sodium soy sauce	30 mL
4 tsp	canola oil, divided	20 mL
	Juice of 1 lime	
1 lb	boneless skinless chicken breasts, trimmed of fat and cut into thin strips	500 g
1 cup	chopped onion	250 mL
1 cup	sliced red bell pepper	250 mL
1 cup	sliced mushrooms	250 mL
1/8 tsp	salt (or to taste)	0.5 mL
	Freshly ground black pepper	

1. In a medium bowl, combine cilantro, chili powder (if using), cumin, soy sauce, 2 tsp (10 mL) of the oil and lime juice. Add chicken and toss to coat. Cover and refrigerate for at least 1 hour or overnight (see tip, at left).

2. In a nonstick skillet, heat the remaining oil over medium-high heat. Sauté onion and red peppers for 2 minutes. Add mushrooms and sauté for 2 minutes or until vegetables are tender. Using a slotted spoon, transfer vegetables to a plate.

3. Add chicken to the skillet and sauté for 6 minutes or until no longer pink inside. Return vegetables and any accumulated juices to the pan and sauté for 1 minute or until vegetables are warmed through. Season with up to 1/8 tsp (0.5 mL) salt and pepper to taste.

Variations

If you do not like cilantro, you can substitute chopped fresh parsley and/or basil. But then you will have to call these Parsley Chicken Fajitas or Basil Chicken Fajitas!

Substitute 2 tbsp (30 mL) freshly squeezed lemon juice for the lime juice.

Baked Chicken Fingers with Cranberry Dipping Sauce

These chicken fingers are healthier than fried, and with homemade Cranberry Dipping Sauce, they are sure to please everyone.

- **Preheat oven to 450°F (230°C)**
- **Baking sheet, lined with parchment paper**

2	boneless skinless chicken breasts (about 12 oz/375 g total), trimmed of fat	2
1	egg	1
1 tbsp	grated light Parmesan cheese	15 mL
1 tbsp	skim milk	15 mL
½ cup	dry whole wheat bread crumbs	125 mL
1 tsp	paprika	5 mL
1 tsp	dried parsley	5 mL
½ tsp	dried oregano	2 mL
	Freshly ground black pepper	
	Cranberry Dipping Sauce (see recipe, opposite)	

1. Cut each chicken breast lengthwise into 4 strips. Set aside.

2. In a bowl, whisk together egg, Parmesan and milk. On a plate, combine bread crumbs, paprika, parsley, oregano and pepper to taste. Dip chicken strips in egg mixture, then in bread crumb mixture, turning to coat evenly and shaking off excess. Place chicken in a single layer on prepared baking sheet. Discard any excess egg mixture and bread crumb mixture.

3. Bake in preheated oven for 15 minutes or until crust is lightly browned and chicken is no longer pink inside. Serve with Cranberry Dipping Sauce.

Nutrients
PER SERVING

Calories	153
Fat	3.3 g
Sodium	247 mg
Carbohydrate	11.8 g
Fiber	1.8 g
Sugar	0.4 g
Protein	17.5 g
Calcium	78 mg
Iron	1.8 mg

Cranberry Dipping Sauce

Prepare this sweet yet low-sugar sauce ahead of time for a cool dip or enjoy it warm.

Kitchen Tip

This dipping sauce can be stored in an airtight container in the refrigerator for up to 3 days.

- **Food processor or immersion blender**

¾ cup	fresh or thawed frozen cranberries	175 mL
2	whole cloves	2
¼ tsp	grated orange zest	1 mL
¼ tsp	grated lime zest	1 mL
⅛ tsp	ground cinnamon	0.5 mL
¼ cup	water	60 mL
2 tbsp	granulated sucralose artificial sweetener, such as Splenda	30 mL

1. In a medium saucepan, combine cranberries, cloves, orange zest, lime zest, cinnamon and water. Bring to a boil over medium-high heat. Boil, stirring occasionally, for 5 minutes. Remove from heat and stir in sweetener. Discard cloves.

2. Transfer cranberry mixture to food processor (or use immersion blender in pot) and purée until smooth.

Nutrients
PER SERVING

Calories	16
Fat	0.1 g
Sodium	2 mg
Carbohydrate	3.8 g
Fiber	1.0 g
Sugar	1.9 g
Protein	0 g
Calcium	5 mg
Iron	0.1 mg

Bran Flake–Crusted Chicken Strips

Makes 4 servings

Serving size: 5 chicken strips

Late Diet Stage 3 to Diet Stage 4

The bran flakes that coat these succulent low-fat chicken strips add fiber while locking in the juices.

- **Preheat oven to 375°F (190°C)**
- **Baking sheet, lined with parchment paper**

2	boneless skinless chicken breasts (about 12 oz/375 g total), trimmed of fat	2
1/4 cup	whole wheat flour	60 mL
1/8 tsp	salt (or to taste)	0.5 mL
	Freshly ground black pepper	
1	egg	1
2 tbsp	skim milk	30 mL
1 tsp	Dijon mustard	5 mL
1 1/2 cups	crushed bran flakes cereal	375 mL
	Peanut Dipping Sauce (see recipe, opposite)	

1. Cut each chicken breast into 10 small strips. Set aside.

2. On a plate, combine flour, up to 1/8 tsp (0.5 mL) salt and pepper to taste. In a bowl, whisk together egg, milk and mustard. Place bran flakes on another plate. Dredge chicken strips in seasoned flour, shaking off excess. Dip in egg mixture, turning to coat evenly and shaking off excess. Coat with bran flakes, patting flakes into the chicken. Place chicken in a single layer on prepared baking sheet. Discard any excess seasoned flour, egg mixture and bran flakes.

3. Bake in preheated oven for 15 minutes or until coating is crispy and chicken is no longer pink inside. Serve with Peanut Dipping Sauce.

Variations

Substitute crushed corn flakes cereal for the bran flakes.

Try these with Cranberry Dipping Sauce (page 231) instead of the Peanut Dipping Sauce.

Nutrients
PER SERVING

Calories	164
Fat	3.0 g
Sodium	248 mg
Carbohydrate	18.0 g
Fiber	3.6 g
Sugar	3.3 g
Protein	17.9 g
Calcium	31 mg
Iron	5.0 mg

Peanut Dipping Sauce

*This easy homemade peanut
sauce makes a deliciously
different dipping sauce for
chicken strips.*

Kitchen Tips

This dipping sauce can
be stored in an airtight
container in the refrigerator
for up to 3 days.

You can also use this sauce
to make chicken satays. Cut
boneless skinless chicken
breasts into cubes, thread
onto wooden skewers and
brush with peanut sauce.
Cover and refrigerate for
at least 1 hour or overnight.
Preheat barbecue grill to
medium-high. Grill, turning
often, until chicken is no
longer pink inside.

Nutrients PER SERVING	
Calories	95
Fat	7.2 g
Sodium	78 mg
Carbohydrate	4.1 g
Fiber	0.8 g
Sugar	1.8 g
Protein	3.5 g
Calcium	23 mg
Iron	0.3 mg

1	clove garlic, minced	1
½ tsp	dry mustard	2 mL
⅓ cup	skim milk	75 mL
3 tbsp	all-natural smooth peanut butter	45 mL
1½ tbsp	reduced-sodium soy sauce	22 mL
2 tsp	freshly squeezed lemon juice	10 mL
1 tsp	sesame oil	5 mL

1. In a small saucepan, combine garlic, mustard, milk, peanut butter, soy sauce, lemon juice and oil. Bring to a boil over medium heat, stirring often. Boil, stirring often, for 5 minutes. Remove from heat and let cool to room temperature before serving.

Variations

Reduce the soy sauce to 1½ tsp (7 mL) and add 1 tbsp (15 mL) fish sauce (nam pla).

If you tolerate spice, add a pinch of cayenne pepper or chili powder.

Classic Chicken Stew

Use up leftover grilled chicken breast to make this creamy stew.

Weight-Loss Surgery Tip

If you are having difficulty eating vegetables, cook them a little longer and/or cut them into smaller pieces so they'll be more tender.

1 tbsp	all-purpose flour	15 mL
½ cup	cold water	125 mL
½ cup	skim milk	125 mL
1 tbsp	olive oil	15 mL
1	onion, chopped	1
1	carrot, chopped	1
1	clove garlic, minced	1
1	chicken bouillon cube	1
½ cup	thawed frozen green peas	125 mL
½ tsp	dried oregano	2 mL
½ tsp	dried thyme	2 mL
1 cup	small mushrooms	250 mL
2 cups	cubed cooked chicken breast (1-inch/2.5 cm cubes)	500 mL
	Freshly ground black pepper	

1. Place flour in a small bowl. Gradually whisk in cold water until smooth. Whisk in milk. Set aside.

2. In a large pot, heat oil over medium heat. Sauté onion and carrot for 4 minutes. Add garlic and sauté for 30 seconds. Stir in bouillon cube, peas, oregano and thyme. Add flour mixture and cook, stirring often, for 4 minutes. Add mushrooms and cook, stirring occasionally, for about 5 minutes or until tender. Add chicken and cook for about 2 minutes or until warmed through. Season to taste with pepper.

Variation

Substitute green beans for the peas.

Nutrients PER SERVING	
Calories	259
Fat	7.9 g
Sodium	346 mg
Carbohydrate	14.1 g
Fiber	2.7 g
Sugar	6.4 g
Protein	31.7 g
Calcium	82 mg
Iron	1.8 mg

Chicken Apple Purée

The simple addition of apple to this recipe makes the puréed chicken sweeter.

Kitchen Tip

Freeze extra purée in an ice cube tray. Once frozen, pop the cubes out and store in an airtight container for up to 3 months.

- **Food processor**

6 oz	boneless skinless chicken breast, trimmed of fat	175 g
¼ tsp	ground cinnamon	1 mL
⅛ tsp	ground cloves	0.5 mL
2	soft apples, such as McIntosh or Gala, peeled and chopped	2
	Chicken Stock (see recipe, page 182) or reduced-sodium low-fat chicken broth (optional)	
	Salt (optional)	

1. In a nonstick skillet, combine chicken, cinnamon and cloves. Add enough water to cover. Bring to a boil over high heat. Reduce heat to medium, cover and simmer for 12 minutes or until chicken is no longer pink inside. Transfer chicken to a cutting board and let cool to room temperature, then cut into chunks. Discard cooking liquid.

2. Meanwhile, place apples in a small saucepan and add enough water to cover. Bring to a boil over high heat. Reduce heat and simmer for 10 minutes or until apples are tender. Drain.

3. Transfer chicken and apples to food processor and purée until smooth. If a thinner consistency is desired, add stock 1 tbsp (15 mL) at a time, pulsing to combine. If desired, season to taste with salt.

Nutrients
PER SERVING

Calories	173
Fat	2.7 g
Sodium	55 mg
Carbohydrate	11.3 g
Fiber	2.7 g
Sugar	8.0 g
Protein	25.4 g
Calcium	15 mg
Iron	1.0 mg

Variations

Substitute turkey for the chicken.

Replace the apples with pears.

Tropical Chicken Purée

Mango and papaya give ordinary chicken purée a tropical twist.

Kitchen Tip

Freeze extra purée in an ice cube tray. Once frozen, pop the cubes out and store in an airtight container for up to 3 months.

- **Food processor**

6 oz	boneless skinless chicken breast, trimmed of fat	175 g
½	mango, peeled and chopped	½
¼ cup	chopped papaya	60 mL
¼ tsp	ground ginger	1 mL
⅛ tsp	ground nutmeg	Pinch
	Chicken Stock (see recipe, page 182) or reduced-sodium low-fat chicken broth (optional)	
	Salt (optional)	

1. Place chicken in a nonstick skillet and add enough water to cover. Bring to a boil over high heat. Reduce heat to medium, cover and simmer for 12 minutes or until chicken is no longer pink inside. Transfer chicken to a cutting board and let cool to room temperature, then cut into chunks. Discard cooking liquid.

2. Meanwhile, in a small saucepan, combine mango, papaya, ginger, nutmeg and 2 tbsp (30 mL) water. Bring to a boil over high heat. Reduce heat and simmer for 2 minutes or until fruit is soft.

3. Transfer chicken and mango mixture to food processor and purée until smooth. If a thinner consistency is desired, add stock 1 tbsp (15 mL) at a time, pulsing to combine. If desired, season to taste with salt.

Variation

Substitute a turkey cutlet for the chicken.

Nutrients
PER SERVING

Calories	175
Fat	3.0 g
Sodium	56 mg
Carbohydrate	10.4 g
Fiber	0.9 g
Sugar	1.8 g
Protein	25.5 g
Calcium	16 mg
Iron	0.8 mg

Sweet Potato and Turkey Purée

Try this high-protein recipe if you are having difficulty eating solid foods. You may need to stick with puréed foods until you are feeling better.

Kitchen Tip

Freeze extra purée in an ice cube tray. Once frozen, pop the cubes out and store in an airtight container for up to 3 months.

- **Food processor**

1 cup	chopped peeled sweet potato	250 mL
6 oz	turkey cutlet	175 g
1	sprig fresh thyme	1
	Chicken Stock (see recipe, page 182) or reduced-sodium low-fat chicken broth (optional)	
	Salt and freshly ground black pepper (optional)	

1. Place sweet potato in a small pot and add enough water to cover. Bring to a boil over high heat. Reduce heat and simmer for 20 minutes or until sweet potato is tender. Drain and set aside.

2. Meanwhile, place turkey and thyme in a nonstick skillet and add enough water to cover. Bring to a boil over high heat. Reduce heat to medium, cover and simmer for 12 minutes or until turkey is no longer pink inside. Transfer turkey to a cutting board and let cool to room temperature, then cut into chunks. Discard cooking liquid.

3. Transfer turkey and sweet potato to food processor and purée until smooth. If a thinner consistency is desired, add stock 1 tbsp (15 mL) at a time, pulsing to combine. If desired, season to taste with salt and pepper.

Variation

Substitute chicken breast for the turkey.

Nutrients
PER SERVING

Calories	81
Fat	0.3 g
Sodium	58 mg
Carbohydrate	4.5 g
Fiber	0.7 g
Sugar	1.4 g
Protein	14.8 g
Calcium	8 mg
Iron	1.0 mg

Turkey Meatloaf Muffins

A muffin pan is an ingenious way to make perfectly portioned mini meatloaves.

Kitchen Tips

These muffins can be cooled, individually wrapped, then frozen in airtight containers for up to 3 months.

You can also use this meat mixture to make meatballs, a regular-size meatloaf or turkey patties.

Weight-Loss Surgery Tip

This is an excellent choice in diet stage 3, when you're introducing solids into your diet.

- **Preheat oven to 350°F (180°C)**
- **12-cup nonstick or silicone muffin pan**

1 lb	extra-lean ground turkey	500 g
1/3 cup	seasoned dry bread crumbs	75 mL
1/4 cup	finely chopped onion	60 mL
1	egg	1
2 tbsp	skim milk	30 mL
2 tbsp	barbecue sauce	30 mL

1. In a large bowl, combine turkey, bread crumbs, onion, egg, milk and barbecue sauce. Knead with your hands until well combined. Spoon about 3 tbsp (45 mL) turkey mixture into each muffin cup.

2. Bake in preheated oven for 20 minutes or until a meat thermometer inserted in the center of a muffin registers 165°F (74°C). Let cool in pan on a wire rack for 10 minutes. Carefully slide a knife around the edges of each meatloaf to loosen, then gently remove from pan using two spoons, draining off any accumulated liquid.

Variations

Substitute any type of extra-lean ground meat, such as chicken or beef.

Top each muffin with a dollop of hot mashed potatoes after baking.

Nutrients
PER SERVING

Calories	149
Fat	5.8 g
Sodium	234 mg
Carbohydrate	7.4 g
Fiber	0.4 g
Sugar	2.5 g
Protein	17.0 g
Calcium	23 mg
Iron	1.9 mg

Turkey Meatballs

These meatballs are packed with nutrition, but they taste so good no one need ever know they're good for you. Try them with your favorite tomato sauce, or add them to low-fat chicken broth for meatball soup.

Kitchen Tips

Wet your hands before rolling the meatballs, to keep them from sticking to your hands.

After rolling the meatballs, freeze them on a baking sheet. Once frozen, store them in an airtight container in the freezer for up to 2 months. Let thaw overnight in the refrigerator.

Use this meat mixture to make meatloaf or mini burgers.

Nutrients
PER SERVING

Calories	140
Fat	5.6 g
Sodium	202 mg
Carbohydrate	6.0 g
Fiber	1.0 g
Sugar	0.8 g
Protein	16.4 g
Calcium	27 mg
Iron	1.8 mg

- **Preheat oven to 400°F (200°C)**
- **Rimmed baking sheet, lined with foil and lightly sprayed with light nonstick cooking spray**

12 oz	extra-lean ground turkey	375 g
¼ cup	finely chopped onion	60 mL
¼ cup	finely diced carrot	60 mL
¼ cup	finely diced celery	60 mL
¼ cup	dry whole wheat bread crumbs	60 mL
⅛ tsp	salt	0.5 mL
⅛ tsp	freshly ground black pepper (optional)	0.5 mL
1	egg	1

1. In a large bowl, combine turkey, onion, carrot, celery, bread crumbs, salt, pepper (if using) and egg. Knead with your hands until well combined.

2. Using about 1 tbsp (15 mL) per meatball, roll turkey mixture into 20 meatballs. Place on prepared baking sheet, making sure they don't touch each other.

3. Bake in preheated oven for 20 minutes or until no longer pink inside.

Variation

Substitute any type of extra-lean ground meat, such as chicken, pork or beef.

Low-Fat Gravy

*Drizzle this low-fat gravy
over meat and poultry dishes
that need a little extra
moisture and flavor.*

Kitchen Tips

If desired, add ¼ tsp (1 mL)
liquid gravy browning.

Store leftovers in an airtight
container in the refrigerator
for up to 3 days.

1 tbsp	all-purpose flour	15 mL
½ cup	evaporated skim milk	125 mL
1 tsp	reduced-sodium beef or chicken bouillon powder	5 mL
⅛ tsp	freshly ground black pepper	0.5 mL
¼ cup	water	60 mL

1. Place flour in a small saucepan and gradually whisk
in milk until smooth. Add bouillon, pepper and water;
bring to a boil over medium-high heat. Reduce heat
and simmer, stirring often, for 5 minutes or until
slightly thickened.

Nutrients
PER SERVING

Calories	17
Fat	0.1 g
Sodium	66 mg
Carbohydrate	2.6 g
Fiber	0 g
Sugar	1.9 g
Protein	1.4 g
Calcium	47 mg
Iron	0.1 mg

Fish and Seafood

Fish and seafood dishes are effortless to make, yet healthy, especially when they are poached, baked or grilled. Try to buy fresh fish more often than frozen, for better flavor and quality. But having some frozen shrimp or seafood mix on hand does make for a quick dinner option when you don't have time to go to the grocery store or fish market. Canned tuna, salmon and crab also make quick alternatives.

Fish and seafood offer many health and nutrition benefits. After weight-loss surgery, fish is a great way to get protein and other important nutrients, including omega-3 fatty acids. When you are learning to introduce solids, fish is usually easy to tolerate, so experiment with the wide array of fish and seafood available.

Fish and Veggies in Foil Parcels

Makes 2 servings

Late Diet Stage 3 to Diet Stage 4

Wrapping food in foil parcels is a convenient, no-mess way to cook. The foil also has the benefit of locking in moisture. Try foil parcels to prepare other fish recipes.

Kitchen Tips

Be careful when opening up the parcels — the steam is very hot!

Any type of fish will do to make these neat little parcels.

- **Preheat oven to 375°F (190°C)**
- **Rimmed baking sheet**

1 tbsp	reduced-sodium soy sauce	15 mL
1 tbsp	rice vinegar	15 mL
6 oz	skinless fish fillet, cut in half	175 g
2	green onions, ends trimmed	2
1	carrot, thinly sliced	1
1 cup	small mushrooms	250 mL
½ cup	snow peas, trimmed	125 mL

1. In a medium bowl, combine soy sauce and vinegar. Add fish and turn to coat. Cover and marinate for 15 minutes.
2. Cut 2 pieces of foil into 12- by 8-inch (30 by 20 cm) rectangles. Arrange one green onion and half each of the carrot, mushrooms and snow peas on each piece of foil. Lay one fish fillet on each pile of vegetables. Gather edges of foil to make a sealed parcel. Lay parcels on baking sheet.
3. Bake in preheated oven for 15 to 20 minutes or until fish is opaque and flakes easily when tested with a fork.

Variation

Be creative with the vegetables you add to the parcels. Try green beans, sliced red bell peppers or sliced white onions.

Nutrients
PER SERVING

Calories	132
Fat	2.3 g
Sodium	340 mg
Carbohydrate	7.0 g
Fiber	2.1 g
Sugar	3.0 g
Protein	20.7 g
Calcium	71 mg
Iron	1.7 mg

Haddock in Tomato Juice

Poaching in tomato juice results in very moist fish with a delicate flavor. Plus, you get a delicious sauce.

Kitchen Tip

"Poaching" means cooking food gently in liquid that is just below the boiling point, also known as a simmer. The surface of the liquid seems to quiver when it is simmering. The skillet is usually covered to keep the steam inside the pan to help cook the food. The food will be infused with some of the flavor of the liquid it is poached in. Poaching is a low-fat cooking method.

Weight-Loss Surgery Tip

This is an excellent recipe to try when you're learning to introduce solids.

Nutrients
PER SERVING

Calories	96
Fat	1.3 g
Sodium	99 mg
Carbohydrate	4.2 g
Fiber	0.8 g
Sugar	2.7 g
Protein	16.2 g
Calcium	42 mg
Iron	1.3 mg

½ tsp	canola oil	2 mL
¼ cup	finely chopped onion	60 mL
1	clove garlic, minced	1
1 cup	reduced-sodium tomato juice	250 mL
1	bay leaf	1
1 tsp	dried oregano	5 mL
	Freshly ground black pepper	
2	skinless haddock fillets (about 11 oz/330 g total)	2

1. In a skillet, heat oil over medium heat. Sauté onions for 1 minute. Add garlic and sauté for 30 seconds. Add tomato juice, bay leaf, oregano and pepper to taste; bring to a simmer. Add haddock, reduce heat to low, cover and poach for 6 to 7 minutes or until fish is opaque and flakes easily when tested with a fork. Discard bay leaf. Using a spatula, transfer fish to serving bowls and pour sauce over top.

Variation

Substitute catfish, tilapia, cod or halibut for the haddock.

Maple-Glazed Barbecue Salmon

Kitchen Tips

The cooking time varies depending on the thickness of the fillet. As a general rule, cook for 10 minutes for every inch (2.5 cm) of thickness.

Instead of grilling, place salmon, skin side down, on a baking sheet lined with foil. Preheat broiler, with the rack about 10 inches (25 cm) from the heat source. Broil salmon for about 10 minutes or until fish is opaque and flakes easily when tested with a fork.

Weight-Loss Surgery Tip

This is an excellent choice when you're learning to introduce solids.

Nutrients PER SERVING	
Calories	143
Fat	5.6 g
Sodium	152 mg
Carbohydrate	6.2 g
Fiber	0 g
Sugar	0 g
Protein	17.5 g
Calcium	11 mg
Iron	0.7 mg

1/4 tsp	Chinese five-spice powder	1 mL
1/8 tsp	freshly ground black pepper	0.5 mL
1/2 tsp	reduced-sodium soy sauce	2 mL
1/2 tsp	Dijon mustard	2 mL
6 oz	skin-on salmon fillet	175 g
1 tbsp	no-sugar-added maple-flavored syrup	15 mL

1. In a bowl, whisk together five-spice powder, pepper, soy sauce and mustard. Add salmon and turn to coat. Cover and refrigerate for at least 1 hour or overnight.

2. Using a paper towel, lightly grease barbecue grill with cooking oil. Preheat grill to medium.

3. Remove salmon from marinade, discarding marinade. Grill salmon, turning once, for 6 to 8 minutes per side or until fish is opaque and flakes easily when tested with a fork. Serve drizzled with syrup.

Lemon Dijon Salmon

1	clove garlic, minced	1
2 tbsp	freshly squeezed lemon juice	30 mL
1 tsp	olive oil	5 mL
1 tsp	Dijon mustard	5 mL
$\frac{1}{2}$ tsp	fat-free mayonnaise	2 mL
6 oz	skin-on salmon fillet	175 g
	Salt and freshly ground black pepper (optional)	

Nutrients
PER SERVING

Calories	152
Fat	7.9 g
Sodium	81 mg
Carbohydrate	2.0 g
Fiber	0.1 g
Sugar	0.5 g
Protein	17.5 g
Calcium	14 mg
Iron	0.7 mg

1. In a bowl, whisk together garlic, lemon juice, olive oil, mustard and mayonnaise. Add salmon and turn to coat. Cover and refrigerate for at least 1 hour or overnight.

2. Using a paper towel, lightly grease barbecue grill with cooking oil. Preheat grill to medium.

3. Remove salmon from marinade, discarding marinade. Grill salmon, turning once, for 6 to 8 minutes per side or until fish is opaque and flakes easily when tested with a fork. Season to taste with salt and pepper (if using).

Simple Sockeye Salmon Salad

1	can (7$\frac{1}{2}$ oz/213 g) sockeye salmon, drained	1
$\frac{1}{4}$ tsp	herbes de Provence	1 mL
	Cayenne pepper (optional)	
1 tsp	rice vinegar	5 mL
$\frac{1}{2}$ tsp	fat-free mayonnaise	2 mL
$\frac{1}{4}$ tsp	Dijon mustard	1 mL

Nutrients
PER SERVING

Calories	188
Fat	11.9 g
Sodium	475 mg
Carbohydrate	0.3 g
Fiber	0.1 g
Sugar	0.1 g
Protein	22.0 g
Calcium	173 mg
Iron	0.7 mg

1. Remove any skin from salmon. In a bowl, using a fork, mash any bones in salmon into very small pieces. Add herbes de Provence, cayenne (if using), vinegar, mayonnaise and mustard; mash to combine.

Mini Salmon Patties

These miniature salmon patties taste delicious topped with a dollop of low-fat plain yogurt.

Kitchen Tips

You can replace the dried dillweed with 1 tsp (5 mL) chopped fresh dill or cilantro.

To prevent the salmon mixture from sticking to your hands when you're forming the patties, wet your hands with cold water. Alternatively, cover and refrigerate the mixture for about 20 minutes; the mixture is easier to work with when it's chilled.

Prepare the salmon mixture and shape the patties the night before, cover and refrigerate.

2	green onions, thinly sliced	2
1	egg, lightly beaten	1
½	slice whole wheat bread, crumbled (or ¼ cup/60 mL dry whole wheat bread crumbs)	½
⅛ tsp	cayenne pepper	0.5 mL
⅛ tsp	dried dillweed	0.5 mL
⅛ tsp	salt (optional)	0.5 mL
1	can (7½ oz/213 g) salmon, drained	1
1 tsp	canola oil	5 mL

1. In a medium bowl, combine green onions, egg, bread crumbs, cayenne, dill and salt (if using).

2. Remove any skin from salmon. Add salmon to onion mixture and mash any bones with a fork, combining with mixture while mashing; let stand for 5 minutes. Form mixture into six ¾-inch (2 cm) thick patties.

3. In a medium nonstick skillet, heat oil over medium-low heat. Cook salmon patties, turning once, for about 5 minutes per side or until golden brown on both sides and hot in the center.

Variation

Substitute ¼ cup (60 mL) quick-cooking rolled oats for the whole wheat bread.

Nutrients
PER SERVING

Calories	74
Fat	3.3 g
Sodium	164 mg
Carbohydrate	1.6 g
Fiber	0.5 g
Sugar	0.4 g
Protein	9.6 g
Calcium	119 mg
Iron	4.0 mg

Swordfish Skewers

These fish skewers are bound to entice your guests at your next barbecue.

Kitchen Tips

The cooking time will depend on the thickness of the fish cubes.

Instead of grilling, lay skewers on a baking sheet. Preheat broiler, with the rack about 10 inches (25 cm) from the heat source. Broil skewers, turning occasionally, for 5 to 10 minutes or until fish is opaque and flakes easily when tested with a fork.

- **Six 12-inch (30 cm) wooden skewers**

1	clove garlic, minced	1
1 tsp	paprika	5 mL
2 tbsp	freshly squeezed lemon juice	30 mL
1 tbsp	olive oil	15 mL
1 lb	skinless swordfish steak, cut into 18 cubes	500 g
12	cherry tomatoes	12
1	small onion, cut into 12 wedges	1
1/8 tsp	salt (or to taste)	0.5 mL
	Freshly ground black pepper	

1. In a medium bowl, whisk together garlic, paprika, lemon juice and oil. Add swordfish and toss to coat. Cover and refrigerate for at least 1 hour or overnight.
2. Soak skewers in water for 30 minutes. Preheat barbecue grill to medium.
3. Remove fish from marinade. Thread a fish cube onto each skewer, followed by a cherry tomato, onion wedge, fish cube, cherry tomato, onion wedge and fish cube. Season skewers with up to 1/8 tsp (0.5 mL) salt and pepper to taste.
4. Grill skewers, turning occasionally, for 5 to 10 minutes or until fish is opaque and flakes easily when tested with a fork.

Variation

Substitute tuna steak or salmon fillet for the swordfish.

Nutrients
PER SERVING

Calories	126
Fat	5.5 g
Sodium	110 mg
Carbohydrate	3.2 g
Fiber	0.8 g
Sugar	1.6 g
Protein	15.5 g
Calcium	11 mg
Iron	0.8 mg

Sea Bass with Red Pepper Sauce

The combination of the bright red sauce, green cilantro and white fish is both beautiful and delectable.

Kitchen Tip

Sea bass can be pricey. If you wish, substitute tilapia, catfish or basa.

- **Preheat broiler**
- **Rimmed baking sheet, lightly sprayed with light nonstick cooking spray**

7 oz	skinless sea bass fillet, cut in half	210 g
1 tbsp	freshly squeezed lemon juice	15 mL
1/8 tsp	salt (or to taste)	0.5 mL
	Freshly ground black pepper	
2 tbsp	Red Pepper Sauce (see recipe, opposite)	30 mL
1 tsp	chopped fresh cilantro	5 mL

1. Place sea bass on prepared baking sheet. Sprinkle with lemon juice and season with up to 1/8 tsp (0.5 mL) salt and pepper to taste.

2. Broil for 4 minutes. Turn fish over and top with red pepper sauce. Broil for 6 to 8 minutes or until fish is opaque and flakes easily when tested with a fork. Serve sprinkled with cilantro.

Nutrients
PER SERVING

Calories	113
Fat	2.5 g
Sodium	219 mg
Carbohydrate	2.0 g
Fiber	0.4 g
Sugar	0.9 g
Protein	19.6 g
Calcium	14 mg
Iron	0.4 mg

Red Pepper Sauce

This roasted red pepper sauce is delightful with fish, as in the recipe opposite, but also makes an excellent spread for Melba toast, topped with shredded low-fat cheese.

Kitchen Tips

If you do not have time to roast the pepper, use 4 pieces of bottled roasted red bell pepper. Drain them well and proceed with step 2, omitting the vinegar.

Red pepper sauce can be stored in an airtight container in the refrigerator for up to 3 days.

- **Preheat broiler**
- **Food processor or blender**

I	red bell pepper	I
I	clove garlic, minced	I
2 tsp	tomato paste	10 mL
½ tsp	olive oil	2 mL
I tsp	cider vinegar	5 mL
⅛ tsp	cayenne pepper (optional)	0.5 mL
	Salt and freshly ground black pepper (optional)	

1. Place red pepper on a baking sheet and broil, turning often, for 8 to 10 minutes or until blackened. Place in a large sealable plastic bag, seal and let cool. When cool enough to handle, slip off skin, remove stem, cut pepper in half and remove seeds.

2. In food processor, purée roasted pepper until smooth. Add garlic, tomato paste, oil, vinegar, cayenne (if using) and, if desired, salt and pepper to taste; process for 1 minute.

Nutrients
PER SERVING

Calories	9
Fat	0.3 g
Sodium	2 mg
Carbohydrate	1.3 g
Fiber	0.4 g
Sugar	0.8 g
Protein	0.2 g
Calcium	2 mg
Iron	0.1 mg

Trout with Herbs and Feta Cheese

Makes 2 servings

Mid Diet Stage 3 to Diet Stage 4

This fish entrée is rich in protein and healthier fats, easy to make and combines the classic flavors of tomato, oregano and feta cheese. Serve with couscous for a nutritious meal.

Weight-Loss Surgery Tip

This is an excellent choice when you're learning to introduce solids.

- **Preheat oven to 400°F (200°C)**
- **6-cup (1.5 L) shallow glass baking dish**

1 tsp	olive oil	5 mL
6 oz	trout fillet, cut in half	175 g
4	slices tomato	4
1 tsp	dried oregano	5 mL
¼ tsp	Italian herb seasoning	1 mL
1 tsp	freshly squeezed lemon juice	5 mL
2 tbsp	crumbled light feta cheese	30 mL

1. Drizzle bottom of baking dish with oil. Arrange trout in a single layer in baking dish. Top each fillet with 2 tomato slices. Sprinkle with oregano, Italian seasoning and lemon juice.

2. Bake in preheated oven for about 15 minutes or until fish is opaque and flakes easily when tested with a fork. Top each fillet with 1 tbsp (15 mL) feta cheese. Bake for 2 minutes or until cheese is warmed through.

Variations

Substitute orange roughy, tilapia or halibut for the trout.

Replace the feta with grated light Parmesan cheese.

Nutrients
PER SERVING

Calories	75
Fat	8.3 g
Sodium	150 mg
Carbohydrate	2.1 g
Fiber	0.8 g
Sugar	0.9 g
Protein	20.4 g
Calcium	98 mg
Iron	0.6 mg

Poached Rainbow Trout

Cooking trout in white wine infuses it with flavor, making this dish rich and delicious.

Weight-Loss Surgery Tip

This is an excellent recipe to try when you're learning to introduce solids.

1	rainbow trout fillet (about 9 oz/270 g)	1
	Salt and freshly ground black pepper (optional)	
1/4	onion	1/4
5	whole black peppercorns	5
1	bay leaf	1
1	sprig fresh thyme	1
1/2 cup	dry white wine	125 mL
1/2 cup	water	125 mL

1. Season trout with salt and pepper (if using). Set aside.

2. In a skillet, combine onion, peppercorns, bay leaf, thyme, wine and water. Bring to a boil over high heat. Turn heat off. Carefully place fish in poaching liquid, cover and poach for about 5 minutes or until fish is opaque and flakes easily when tested with a fork. Using a slotted spatula, remove fish from poaching liquid, draining well. Discard poaching liquid.

Variations

Any type of fish will work in place of the trout in this recipe. The cooking time will vary depending on the thickness of the fish.

Vary the flavor of the poaching liquid by adding your choice of aromatic vegetables, such as leeks, green onions, garlic, celery and/or carrots.

Nutrients
PER SERVING

Calories	160
Fat	4.9 g
Sodium	38 mg
Carbohydrate	1.9 g
Fiber	0.2 g
Sugar	0.8 g
Protein	18.9 g
Calcium	68 mg
Iron	0.4 mg

Cold Shrimp Spring Rolls

Makes 2 servings

Serving size: 1 wrap

Diet Stage 4

These fresh spring rolls are as much a delight to the eyes as they are to the palate. Serve with additional Thai Red Chili Sauce (see recipe, opposite) for dipping.

Kitchen Tips

You can find rice paper in the Asian foods aisle of your grocery store or at an Asian market. If you cannot find it, use whole wheat flour tortillas.

The damp tea towel helps keep the delicate rice paper from drying out and makes it easier to work with.

Nutrients
PER SERVING

Calories	140
Fat	5.0 g
Sodium	91 mg
Carbohydrate	14.4 g
Fiber	0.7 g
Sugar	0.8 g
Protein	13.8 g
Calcium	63 mg
Iron	0.9 mg

- **8-inch (20 cm) pie plate**

1 cup	boiling water	250 mL
2	9-inch (23 cm) round rice paper wraps	2
6	cooked large shrimp, tails removed	6
1 cup	bean sprouts, steamed	250 mL
1/2 cup	shredded iceberg lettuce	125 mL
2 tbsp	chopped fresh cilantro or basil	30 mL
2 tsp	Thai Red Chili Sauce (see recipe, opposite)	10 mL

1. Cover a cutting board with a damp tea towel. Pour boiling water into pie plate. Carefully slip 1 rice paper wrap into the pie plate and let soften for 30 seconds. Carefully remove wrap and place flat on tea towel. Lay 3 shrimp in a line across wrap, about 1 inch (2.5 cm) from the edge closest to you. Top shrimp with half the bean sprouts, lettuce and cilantro. Drizzle half the chili sauce over top.

2. Carefully roll up bottom edge of rice paper tightly over filling. When you're about 1 inch (2.5 cm) away from the end, fold the two sides of the rice paper toward the center. Continue rolling wrap to the end. Repeat with the other rice paper wrap, using the remaining ingredients. Cut in half on a diagonal. Serve immediately.

Variations

If you tolerate peanuts, add 1/4 tsp (1 mL) crushed peanuts to each wrap, or add them to the Thai Red Chili Sauce.

In place of the shrimp, use 1/2 cup (125 mL) shredded cooked chicken breast.

Use any vegetables you like, such as julienned cucumbers, carrots and/or red bell peppers.

Thai Red Chili Sauce

*My version of the popular
Thai Red Chili Sauce is
lower in sugar thanks to the
sweetener and is thickened
with cornstarch. Use in
Cold Shrimp Spring Rolls
(opposite) or as a dipping
sauce for cocktail shrimp,
tofu, fish or chicken.*

Kitchen Tips

If desired, add a couple of
drops of red food coloring.

Adjust the spiciness to your
tolerance by using more or
less Thai red chile pepper or
hot pepper flakes.

This sauce can be stored in
an airtight container in the
refrigerator for up to 1 week.

Nutrients
PER SERVING

Calories	8
Fat	0 g
Sodium	78 mg
Carbohydrate	2.0 g
Fiber	0.1 g
Sugar	0.3 g
Protein	0.1 g
Calcium	2 mg
Iron	0.1 mg

- **Mini chopper (optional)**

1	small Thai red chile pepper (or ½ tsp/2 mL hot pepper flakes)	1
1	clove garlic	1
¼ cup	granulated sucralose artificial sweetener, such as Splenda	60 mL
½ cup	water	125 mL
1 tbsp	white vinegar	15 mL
1 tbsp	freshly squeezed lime juice	15 mL
2 tsp	fish sauce (nam pla)	10 mL
2 tsp	cornstarch	10 mL
2 tsp	cold water	10 mL

1. In mini chopper, finely chop chile pepper and garlic (or simply chop them by hand). Add sweetener, ½ cup (125 mL) water, vinegar, lime juice and fish sauce; process until well combined.

2. Pour into a small saucepan and bring to a simmer over medium-heat. Simmer, stirring occasionally, for 3 minutes.

3. In a small bowl, whisk cornstarch and cold water until smooth. Stir into saucepan and simmer, stirring often, for 1 minute. Let cool for about 20 minutes before using.

Shrimp with White Wine

Dinner is ready in under 30 minutes with this quick dish. Serve some steamed veggies and Oregano Potato Chips (page 297) alongside. Or, if you tolerate rice or pasta, serve this shrimp over top.

Kitchen Tips

If using frozen shrimp, thaw them overnight in the refrigerator first and drain well.

When cooking shrimp, let them sizzle for about 30 seconds, then stir, let them sizzle, then stir again. Make sure they're evenly cooked, but avoid overcooking.

1 tsp	olive oil	5 mL
1	shallot, minced	1
1	clove garlic, minced	1
3 tbsp	dry white wine	45 mL
12 oz	large shrimp, peeled and deveined	375 g
1 tbsp	chopped fresh parsley	15 mL
1/8 tsp	salt (or to taste)	0.5 mL
	Freshly ground black pepper	

1. In a medium nonstick skillet, heat oil over medium-high heat. Sauté shallot and garlic for 1 minute. Add wine and simmer for 30 seconds. Stir in shrimp and simmer, stirring often, for 2 minutes or until pink and opaque. Remove from heat and stir in parsley. Season with up to 1/8 tsp (0.5 mL) salt and pepper to taste.

Nutrients
PER SERVING

Calories	128
Fat	2.8 g
Sodium	200 mg
Carbohydrate	3.2 g
Fiber	0.1 g
Sugar	0.4 g
Protein	19.4 g
Calcium	56 mg
Iron	2.5 mg

Seafood Medley

The tarragon adds the finishing touch to this nourishing and tasty assortment of seafood.

Kitchen Tips

Thaw frozen seafood overnight in the refrigerator.

If you can't find reduced-sodium fish stock, substitute Vegetable Stock (page 181) or reduced-sodium vegetable broth.

This dish freezes well. Transfer individual portions to airtight containers and freeze for up to 4 months. Be sure to leave some room for expansion.

1 tbsp	olive oil	15 mL
½ cup	finely chopped onion	125 mL
½ cup	finely chopped celery	125 mL
1½ tbsp	all-purpose flour	22 mL
3 cups	reduced-sodium fish stock	750 mL
3	cloves garlic, minced	3
3 tbsp	tomato paste	45 mL
1 lb	frozen mixed seafood, thawed and rinsed	500 g
2 tsp	chopped fresh tarragon	10 mL
	Freshly ground black pepper	

1. In a pot, heat oil over medium heat. Sauté onion and celery for 2 minutes or until starting to soften. Sprinkle with flour and cook, stirring constantly, for 30 seconds.

2. Gradually stir in stock. Stir in garlic and tomato paste; bring to a boil. Reduce heat and simmer, stirring often, for 5 minutes. Add seafood and simmer, stirring occasionally, for 8 minutes. Add tarragon and pepper to taste; simmer for 2 minutes or until seafood is firm and opaque.

Variations

You can add fresh mussels in the shell with the mixed seafood. Mussels are cooked when the shells open (discard any that do not open). Sprinkle each serving with chopped fresh parsley

Add ½ cup (125 mL) thawed frozen corn kernels with the seafood.

Nutrients
PER SERVING

Calories	239
Fat	7.7 g
Sodium	194 mg
Carbohydrate	14.7 g
Fiber	2.7 g
Sugar	4.2 g
Protein	27.0 g
Calcium	107 mg
Iron	2.4 mg

Curried Seafood

Makes 6 servings

Diet Stage 4

Curry powder, a blend of up to 20 ground spices, varies in its degree of spiciness. Using mild curry powder in this seafood medley means it's packed with flavor but not too spicy. If you tolerate spice, you can use a spicier curry powder.

Kitchen Tips

This curry freezes well. Transfer individual portions to airtight containers and freeze for up to 4 months. Be sure to leave some room for expansion.

If you can't find reduced-sodium fish stock, substitute Vegetable Stock (page 181) or reduced-sodium vegetable broth.

2 tsp	canola oil	10 mL
½ cup	sliced leek (white and light green part only)	125 mL
½ cup	diced peeled potato	125 mL
3 tbsp	mild curry powder	45 mL
1 tsp	dried parsley	5 mL
¼ tsp	ground fennel seeds	1 mL
1½ cups	reduced-sodium fish stock	375 mL
2 tsp	freshly squeezed lemon juice	10 mL
1 lb	frozen mixed seafood, thawed and rinsed	500 g
¾ cup	thawed frozen corn kernels (optional)	175 mL
1½ tbsp	cornstarch	22 mL
¾ cup	skim milk	175 mL
	Freshly ground black pepper	

1. In a large pot, heat oil over medium-high heat. Sauté leeks for 1 minute. Add potato, curry powder, parsley, fennel, fish stock and lemon juice; bring to a boil. Reduce heat and simmer for 15 minutes or until potatoes start to soften.

2. Stir in seafood and corn (if using); increase heat to medium-high and bring to a boil. Reduce heat and simmer, stirring occasionally, for 10 minutes or until seafood is firm and opaque.

3. Place cornstarch in a small bowl. Gradually add milk, whisking until smooth. Stir into pot, increase heat to medium and cook, stirring often, for 2 minutes or until sauce thickens. Season to taste with pepper.

Nutrients
PER SERVING

Calories	158
Fat	4.4 g
Sodium	144 mg
Carbohydrate	11.2 g
Fiber	2.0 g
Sugar	2.7 g
Protein	18.5 g
Calcium	99 mg
Iron	2.2 mg

Vegetarian and Vegan Entrées

Some people choose to become vegetarian; others are raised to eat vegetarian foods for cultural or religious reasons. A vegetarian diet can be healthy as long as some general guidelines are followed. Refer to page 65 for tips on ensuring a nutritious vegetarian diet.

Even those who are not vegetarian can enjoy vegetarian meals as part of a well-balanced diet. After weight-loss surgery, vegetarian options provide an alternative to meat and poultry dishes, which can be difficult to tolerate.

Basic Instructions for Cooking Dried Beans

Pick through beans to remove any stones or foreign objects. Place beans in a strainer and rinse thoroughly with cold water. Transfer beans to a bowl of fresh cold water (enough to cover the beans), cover and let soak at room temperature for at least 3 hours or overnight. Drain water and rinse beans well. Place beans in a saucepan and add enough water to cover the beans by 2 inches (5 cm). Bring to a boil, then reduce heat to low and simmer for 1 to 2 hours or until beans are tender. (The cooking time will depend on how long the beans were soaked, the size of the beans and the type of bean.) Drain and rinse well.

Vegetarian Chili

Your family and friends will never guess that this chili is vegetarian — and so good for you!

Kitchen Tips

One 19-oz (540 mL) can of kidney beans yields about 2 cups (500 mL).

This chili freezes well. Let cool, then transfer individual portions to airtight containers and freeze for up to 4 months. Be sure to leave some room for expansion.

Weight-Loss Surgery Tip

To add more protein, stir 1 scoop of unflavored protein powder into each serving.

2 tsp	olive oil	10 mL
2	cloves garlic, minced	2
1	onion, chopped	1
1	zucchini, peeled, seeded and chopped	1
1	green or red bell pepper, chopped	1
1	can (28 oz/796 mL) reduced-sodium diced tomatoes	1
2 tsp	chili powder	10 mL
1 tsp	ground cumin	5 mL
½ tsp	dried oregano	2 mL
½ tsp	freshly ground black pepper	2 mL
2 cups	drained rinsed canned red kidney beans	500 mL
¾ cup	thawed frozen corn kernels	175 mL
1	package (12 oz/340 g) simulated ground beef (such as Veggie Ground Round)	1

1. In a large pot, heat oil over medium heat. Sauté garlic, onion, zucchini and green pepper for 6 minutes or until tender.

2. Stir in tomatoes, chili powder, cumin, oregano and pepper; bring to a gentle boil. Reduce heat and simmer, stirring occasionally, for 10 minutes. Add beans and corn; simmer, stirring occasionally, for 8 minutes. Add simulated beef and simmer, stirring occasionally, for 2 minutes.

Nutrients
PER SERVING

Calories	93
Fat	1.4 g
Sodium	16 mg
Carbohydrate	16.1 g
Fiber	5.9 g
Sugar	2.7 g
Protein	4.7 g
Calcium	12 mg
Iron	0.4 mg

Baby Lima Bean Stew

*People tend to shy away
from dried beans, thinking
they are too difficult to
prepare. This recipe is
easy to make — you just
need some time to let the
beans soak.*

Kitchen Tips

Lima beans contain protein,
iron, potassium and fiber.
They are also known as
butter beans, because they
have a nice, natural buttery
taste to them. If you cannot
find baby lima beans, use
large lima beans instead (you
may need to increase the
cooking time slightly).

The time it takes to cook the
beans depends on how long
they are soaked, so keep
checking them for doneness
as they cook.

1 cup	dried baby lima beans	250 mL
1 tsp	canola oil	5 mL
1	large onion, chopped	1
1	carrot, sliced	1
1	potato, peeled and chopped	1
1	clove garlic, minced	1
2 tbsp	tomato paste	30 mL
2 tbsp	chopped fresh parsley	30 mL
1/4 tsp	salt (or to taste)	1 mL
	Freshly ground black pepper	

1. Place beans in a large bowl and add enough cold water to cover by at least 3 inches (7.5 cm). Cover and let soak overnight.

2. Drain beans and transfer beans to a large pot. Add enough fresh water to cover beans by 2 inches (5 cm). Bring to a boil over high heat. Reduce heat and simmer for 45 to 60 minutes or until beans are tender. Drain and rinse.

3. Meanwhile, in a large nonstick skillet, heat oil over medium heat. Sauté onion, carrot and potato for about 5 minutes or until onion is softened. Stir in garlic, 1/4 cup (60 mL) water and tomato paste. Cook, stirring often and adding 1/4 cup (60 mL) water every 5 minutes, for about 40 minutes or until vegetables are soft but sauce remains somewhat thick.

4. Add cooked beans to vegetable mixture and remove from heat. Stir in parsley. Season with up to 1/4 tsp (1 mL) salt and pepper to taste.

Nutrients
PER SERVING

Calories	157
Fat	1.2 g
Sodium	116 mg
Carbohydrate	29.9 g
Fiber	8.3 g
Sugar	5.1 g
Protein	8.0 g
Calcium	43 mg
Iron	2.5 mg

Cuban Black Beans

Makes 6 servings

Mid Diet Stage 3 to
Diet Stage 4

*Beans are a culinary
element found throughout
the Caribbean. Serve this
dish on its own or alongside
some steamed rice for a
traditional tropical meal.*

Kitchen Tips

One 19-oz (540 mL)
can of black beans yields
about 2 cups (500 mL). If
you use 2 smaller cans or
1 larger can, measure 2 cups
(500 mL), then refrigerate
any extras in an airtight
container for up to 3 days or
freeze for up to 3 months.

Instead of canned black
beans, use the instructions
on page 257 to cook dried
black beans. You'll need
about 1 cup (250 mL)
dried beans to make 2 cups
(500 mL) cooked.

Nutrients PER SERVING	
Calories	97
Fat	2.2 g
Sodium	272 mg
Carbohydrate	14.6 g
Fiber	4.3 g
Sugar	1.2 g
Protein	4.5 g
Calcium	50 mg
Iron	1.5 mg

2 tsp	olive oil	10 mL
1	small onion, chopped	1
½	red bell pepper, chopped	½
2	cloves garlic, minced	2
1 tbsp	dried oregano	15 mL
1 tbsp	white vinegar	15 mL
2 cups	drained rinsed canned black beans	500 mL
½ cup	Vegetable Stock (see recipe, page 181) or reduced-sodium vegetable broth	125 mL
	Salt and freshly ground black pepper (optional)	

1. In a large nonstick skillet, heat oil over medium heat. Sauté onion and red pepper for 4 minutes. Add garlic and oregano; sauté for 30 seconds. Add vinegar and cook, stirring, for 30 seconds.
2. Stir in beans and stock; reduce heat and simmer, stirring occasionally, for about 10 minutes or until beans are hot and mixture is slightly thickened. If desired, season to taste with salt and pepper to taste.

Black Beans with Sweet Potato

Late Diet Stage 3 to Diet Stage 4

This economical dish is packed with protein and fiber, easy to make and tastes great.

1 tsp	canola oil	5 mL
2½ cups	diced peeled sweet potatoes	625 mL
1	onion, chopped	1
⅓ cup	water	75 mL
2 cups	drained rinsed canned black beans (see tips, page 260)	500 mL
1 tsp	ground cumin	5 mL
½ tsp	ground coriander	2 mL
½ tsp	ground cinnamon	2 mL
⅛ tsp	salt (optional)	0.5 mL

1. In a large nonstick skillet, heat oil over medium heat. Sauté sweet potatoes and onion for 10 minutes or until potatoes start to soften. Add water and boil for about 10 minutes or until sweet potatoes are tender. Drain off any excess water.

2. Stir in beans, cumin, coriander and cinnamon; cook, stirring occasionally, for 5 minutes or until beans are heated through. If desired, season with up to ⅛ tsp (0.5 mL) salt.

Variation

During diet stage 4, turn this recipe into a wrap. Spoon about ¼ cup (60 mL) bean mixture down the center of a small whole wheat flour tortilla. Sprinkle with 1 tbsp (15 mL) shredded light Cheddar cheese and roll up. Place on a baking sheet lined with foil and bake in a 350°F (180°C) oven for 5 to 7 minutes or until wrap is warmed and cheese is melted.

Nutrients
PER SERVING

Calories	196
Fat	1.8 g
Sodium	448 mg
Carbohydrate	36.8 g
Fiber	8.3 g
Sugar	4.7 g
Protein	7.7 g
Calcium	79 mg
Iron	2.2 mg

Mixed Bean Salad with Hemp

Makes 4 servings

Diet Stage 4

Hemp seed oil is rich in omega-3 and omega-6 fatty acids and provides a pleasant, nutty flavor — the perfect finishing touch to this mixed bean salad, which tastes even better the next day.

Kitchen Tip

One 19-oz (540 mL) can of mixed beans yields about 2 cups (500 mL). If you use 2 smaller cans or 1 larger can, measure 2 cups (500 mL), then refrigerate any extras in an airtight container for up to 3 days or freeze for up to 3 months.

2 tsp	balsamic vinegar	10 mL
2 tsp	hemp seed oil	10 mL
1 tsp	olive oil	5 mL
½ tsp	ground cumin	2 mL
3	green onions, thinly sliced	3
3	stalks celery, diced	3
1	carrot, diced	1
¼ cup	finely chopped red onion	60 mL
2 tbsp	finely chopped fresh cilantro or parsley	30 mL
2 cups	drained rinsed canned mixed beans	500 mL
	Salt and freshly ground black pepper (optional)	

1. In a medium bowl, whisk together vinegar, hemp seed oil, olive oil and cumin. Stir in green onions, celery, carrot, red onion and cilantro. Stir in beans. If desired, season to taste with salt and pepper. Cover and refrigerate for at least 1 hour or overnight to blend the flavors.

Variation

This recipe is versatile: use any type of bean and sub in different vegetables to make a variety of delicious bean salads. For the veggies, try chopped cooked yellow or green beans, diced zucchini, diced red or green bell peppers and/or chopped tomatoes.

Nutrients
PER SERVING

Calories	184
Fat	4.6 g
Sodium	481 mg
Carbohydrate	28.2 g
Fiber	8.6 g
Sugar	2.6 g
Protein	8.8 g
Calcium	71 mg
Iron	2.2 mg

Lentil-Stuffed Zucchini

Late Diet Stage 3 to
Diet Stage 4

These lentil-stuffed zucchini boats are a pleasure to serve and a cinch to make.

Kitchen Tips

Save the flesh you scoop out of the zucchini and add it to your favorite soup or stew.

If desired, you can gently mash the lentil mixture before filling the zucchini.

- **Preheat oven to 350°F (180°C)**
- **11- by 7-inch (28 by 18 cm) glass baking dish, lightly sprayed with light nonstick cooking spray**

4	zucchini, cut in half lengthwise	4
¾ cup	cooked brown lentils	175 mL
½ cup	diced tomato	125 mL
¼ cup	finely chopped onion	60 mL
1 tsp	chopped fresh parsley	5 mL
¼ tsp	mild curry powder	1 mL
¼ tsp	salt (or to taste)	1 mL

1. Using a teaspoon or melon baller, scoop out the center of each zucchini half, leaving ¼-inch (0.5 cm) thick walls. Set aside.

2. In a medium bowl, combine lentils, tomato, onion, parsley and curry powder. Season with up to ¼ tsp (1 mL) salt.

3. Divide lentil mixture evenly among zucchini halves. Arrange in a single layer in prepared baking dish.

4. Cover and bake in preheated oven for 1 hour or until zucchini are tender.

Variations

Sprinkle with 3 tbsp (45 mL) seasoned dry bread crumbs before baking.

Sprinkle each stuffed zucchini with about ¼ tsp (1 mL) grated light Parmesan cheese just before serving.

Substitute garlic powder or ground cumin for the curry powder.

Add 1 minced garlic clove to the lentil mixture.

Nutrients
PER SERVING

Calories	62
Fat	0.4 g
Sodium	220 mg
Carbohydrate	11.1 g
Fiber	2.1 g
Sugar	1.4 g
Protein	4.2 g
Calcium	16 mg
Iron	1.4 mg

Edamame with Yellow Pepper and Radish

Edamame are fresh soybeans. This cold vegetarian dish is hearty and packed with nutrition, so it makes a great meal all on its own.

Kitchen Tips

Wasabi powder can be found in the Asian foods aisle of well-stocked grocery stores and at Asian markets.

Omit the wasabi powder if it is too spicy for you to tolerate.

2 cups	water	500 mL
I cup	frozen shelled edamame	250 mL
	Salt	
I tsp	minced gingerroot	5 mL
¼ tsp	wasabi powder (optional)	I mL
I tbsp	rice vinegar	15 mL
I tsp	sesame oil	5 mL
I tsp	canola oil	5 mL
3	radishes, thinly sliced	3
I	green onion, thinly sliced	I
½ cup	finely chopped yellow bell pepper	125 mL
¼ cup	diced celery	60 mL

1. In a small pot, bring water to a boil over high heat. Add edamame and ⅛ tsp (0.5 mL) salt; reduce heat and simmer for about 10 minutes or until edamame are tender. Drain and set aside.

2. In a medium bowl, combine ginger, wasabi powder (if using), vinegar, sesame oil and canola oil. Add cooked edamame, radishes, green onion, yellow pepper and celery; toss to coat. If desired, season to taste with salt. Cover and refrigerate for at least 1 hour or overnight to blend the flavors.

Nutrients
PER SERVING

Calories	69
Fat	3.5 g
Sodium	117 mg
Carbohydrate	5.9 g
Fiber	2.3 g
Sugar	2.1 g
Protein	4.4 g
Calcium	35 mg
Iron	1.0 mg

Szechuan Tofu Stir-Fry

Coating the tofu in cornstarch before cooking gives it a light and crispy crust. The tofu takes on the flavor of the low-sugar Szechuan sauce.

Kitchen Tip

Another way to coat the tofu with cornstarch is to add both to a sealable food storage bag, seal and shake.

Szechuan Sauce

2 tsp	granulated sucralose artificial sweetener, such as Splenda	10 mL
1 tsp	cornstarch	5 mL
1/4 tsp	hot pepper flakes	1 mL
1/4 cup	reduced-sodium soy sauce	60 mL
1/4 cup	water	60 mL
1 tbsp	tomato paste	15 mL
2 tsp	balsamic vinegar	10 mL

Stir-Fry

2 tbsp	cornstarch	30 mL
1	package (14 oz/400 g) extra-firm tofu, drained and cut into 1-inch (2.5 cm) cubes	1
2 tsp	canola oil, divided	10 mL
3	cloves garlic, minced	3
2 1/2 cups	green beans	625 mL
2 tsp	minced gingerroot	10 mL
1/4 cup	water	60 mL

1. *Sauce:* In a small bowl, whisk together sweetener, cornstarch, hot pepper flakes, soy sauce, water, tomato paste and vinegar. Set aside.

2. *Stir-fry:* Place cornstarch on a large plate. Add tofu and turn to coat.

3. In a large nonstick skillet, heat 1 tsp (5 mL) oil over medium-high heat. Arrange tofu in a single layer and cook, undisturbed, for 2 minutes. Turn tofu over and cook, gently stirring occasionally, for 2 to 3 minutes or until golden brown on all sides. Transfer tofu to a plate.

4. Add the remaining oil to the skillet and heat over medium-high heat. Stir-fry garlic, green beans and ginger for 1 minute. Add water, cover and cook for 2 to 4 minutes or until beans are tender-crisp. Add reserved sauce and cook, stirring often, for 1 minute or until thickened. Return tofu to the pan and stir-fry for about 1 minute or until heated through.

Nutrients
PER SERVING

Calories	166
Fat	7.5 g
Sodium	544 mg
Carbohydrate	15.2 g
Fiber	4.0 g
Sugar	1.8 g
Protein	11.3 g
Calcium	225 mg
Iron	3.1 mg

Eggplant, Tofu and Spinach Lasagna

Makes 8 servings

Late Diet Stage 3 to Diet Stage 4

While you're waiting for the eggplant to soften, go outside for a 20-minute walk. When you get home, you'll be ready to make this nutrient-rich vegan lasagna.

- **Preheat oven to 375°F (190°C)**
- **Food processor or immersion blender**
- **11- by 7-inch (28 by 18 cm) glass baking dish, lightly sprayed with light nonstick cooking spray**

1	eggplant	1
1 tsp	salt	5 mL
8 oz	firm tofu, drained	250 g
5 oz	frozen spinach, thawed and excess water squeezed out	150 g
1	clove garlic	1
½ tsp	dried oregano	2 mL
½ tsp	dried basil	2 mL
⅛ tsp	salt (or to taste)	0.5 mL
	Freshly ground black pepper	
1½ cups	Tomato Basil Sauce (see recipe, page 272)	375 mL

1. Cut off stems and slice eggplant lengthwise into ¼-inch (0.5 cm) thick slices. Sprinkle each slice with salt and place in a large bowl. Let stand for 1 hour. Dry eggplant with a paper towel.

2. In a food processor or using an immersion blender, process tofu, spinach, garlic, oregano and basil until combined. Season with up to ⅛ tsp (0.5 mL) salt and pepper to taste.

3. Pour half the tomato sauce into prepared baking dish. Arrange one-third of the eggplant slices on top, trimming to fit as necessary. Spread half the tofu mixture over eggplant. Repeat layers. Arrange the remaining eggplant on top. Top with the remaining tomato sauce.

4. Cover and bake in preheated oven for 30 minutes. Uncover and bake for 10 to 20 minutes or until eggplant is tender.

Nutrients
PER SERVING

Calories	61
Fat	1.9 g
Sodium	425 mg
Carbohydrate	7.6 g
Fiber	3.0 g
Sugar	1.9 g
Protein	4.3 g
Calcium	93 mg
Iron	1.2 mg

Tofu Patties

These patties are completely vegan and packed with nutrition.

Kitchen Tip

Look for tofu enriched with calcium.

- **Preheat oven to 325°F (160°C)**
- **Rimmed baking sheet, lightly sprayed with light nonstick cooking spray**

10 oz	firm tofu, drained and mashed	300 g
¾ cup	quick-cooking rolled oats	175 mL
2 tbsp	reduced-sodium soy sauce	30 mL
½ tsp	dried basil	2 mL
½ tsp	dried oregano	2 mL
½ tsp	garlic powder	2 mL
½ tsp	onion powder	2 mL
	Freshly ground black pepper	

1. In a medium bowl, combine tofu, oats, soy sauce, basil, oregano, garlic powder, onion powder and pepper to taste. Knead for a few minutes. Shape into 6 patties, about 1 inch (2.5 cm) thick. Place on prepared baking sheet.

2. Bake in preheated oven for 20 to 25 minutes, flipping patties halfway through, until lightly browned.

Nutrients
PER SERVING

Calories	91
Fat	3.3 g
Sodium	178 mg
Carbohydrate	9.3 g
Fiber	1.4 g
Sugar	0.5 g
Protein	6.3 g
Calcium	106 mg
Iron	1.5 mg

Portobello Mushroom Burgers

These burgers are moist and packed with flavor.

Kitchen Tips

If desired, top each burger with 1 tbsp (15 mL) light shredded cheese.

These burgers can also be grilled on the barbecue. Spray the grill with light nonstick cooking spray and preheat to medium-high. Grill, turning once, for 3 minutes per side or until firm and hot in the center.

You can use seasoned dry bread crumbs in place of the whole wheat bread crumbs.

For more information on texturized vegetable protein, see page 97.

Nutrients
PER SERVING

Calories	137
Fat	4.3 g
Sodium	353 mg
Carbohydrate	15.1 g
Fiber	3.0 g
Sugar	2.9 g
Protein	9.3 g
Calcium	73 mg
Iron	2.5 mg

- **Preheat oven to 350°F (180°C)**
- **Food processor**
- **Rimmed baking sheet, lightly sprayed with light nonstick cooking spray**

1/2 cup	texturized vegetable protein (TVP) granules	125 mL
1/4 cup	boiling water	60 mL
1 tbsp	canola oil	15 mL
1/4 cup	chopped onion	60 mL
1	portobello mushroom, stem removed, chopped	1
1	egg white, lightly beaten	1
1 tbsp	chopped fresh parsley	15 mL
1/4 tsp	dried thyme	1 mL
1/8 tsp	garlic powder	0.5 mL
1/8 tsp	dried oregano	0.5 mL
1/2 cup	dry whole wheat bread crumbs	125 mL
1/8 tsp	salt (or to taste)	0.5 mL
	Freshly ground black pepper	

1. In a small bowl, combine TVP and boiling water. Let stand for 5 minutes or until TVP is rehydrated.

2. Meanwhile, in a nonstick skillet, heat oil over medium heat. Sauté onion for 2 minutes. Add mushroom and sauté for 2 minutes.

3. In food processor, pulse TVP, onion mixture, egg white, parsley, thyme, garlic powder and oregano until combined. Transfer to a large bowl and stir in bread crumbs. Season with up to 1/8 tsp (0.5 mL) salt and pepper to taste. Shape into 8 small patties, about 3/4 inch (2 cm) thick. Place on prepared baking sheet

4. Bake in preheated oven for 20 minutes, flipping patties halfway through, until firm and hot in the center.

Mini Crustless Broccoli and Cheese Quiche

Although by definition a quiche requires a crust, by eliminating the crust you save tons of fat and calories, making this vegetarian recipe that much healthier.

Kitchen Tip

You can also use twelve ¾-cup (175 mL) custard cups, sprayed with light cooking spray and lightly floured, in place of the muffin pan to bake these mini quiches. Adjust the cooking time to 35 to 40 minutes.

- **Preheat oven to 350°F (180°C)**
- **12-cup nonstick muffin pan, sprayed with light nonstick cooking spray and lightly floured**

2 tbsp	all-purpose flour	30 mL
1½ cups	skim milk	375 mL
3	eggs	3
2	egg whites	2
2 cups	frozen broccoli, thawed, drained and chopped	500 mL
1½ cups	shredded light Cheddar cheese	375 mL
½ cup	finely chopped red bell pepper	125 mL
⅛ tsp	ground nutmeg	0.5 mL
	Freshly ground black pepper	

1. Place flour in a large bowl and gradually add milk, whisking until smooth. Whisk in eggs and egg whites. Stir in broccoli, cheese, red pepper, nutmeg and pepper to taste.

2. Divide egg mixture equally among prepared muffin cups. Bake in preheated oven for 25 to 30 minutes or until a tester inserted in the center comes out clean. Let cool in pan on a wire rack for 10 minutes. Slide a knife around the edges of each muffin cup and gently remove quiches from pan.

Nutrients
PER SERVING

Calories	154
Fat	6.8 g
Sodium	298 mg
Carbohydrate	9.0 g
Fiber	1.3 g
Sugar	4.4 g
Protein	14.9 g
Calcium	300 mg
Iron	0.6 mg

Variations

Any type of vegetable will work in these quiches. Try 1 cup (250 mL) total of any combination of the following: chopped spinach, mushrooms, onions and/or green bell peppers.

Experiment with different low-fat or light cheeses, such as Havarti or Swiss.

Spinach and Leek Oven Frittata

A frittata is an oven-baked omelet with the ingredients mixed right into the egg rather than folded inside. This easy dish makes for a quick vegetarian dinner.

- **Preheat oven to 350°F (180°C)**
- **6-cup (1.5 L) baking dish, sprayed with light nonstick cooking spray**

1 tsp	olive oil	5 mL
1 cup	chopped leek (white and light green parts only)	250 mL
1/3 cup	chopped onion	75 mL
1 cup	chopped spinach	250 mL
1 tbsp	all-purpose flour	15 mL
3 tbsp	skim milk	45 mL
6	eggs, lightly beaten	6
1/3 cup	shredded light Cheddar cheese	75 mL
	Freshly ground black pepper	

1. In a medium nonstick skillet, heat oil over medium-high heat. Sauté leek and onion for 1 minute. Add spinach and sauté for about 1 minute or until starting to wilt. Remove from heat and set aside.

2. Place flour in a large bowl and gradually add milk, whisking until a smooth paste forms. Stir in eggs. Stir in leek mixture, cheese and pepper to taste. Pour into prepared baking dish.

3. Bake in preheated oven for about 30 minutes or until a tester inserted in the center comes out clean.

Nutrients
PER SERVING

Calories	107
Fat	6.2 g
Sodium	112 mg
Carbohydrate	5.3 g
Fiber	0.7 g
Sugar	1.7 g
Protein	8.1 g
Calcium	91 mg
Iron	1.3 mg

Pasta, Rice and Grains

Pasta, rice and grains provide important nutrition. Although some of these foods can initially be difficult to tolerate after weight-loss surgery, in the long term they can be enjoyed as part of a healthy, well-balanced diet. The recipes in this chapter will give you ideas on how to cook and prepare a variety of nutritious grains. Use the chart below as a guide to cooking rice and whole grains, and create your own interesting and delicious recipes.

Cooking with Rice and Whole Grains

To cook 1 cup (250 mL) of dry grains, combine the grains with the specified amount of water. Bring to a boil over high heat, then reduce heat to low, cover and simmer for the specified amount of time. Drain excess water, if necessary.

GRAIN (1 CUP/250 ML)	WATER	COOKING TIME
Barley, hulled (whole-grain)	3 cups (750 mL)	55 minutes
Barley, pearl	3 cups (750 mL)	45 minutes
Barley, pot	2 cups (500 mL)	35 minutes
Bulgur	2 cups (500 mL)	15 minutes
Millet	2½ cups (625 mL)	20 minutes
Oats, quick-cooking	2 cups (500 mL)	5 minutes
Oats, old-fashioned (large-flake)	4 cups (1 L)	5 minutes
Quinoa	2 cups (500 mL)	15 minutes
Rice, long-grain white	2 cups (500 mL)	25 minutes
Rice, long-grain brown	2½ cups (625 mL)	40 minutes
Rice, short-grain brown	2 cups (500 mL)	45 minutes
Wheat berries	3 cups (750 mL)	90 minutes
Wild rice	3 cups (750 mL)	45 minutes

Tomato Basil Sauce

Vegetables enhance both the flavor and the nutrition of this tomato sauce.

Kitchen Tips

For a quick dinner in diet stage 4, cook some whole wheat, brown rice or spelt pasta (such as penne). Top with sauce and sprinkle with grated light Parmesan cheese. Leftover pasta is delicious baked in the oven with some shredded light mozzarella cheese over top.

This sauce freezes well. Let the sauce cool, then transfer individual portions to airtight containers and freeze for up to 4 months. Be sure to leave room for expansion.

Nutrients PER SERVING	
Calories	21
Fat	0.4 g
Sodium	94 mg
Carbohydrate	4.4 g
Fiber	1.1 g
Sugar	0.6 g
Protein	0.9 g
Calcium	20 mg
Iron	0.6 mg

- **Food processor, blender or immersion blender**

1 tsp	olive oil	5 mL
3	cloves garlic, minced	3
1	large onion, finely chopped	1
1	carrot, finely chopped	1
1	stalk celery, finely chopped	1
1	can (28 oz/796 mL) reduced-sodium crushed tomatoes	1
3 tbsp	chopped fresh basil	45 mL
1 tbsp	Italian herb seasoning	15 mL
1/4 cup	water	60 mL
1 tbsp	tomato paste	15 mL
1/4 tsp	salt (or to taste)	1 mL
	Freshly ground black pepper	

1. In a large saucepan, heat oil over medium heat. Sauté garlic, onion, carrot and celery for 2 minutes.

2. Stir in tomatoes, basil, Italian seasoning, water and tomato paste; reduce heat to low, cover and simmer, stirring occasionally, for 30 minutes or until vegetables are soft and sauce is slightly thickened. Remove from heat and let cool for 20 minutes.

3. Working in batches, transfer soup to food processor (or use immersion blender in pot) and purée until smooth. Return to pot (if necessary) and season with up to 1/4 tsp (1 mL) salt and pepper to taste.

Variation

Substitute 1/2 cup (125 mL) chopped mushrooms or 1/2 cup (125 mL) chopped red bell pepper for either the carrot or the celery.

Tomato and Meat Sauce

*This tomato and meat sauce
is a tradition in my family.*

Kitchen Tips

In addition to using this
sauce for spaghetti or
lasagna, try serving it
over rice for a twist on
traditional rice.

This sauce freezes well. Let
the sauce cool, then transfer
individual portions to airtight
containers and freeze for
up to 2 months. Be sure to
leave room for expansion.

1 tsp	olive oil	5 mL
1	large onion, finely chopped	1
1 lb	extra-lean ground beef	500 g
1 cup	chopped mushrooms	250 mL
3	cloves garlic, minced	3
1	can (28 oz/796 mL) reduced-sodium crushed tomatoes	1
1 tbsp	Italian herb seasoning	15 mL
½ cup	water	125 mL
1 tbsp	tomato paste	15 mL
¼ tsp	salt (or to taste)	1 mL
	Freshly ground black pepper	

1. In a large saucepan, heat oil over medium-high heat. Sauté onion for 1 minute. Add beef and mushrooms; cook, breaking beef up with the back of a wooden spoon, for about 8 minutes or until beef is no longer pink.

2. Stir in garlic, tomatoes, Italian seasoning, water and tomato paste; reduce heat to low, cover and simmer, stirring occasionally, for 30 minutes or until sauce is thick. Season with up to ¼ tsp (1 mL) salt and pepper to taste.

Variation

Use any type of extra-lean ground meat in place of the ground beef.

Nutrients
PER SERVING

Calories	28
Fat	1.0 g
Sodium	41 mg
Carbohydrate	1.1 g
Fiber	0.3 g
Sugar	0.4 g
Protein	3.9 g
Calcium	6 mg
Iron	0.5 mg

Pad Thai with Brown Rice Noodles

Makes 6 servings

Diet Stage 4

Using brown rice noodles increases the fiber content of the classic pad Thai recipe. I've also reduced the fat by using tofu and egg whites, and reduced the sugar by using artificial sweetener. The result is a healthy lifelong meal choice. Leftovers taste even better.

Kitchen Tip

Make sure to use granulated sucralose artificial sweetener that measures like sugar, not the packets.

Nutrients PER SERVING	
Calories	206
Fat	6.9 g
Sodium	576 mg
Carbohydrate	21.5 g
Fiber	2.5 g
Sugar	1.4 g
Protein	16.9 g
Calcium	154 mg
Iron	2.0 mg

4 oz	brown rice noodles (see tip, at left)	125 g
4 cups	very warm water	1 L
3 tbsp	granulated sucralose artificial sweetener, such as Splenda	45 mL
1/4 tsp	hot pepper flakes (optional)	1 mL
1/4 cup	water	60 mL
2 tbsp	freshly squeezed lime juice	30 mL
1 1/2 tbsp	tomato paste	22 mL
1 1/2 tbsp	fish sauce (nam pla)	22 mL
1 tbsp	sesame oil	15 mL
1	package (14 oz/400 g) extra-firm tofu, drained and cut into 3/4-inch (2 cm) cubes	1
2	egg whites, lightly beaten	2
1	clove garlic, minced	1
3	green onions, thinly sliced	3
1 cup	bean sprouts	250 mL
2 tbsp	chopped unsalted peanuts (optional)	30 mL
2 tbsp	chopped fresh cilantro	30 mL
	Salt and freshly ground pepper (optional)	

1. In a large bowl, soak brown rice noodles in very warm water for about 30 minutes or until noodles are tender but not too soft. Drain and set aside.

2. Meanwhile, in a small bowl, combine sweetener, hot pepper flakes (if using), 1/4 cup (60 mL) water, lime juice, tomato paste and fish sauce. Set aside.

3. In a large nonstick skillet, heat oil over medium-high heat. Arrange tofu in a single layer and cook, undisturbed, for 2 minutes. Turn tofu over and cook, gently stirring occasionally, for 2 to 3 minutes or until golden brown on all sides. Transfer tofu to a large plate.

Kitchen Tip

Use the wider flat brown rice noodles. If you cannot find brown rice noodles in the Asian foods section of your grocery store, try a health food store or an Asian specialty market. Otherwise, use plain white rice noodles, vermicelli noodles, spelt noodles or whole wheat pasta, cooking them according to package directions.

Weight-Loss Surgery Tip

In the long term, most people can enjoy some amount of pasta or noodles after weight-loss surgery.

4. Add egg whites and garlic to the skillet and cook over medium heat, using a wooden spoon to scramble the eggs, for 1 to 2 minutes or until eggs are set. Add drained noodles and fish sauce mixture; cook, stirring often, for about 3 minutes or until noodles are tender. If the mixture is too dry, add water, 1 tbsp (15 mL) at a time, until the desired consistency is achieved.

5. Return tofu to the pan and stir in green onions, bean sprouts and peanuts (if using); cook, stirring, for 1 minute. Remove from heat and stir in cilantro. If desired, season to taste with salt and pepper.

Variations

Substitute 1 cup (250 mL) shredded cooked chicken or shrimp for the tofu and omit step 3.

Replace half the bean sprouts with $1/2$ cup (125 mL) shredded carrots.

Brown Rice with Black-Eyed Peas

This recipe is a variation on a traditional East Indian dish that combines rice and peas. Made with brown rice, vegetable stock and black-eyed peas, it makes an excellent accompaniment to your meal.

Kitchen Tip

For convenience, you can use rinsed drained canned black-eyed peas rather than cooking your own; heat before adding to rice.

I tsp	olive oil	5 mL
I	small onion, finely chopped	I
½ cup	long-grain brown rice	125 mL
I¼ cups	Vegetable Stock (see recipe, page 181) or reduced-sodium vegetable broth	300 mL
½ cup	dried black-eyed peas, cooked (see page 257) and hot	125 mL
⅛ tsp	salt (or to taste)	0.5 mL

1. In a medium saucepan, heat oil over medium heat. Sauté onion for 2 minutes or until lightly browned.

2. Stir in rice and stock; bring to a boil. Reduce heat to low, cover and simmer for 35 to 40 minutes or until stock is absorbed and rice is tender. Let stand for 10 minutes. Fluff rice with a fork, then gently stir in peas. Season with up to ⅛ tsp (0.5 mL) salt.

Variation

Any variety of rice and any type of beans can be used to make this recipe. See the chart on page 271 to determine the length of time and the amount of liquid you'll need to cook the rice. See page 257 for instructions on cooking dried beans.

Nutrients
PER SERVING

Calories	117
Fat	2.2 g
Sodium	77 mg
Carbohydrate	21.1 g
Fiber	3.0 g
Sugar	2.0 g
Protein	3.4 g
Calcium	26 mg
Iron	0.9 mg

Cucumber Mint Quinoa

The cucumber, mint and ginger in this recipe give the quinoa a refreshing and zingy flavor, making it a wonderful side dish on a warm summer day.

Kitchen Tips

Quinoa (pronounced *KEEN-wah*) is an ancient grain that has become popular because of its superior nutritional quality. Of all grains, it is the highest in protein.

You will need ⅓ cup (75 mL) raw quinoa and ⅔ cup (150 mL) water to make 1 cup (250 mL) cooked quinoa.

I	green onion, finely sliced	I
I tsp	minced gingerroot	5 mL
I tbsp	freshly squeezed lime juice	15 mL
2 tsp	olive oil	10 mL
I	small cucumber, peeled, seeded and diced	I
I cup	cooked quinoa (see page 271)	250 mL
I tbsp	finely chopped fresh mint	15 mL
¼ tsp	salt (or to taste)	1 mL

1. In a medium bowl, combine green onion, ginger, lime juice and oil. Stir in cucumber, quinoa and mint. Season with up to ¼ tsp (1 mL) salt. Cover and refrigerate for at least 1 hour or overnight to blend the flavors.

Variation

Use cooked couscous in place of the quinoa.

Add ½ cup (125 mL) cooked or rinsed drained canned chickpeas, firm tofu or cooked chicken breast to add protein.

Nutrients
PER SERVING

Calories	112
Fat	4.4 g
Sodium	200 mg
Carbohydrate	15.2 g
Fiber	2.3 g
Sugar	0.9 g
Protein	3.2 g
Calcium	23 mg
Iron	1.1 mg

Chickpea Couscous

Makes 4 servings

Diet Stage 4

This dish is filling enough to be enjoyed as a lunch meal on its own. Or reduce the portion and enjoy it alongside grilled chicken.

Kitchen Tips

Couscous is inexpensive, versatile and quick to prepare. Look for it with the pasta or the rice in your grocery store or bulk food store. It comes in both regular and whole wheat, and can be eaten cold, as in a salad, or warm, as in a stew. Prepared couscous is light and fluffy and takes on the flavors of the foods and spices it is cooked with.

Adjust the flavoring to your liking by increasing or decreasing the amount of cumin, paprika and lemon juice to taste.

Nutrients
PER SERVING

Calories	153
Fat	3.3 g
Sodium	214 mg
Carbohydrate	25.4 g
Fiber	3.5 g
Sugar	2.3 g
Protein	5.4 g
Calcium	33 mg
Iron	1.1 mg

• **6-cup (1.5 L) casserole dish or heatproof bowl with cover**

½ cup	couscous	125 mL
⅛ tsp	salt	0.5 mL
½ cup	boiling water	125 mL
1	small carrot, chopped	1
¼	red bell pepper, coarsely chopped	¼
¾ cup	coarsely chopped cooked or rinsed drained canned chickpeas	175 mL
1 tbsp	finely chopped red onion	15 mL
1 tbsp	finely chopped fresh cilantro	15 mL
1 ½ tsp	ground cumin	7 mL
¼ tsp	paprika	1 mL
1 tbsp	freshly squeezed lemon juice	15 mL
2 tsp	olive oil	10 mL

1. In casserole dish, combine couscous, salt and boiling water. Cover and let stand for about 5 minutes or until water is absorbed and couscous is tender. Fluff with a fork.

2. Stir in carrot, red pepper, chickpeas, red onion, cilantro, cumin, paprika, lemon juice and oil. Cover and refrigerate for at least 1 hour or overnight to blend the flavors.

Variation

Substitute other vegetables, such as chopped zucchini, tomato and/or green bell peppers for the carrot and red pepper.

Barley Pilaf with Onions and Mushrooms

Makes 4 servings

Diet Stage 4

Barley has been used for years in breads, cereal and soups. Hulled barley, also known as whole-grain barley, is the most nutritious variety, but it takes a long time to cook and is sometimes difficult to find. Pot barley is more widely available and still provides great nutrition. For this recipe, experiment with different varieties of barley, making sure to adjust the cooking time accordingly.

Kitchen Tips

Leave barley undisturbed while it's cooking.

Use any variety of mushrooms, such as cremini, oyster or shiitake, or a combination.

Nutrients PER SERVING	
Calories	94
Fat	2.3 g
Sodium	45 mg
Carbohydrate	13.9 g
Fiber	1.9 g
Sugar	4.4 g
Protein	5.3 g
Calcium	70 mg
Iron	0.6 mg

I tsp	olive oil	5 mL
I	small onion, finely chopped	I
I ½ cups	chopped mushrooms	375 mL
½ cup	pot barley	125 mL
I cup	Chicken Stock (see recipe, page 182) or reduced-sodium low-fat chicken broth	250 mL
	Salt and freshly ground black pepper (optional)	

1. In a medium saucepan, heat oil over medium heat. Sauté onion for 2 minutes. Add mushrooms and sauté for about 5 minutes or until starting to soften.

2. Stir in barley and stock; bring to a boil. Reduce heat to low, cover and simmer for 35 minutes or until barley is tender. Remove from heat and let stand for 10 minutes. Season to taste with salt and pepper (if using).

Khorasan Wheat with Bell Peppers

Makes 5 servings

Diet Stage 4

Khorasan is an ancient wheat grain, commonly known as Kamut, that is high in fiber and a good source of the antioxidant selenium. You can find khorasan wheat berries in the health-food section of your grocery store or in a specialty health food store.

Kitchen Tips

Try using tamari, a dark, rich fermented soy sauce in place of the soy sauce in this recipe.

Store leftovers in an airtight container in the refrigerator for up to 3 days. Enjoy cold or reheat leftovers in a small saucepan over medium-low heat for 3 to 4 minutes or until warmed through.

Nutrients
PER SERVING

Calories	87
Fat	1.4 g
Sodium	219 mg
Carbohydrate	16.1 g
Fiber	3.1 g
Sugar	1.1 g
Protein	3.7 g
Calcium	22 mg
Iron	1.2 mg

1 ½ cups	water	375 mL
½ cup	khorasan wheat berries (such as Kamut)	125 mL
1 tsp	olive oil	5 mL
½	red bell pepper, finely chopped	½
½	yellow bell pepper, finely chopped	½
½	small zucchini, finely chopped	½
2	green onions, thinly sliced	2
2 tbsp	reduced-sodium soy sauce	30 mL
2 tbsp	chopped fresh parsley or cilantro	30 mL

1. In a small pot, bring water to a boil over high heat. Add wheat berries, reduce heat to low, cover and simmer for about 45 minutes or until tender. Drain and set aside.

2. In a medium nonstick skillet, heat oil over medium-high heat. Sauté red pepper and yellow pepper for about 2 minutes or until starting to soften. Add zucchini and sauté for 1 to 2 minutes or until vegetables are tender. Stir in cooked wheat berries, green onions and soy sauce; cook, stirring, for 1 minute. Serve garnished with parsley.

Variation

Substitute 1 cup (250 mL) cooked hulled barley for the khorasan wheat berries. For instructions on cooking barley, see page 271.

Spinach Pinwheels

These vibrant little pinwheel sandwiches will impress guests, friends and family.

Kitchen Tips

These pinwheels make wonderful hors d'oeuvres. For an added touch, insert a small decorative wooden skewer in each.

If you cannot find unsweetened dried cranberries, use the sweetened variety. At the recommended serving size, your sugar intake will still be relatively low. As an alternative, try substituting dried goji berries (also known as wolfberries), which can be found in bulk or health food stores.

½ cup	chopped baby spinach	125 mL
¼ cup	light cream cheese, softened	60 mL
¼ cup	light ricotta cheese	60 mL
3 tbsp	chopped dried cranberries (preferably unsweetened)	45 mL
2 tbsp	chopped fresh chives	30 mL
2	10-inch (25 cm) spinach-flavored flour tortillas	2

1. In a bowl, combine spinach, cream cheese, ricotta cheese, cranberries and chives.

2. Lay tortillas on a cutting board. Spread half the spinach mixture over each tortilla. Tightly roll up tortillas. Using a very sharp knife, cut off the uneven edges and discard. Cut each rolled tortilla into 6 pinwheels, about $1\frac{1}{2}$ inches (4 cm) thick.

Variations

Use any flavor of flour tortilla, such as whole wheat or sun-dried tomato.

For more protein, lay 3 oz (90 g) thinly sliced deli smoked turkey over each tortilla before adding the spinach filling.

If you cannot tolerate the texture of dried cranberries, substitute any flavor of no-sugar-added fruit spread.

Nutrients
PER SERVING

Calories	111
Fat	4.7 g
Sodium	192 mg
Carbohydrate	12.9 g
Fiber	1.1 g
Sugar	4.0 g
Protein	4.6 g
Calcium	106 mg
Iron	0.3 mg

Greek Salad Pita Pockets

Makes 4 servings

Serving size: 2 pita pockets

Diet Stage 4

Serve these mini pita pockets alongside grilled chicken for a complete meal.

3 tbsp	Greek-style low-fat plain yogurt	45 mL
2 tsp	chopped fresh mint	10 mL
1	green onion, thinly sliced	1
1/4 cup	finely chopped tomato	60 mL
1/4 cup	finely chopped cucumber, peeled and seeded	60 mL
3 tbsp	crumbled light feta cheese	45 mL
1/4 tsp	olive oil	1 mL
1/8 tsp	dried oregano	0.5 mL
8	2-inch (5 cm) mini whole wheat pita pockets	8

1. In a small bowl, combine yogurt and mint. Set aside.
2. In a medium bowl, combine green onion, tomato, cucumber, feta, oil and oregano.
3. Make a small opening in each pita pocket. Spread yogurt mixture evenly in each pocket, coating both sides. Using a small spoon, fill each pocket with green onion mixture, dividing evenly. Serve immediately.

Variations

Instead of filling mini pita pockets, spread the yogurt mixture and green onion mixture over 7-inch (18 cm) whole wheat flour tortillas and make wraps.

For a Greek-style cold couscous salad, omit the pita pockets and combine all the other ingredients in a bowl with 1 cup (250 mL) cooled cooked couscous.

Nutrients
PER SERVING

Calories	103
Fat	2.1 g
Sodium	248 mg
Carbohydrate	17.5 g
Fiber	2.5 g
Sugar	1.5 g
Protein	4.8 g
Calcium	48 mg
Iron	1.0 mg

Side Dishes

Vegetables provide important nutrients and fiber, but most people find it time-consuming to prepare vegetable dishes other than peas, corn and carrots. With the recipes in this chapter, you will soon discover that vegetables are easy to make and can be quite flavorful. Aim to enjoy a variety of colorful vegetables daily for optimal nutrition.

When preparing vegetables to use in a recipe, plan ahead and chop a little extra. Store extra chopped veggies in an airtight container to use the next day in another recipe, to add to a salad or to enjoy as a snack. If you are in a rush, frozen vegetables or precut fresh vegetables can be substituted in the recipes.

If you choose to eat a starchy vegetable, such as potatoes, sweet potatoes or yams, at a meal, consider this your starch choice and avoid having another starch or grain, such as rice, pasta or bread.

The portion sizes in these recipes are set at about $\frac{1}{4}$ cup (60 mL); however, you can adjust the serving size depending on what else you are eating at a particular meal. For example, if you are having a 3-oz (90 g) serving of a protein-rich food and no starch, you can up your vegetable side dish portion to about $\frac{1}{2}$ cup (125 mL). But if you're having both a starch and a vegetable on the side, stick to $\frac{1}{4}$ cup (60 mL) of each. Remember, too, that the serving sizes are guidelines only; adjust them based on your needs.

When adding salt to taste, keep in mind that $\frac{1}{8}$ tsp (0.5 mL) contains 290 mg of sodium — that's 12% of the recommended daily maximum of 2,400 mg.

Beets with Parsley

Makes 8 servings

Diet Stage 4

Add color to your plate with this ruby red dish.

Kitchen Tips

Instead of using canned beets, you can steam 1¾ cups (425 mL) thinly sliced peeled fresh beets (about 1 large) for about 10 minutes or until tender.

For a slightly different flavor, try balsamic vinegar or freshly squeezed lemon juice in place of the red wine vinegar.

1	can (14 oz/398 mL) sliced beets, drained	1
½	red onion, thinly sliced	½
2 tbsp	red wine vinegar	30 mL
2 tsp	chopped fresh parsley	10 mL
	Salt and freshly ground black pepper (optional)	

1. In a medium bowl, combine beets, red onion, vinegar and parsley, tossing to coat. If desired, season to taste with salt and pepper. Cover and refrigerate for at least 1 hour, until chilled, or for up to 3 days.

Nutrients
PER SERVING

Calories	19
Fat	0.1 g
Sodium	28 mg
Carbohydrate	4.2 g
Fiber	0.8 g
Sugar	3.1 g
Protein	0.7 g
Calcium	8 mg
Iron	0.3 mg

Broccoli and Mushroom Stir-Fry

Enhance any entrée with this easy side dish that is filled with a multitude of vitamins and minerals.

Kitchen Tip

If you do not have a steamer basket, simply boil the broccoli in the same amount of water in a medium saucepan with a tight-fitting lid.

Weight-Loss Surgery Tip

Steam the broccoli a little longer if you require a softer texture.

- **Steamer basket**

1 cup	small florets broccoli (about 1 small head)	250 mL
½ tsp	canola oil	2 mL
¼	small onion, sliced	¼
1 cup	sliced mushrooms	250 mL
2 tsp	sliced gingerroot	10 mL
2 tsp	finely chopped fresh parsley	10 mL
	Salt and freshly ground black pepper (optional)	

1. In a pot, bring 1 inch (2.5 cm) of water to a boil over high heat. Place broccoli in steamer basket and set over boiling water. Cover and steam for 6 to 7 minutes or until tender.

2. Meanwhile, in a large nonstick skillet, heat oil over medium-high heat. Sauté onion for 2 minutes. Add mushrooms and ginger; sauté for about 4 minutes or until mushrooms are tender. Remove from heat and stir in broccoli and parsley. If desired, season to taste with salt and pepper.

Variation

Use cauliflower in place of the broccoli.

Nutrients
PER SERVING

Calories	11
Fat	0.5 g
Sodium	4 mg
Carbohydrate	1.4 g
Fiber	0.6 g
Sugar	0.3 g
Protein	0.8 g
Calcium	7 mg
Iron	0.2 mg

Cinnamon-Glazed Carrot Coins

The whole family will love these bright coins with their fun shape and scrumptious taste.

Kitchen Tips

The cooking time will vary depending on the size of the coins.

Try cutting the carrots on the diagonal for an elegant look.

Weight-Loss Surgery Tip

Steam the carrots a little longer if you require a softer texture.

• **Steamer basket**

8 oz	carrots, sliced into coins (about 1¼ cups/300 mL)	250 g
¼ tsp	ground cinnamon	1 mL
⅛ tsp	ground nutmeg	0.5 mL
½ tsp	margarine	2 mL

1. In a pot, bring 1 inch (2.5 cm) of water to a boil over high heat. Place carrots in steamer basket and set over boiling water. Reduce heat to medium, cover and steam for about 15 minutes or until tender.

2. Transfer carrots to a serving dish and stir in cinnamon, nutmeg and margarine.

Variation

Substitute parsnips for the carrots, or use half parsnips and half carrots.

Nutrients
PER SERVING

Calories	31
Fat	0.6 g
Sodium	48 mg
Carbohydrate	6.2 g
Fiber	1.9 g
Sugar	3.0 g
Protein	0.6 g
Calcium	22 mg
Iron	0.2 mg

Oven-Roasted Cauliflower

Simply delicious cauliflower is packed with fiber and vitamin C. For added fun and color, look for orange, green or purple varieties.

Kitchen Tip

Not drying off the cauliflower helps the seasonings coat it better.

- **Preheat oven to 425°F (220°C)**
- **Large rimmed baking sheet, lightly sprayed with light nonstick cooking spray**

3 cups	small cauliflower florets (about ¼ of a small head)	750 mL
I	clove garlic, minced	I
¼ cup	chopped onion	60 mL
¼ tsp	ground turmeric	I mL
¼ tsp	paprika	I mL
I tsp	olive oil	5 mL
	Salt and freshly ground black pepper (optional)	

1. Rinse cauliflower under cold running water, and do not dry. Place in a large bowl and add garlic, onion, turmeric, paprika and oil; toss to coat. Spread out in a single layer on prepared baking sheet.

2. Bake in preheated oven for 20 to 25 minutes, turning halfway through, until golden brown and tender. If desired, season to taste with salt and pepper.

Nutrients PER SERVING	
Calories	23
Fat	0.9 g
Sodium	15 mg
Carbohydrate	3.6 g
Fiber	1.4 g
Sugar	1.5 g
Protein	1.1 g
Calcium	14 mg
Iron	0.3 mg

Steamed Green Beans

This yummy, nutritious side dish is ready to eat in under 10 minutes.

Kitchen Tips

Serve these green beans warm or cold.

Instead of chopping the green beans, you can steam them whole, if you prefer.

Weight-Loss Surgery Tip

Steam the green beans a little longer if you require a softer texture.

- **Steamer basket**

8 oz	green beans, trimmed and cut into 1-inch (2.5 cm) pieces	250 g
1	clove garlic, minced (optional)	1
1 tsp	grated lemon zest	5 mL
1 tsp	freshly squeezed lemon juice	5 mL
	Salt and freshly ground black pepper (optional)	

1. In a pot, bring 1 inch (2.5 cm) of water to a boil over high heat. Place green beans in steamer basket and set over boiling water. Cover and steam for about 5 to 6 minutes or until tender-crisp.

2. Transfer green beans to a serving dish and stir in garlic (if using), lemon zest and lemon juice. If desired, season to taste with salt and pepper.

Nutrients
PER SERVING

Calories	19
Fat	0.1 g
Sodium	2 mg
Carbohydrate	4.5 g
Fiber	1.5 g
Sugar	2.0 g
Protein	1.0 g
Calcium	29 mg
Iron	0.6 mg

Herbed Parsnips

*Once you try these
appetizing parsnips, you are
sure to make them often.*

Kitchen Tips

Chop parsnips into 1-inch
(2.5 cm) pieces.

To make a simple parsnip
soup, transfer the cooked
parsnips to a blender
and add 1 cup (250 mL)
Vegetable Stock (see recipe,
page 181) or store-bought
reduced-sodium vegetable
broth; purée until smooth.
Transfer to a saucepan and
simmer over low heat until
warmed through.

- **Preheat oven to 425°F (220°C)**
- **4-cup (1 L) baking dish, lightly sprayed with light nonstick cooking spray**

8 oz	parsnips, chopped (about 1⅓ cups/325 mL)	250 g
1	clove garlic, minced	1
½ tsp	dried thyme	2 mL
½ tsp	canola oil	2 mL
	Salt and freshly ground black pepper (optional)	
1 tsp	no-sugar-added maple-flavored syrup	5 mL

1. In prepared baking dish, combine parsnips, garlic, thyme and oil, tossing to coat. If desired, season to taste with salt and pepper.
2. Cover and bake in preheated oven for 30 minutes or until parsnips are almost tender. Carefully turn parsnips and stir in syrup. Bake, uncovered, for 10 minutes or until golden brown and tender.

Variation

Substitute carrots for the parsnips.

Nutrients
PER SERVING

Calories	56
Fat	0.8 g
Sodium	9 mg
Carbohydrate	12.6 g
Fiber	2.2 g
Sugar	3.0 g
Protein	0.8 g
Calcium	26 mg
Iron	0.5 mg

Rapini with Garlic

Makes 8 servings

Diet Stage 4

Rapini, also known as Italian broccoli or rabe, has a distinct bitter flavor that makes this dish unique. It's a nice change from everyday greens.

Kitchen Tip

To prepare the rapini, cut off the tough stalks about 2 inches (5 cm) from the end. Roughly chop rapini into large pieces about 2 inches (5 cm) long.

Weight-Loss Surgery Tip

The tough, stringy rapini stalks may be difficult to tolerate initially. The florets should be okay when you're introducing cooked vegetables.

4 cups	water	1 L
1 lb	rapini, roughly chopped (see tip, at left)	500 g
1 tsp	olive oil	5 mL
3	cloves garlic, minced	3
	Hot pepper flakes (optional)	
	Salt and freshly ground black pepper (optional)	

1. In a pot, bring water to a boil over high heat. Add rapini, reduce heat and simmer for 8 minutes or until tender-crisp. Drain and rinse under cold water. Squeeze out as much excess water as you can.

2. In a large nonstick skillet, heat oil over medium-high heat. Sauté garlic for 30 seconds. Stir in rapini and sauté for about 2 minutes or until warmed through. If desired, season to taste with hot pepper flakes, salt and black pepper.

Variation

Sauté $1/2$ onion, thinly sliced, for 2 minutes before adding the garlic.

Nutrients
PER SERVING

Calories	25
Fat	0.6 g
Sodium	22 mg
Carbohydrate	3.3 g
Fiber	0 g
Sugar	0.8 g
Protein	2.3 g
Calcium	35 mg
Iron	0.6 mg

Root Medley

*Toss these tubers together
and bring this dish to
a potluck — everyone
will rave!*

Kitchen Tips

If you do not have a lid for
your baking dish, use foil to
cover it.

To use up leftovers and
make a simple root soup
that is beet red, transfer
1½ cups (325 mL) cooked
roots to a blender and
add 1 cup (250 mL)
Vegetable Stock (see recipe,
page 181) or store-bought
reduced-sodium vegetable
broth; purée until smooth.
Transfer to a saucepan and
simmer over low heat until
warmed through.

Nutrients
PER SERVING

Calories	28
Fat	0.8 g
Sodium	60 mg
Carbohydrate	5.3 g
Fiber	0.8 g
Sugar	1.7 g
Protein	0.5 g
Calcium	11 mg
Iron	0.2 mg

- **Preheat oven to 400°F (200°C)**
- **12-cup (3 L) casserole dish**

6	white pearl onions, peeled	6
3	cloves garlic, minced	3
1	turnip, peeled and cut into ¾-inch (2 cm) cubes	1
1	parsnip, peeled and cut into ¾-inch (2 cm) thick slices	1
1	large beet, peeled and cut into thick wedges	1
1 cup	baby carrots	250 mL
1½ tsp	dried herbes de Provence	7 mL
1 tbsp	no-sugar-added maple-flavored syrup	15 mL
2 tsp	olive oil	10 mL
	Salt and freshly ground black pepper (optional)	

1. In casserole dish, combine onions, garlic, turnip, parsnip, beet, carrots, herbes de Provence, syrup and oil.

2. Cover and bake in preheated oven for 40 minutes or until tender. Uncover and broil for 3 to 5 minutes or until golden brown. If desired, season to taste with salt and pepper.

Variation

Use any combination of root and/or tuber vegetables. Try rutabaga, yams, sweet potato and/or cassava.

Rutabaga Fries

*Crispy with a bite, these
fries will quickly become
your favorite side dish.*

- **Preheat oven to 400°F (200°C)**
- **Steamer basket**
- **Large rimmed baking sheet, lightly sprayed
  with light nonstick cooking spray**

I lb	rutabaga, peeled and cut into ½-inch (1 cm) thick spears	500 g
⅛ tsp	garlic powder	0.5 mL
I tsp	olive oil	5 mL
⅛ tsp	coarse sea salt (or to taste)	0.5 mL

1. In a pot, bring 1 inch (2.5 cm) of water to a boil over high heat. Place rutabaga in steamer basket and set over boiling water. Cover and steam for 10 minutes or until starting to soften.

2. Transfer to a large bowl and, using a paper towel, pat rutabaga dry. Add garlic powder and oil; toss to coat. Spread out in a single layer on prepared baking sheet.

3. Bake in preheated oven for 30 minutes, turning halfway through, until golden brown and tender. Season with up to ⅛ tsp (0.5 mL) salt.

Variation

Use any herb or spice of your choice, such as dried oregano, ground turmeric, paprika, dried herbes de Provence or Chinese five-spice powder, in place of the garlic powder.

Nutrients
PER SERVING

Calories	26
Fat	0.7 g
Sodium	61 mg
Carbohydrate	4.6 g
Fiber	1.4 g
Sugar	3.2 g
Protein	0.7 g
Calcium	27 mg
Iron	0.3 mg

Oven-Baked Sweet Potatoes

Late Diet Stage 3 to Diet Stage 4

These cubed sweet potatoes are just the thing to serve with any meat entrée.

- **Preheat oven to 400°F (200°C)**
- **Small rimmed baking sheet, lightly sprayed with light nonstick cooking spray**

1 ½ cups	cubed peeled sweet potato (1-inch/2.5 cm cubes)	375 mL
⅛ tsp	ground nutmeg	0.5 mL
½ tsp	freshly squeezed lemon juice	2 mL
¼ tsp	olive oil	1 mL
1 tbsp	no-sugar-added maple-flavored syrup	15 mL
⅛ tsp	grated orange zest	0.5 mL

1. In a medium bowl, combine sweet potato, nutmeg, lemon juice and oil, tossing to coat. Spread out in a single layer on prepared baking sheet.

2. Cover with foil and bake in preheated oven for 15 minutes. Remove foil and bake for 30 minutes, turning halfway through, until golden brown and tender.

3. Transfer sweet potatoes to a serving dish, drizzle with syrup and sprinkle with orange zest.

Nutrients
PER SERVING

Calories	22
Fat	0.2 g
Sodium	14 mg
Carbohydrate	5.4 g
Fiber	0.5 g
Sugar	0.7 g
Protein	0.3 g
Calcium	5 mg
Iron	0.1 mg

Cauliflower Mashed Potatoes

2	potatoes, peeled and cubed	2
4 cups	cold water	1 L
1/4 cup	Cauliflower Purée (see recipe, below)	60 mL
1/4 cup	skim milk	60 mL
1 tbsp	margarine	15 mL
1 tbsp	chopped fresh chives (optional)	15 mL
	Salt and freshly ground black pepper (optional)	

1. In a medium saucepan, combine potatoes and cold water. Bring to a boil over high heat. Reduce heat to medium and cook for about 20 minutes or until potatoes are tender. Drain and return to pot.
2. Add cauliflower purée, milk and margarine. Mash together with a potato masher. Stir in chives (if using). If desired, season to taste with salt and pepper.

Cauliflower Purée

• **Blender or food processor**

1/2 cup	water	125 mL
1 cup	cauliflower florets	250 mL

1. In a small saucepan, bring water to a boil over high heat. Add cauliflower, cover and boil for 10 minutes or until very soft.
2. Using a slotted spoon, transfer cauliflower to blender, reserving cooking water. Process until smooth, about the texture of applesauce. To make smoother, blend in reserved cooking water 1 tsp (5 mL) at a time until desired texture is achieved.

Herbed Mashed Potatoes

Carrots and fresh herbs enhance the color and flavor of ordinary mashed potatoes. The low-fat yogurt adds protein and zing.

Kitchen Tips

Russet potatoes work best for mashing.

When serving, top scoops of mashed potato with 1 tbsp (15 mL) shredded light Cheddar cheese

If you don't have fresh herbs on hand, you can use ½ tsp (2 mL) dried dillweed and ¼ tsp (1 mL) dried parsley.

1	large potato, peeled and cubed	1
½	carrot, chopped	½
4 cups	cold water	1 L
1 tsp	finely chopped fresh chives	5 mL
1 tsp	finely chopped fresh dill	5 mL
1 tsp	finely chopped fresh parsley	5 mL
2 tbsp	Greek-style low-fat plain yogurt	30 mL
1½ tbsp	skim milk	22 mL
⅛ tsp	salt (or to taste)	0.5 mL
	Freshly ground black pepper	

1. In a medium saucepan, combine potato, carrot and cold water. Bring to a boil over high heat. Reduce heat to medium and cook for about 20 minutes or until vegetables are tender. Drain and return to pot.

2. Mash potatoes and carrots with a potato masher. Stir in chives, dill, parsley, yogurt and milk. Season with up to ⅛ tsp (0.5 mL) salt and pepper to taste.

Nutrients PER SERVING	
Calories	48
Fat	0.1 g
Sodium	63 mg
Carbohydrate	10.9 g
Fiber	1.1 g
Sugar	1.0 g
Protein	1.2 g
Calcium	19 mg
Iron	0.2 mg

Boiled Mini Potatoes

Makes 4 servings

Late Diet Stage 3 to Diet Stage 4

This recipe is the perfect side when you have limited time for food preparation.

Kitchen Tip

If using salt, try using a specialty salt, such as fleur de sel or coarse sea salt.

8 oz	red-skinned mini potatoes	250 g
4 cups	cold water	1 L
2 tsp	chopped fresh parsley	10 mL
1/2 tsp	olive oil	2 mL
	Salt and freshly ground black pepper (optional)	

1. In a medium saucepan, combine potatoes and cold water. Bring to a boil over high heat. Reduce heat to medium and cook for about 25 minutes or until potatoes are tender. Drain and transfer to a serving bowl.

2. Add parsley and oil, tossing to coat. If desired, season to taste with salt and pepper.

Nutrients
PER SERVING

Calories	54
Fat	0.6 g
Sodium	11 mg
Carbohydrate	11.0 g
Fiber	1.4 g
Sugar	0.5 g
Protein	1.3 g
Calcium	15 mg
Iron	0.5 mg

Oregano Potato Chips

Late Diet Stage 3 to
Diet Stage 4

*These thinly sliced roasted
potatoes are a healthier
alternative to store-bought
potato chips. Serve
alongside a protein dish of
your choice and steamed
vegetables.*

Kitchen Tips

Use a mandolin to slice the
potatoes thinly and evenly.

Keep the oven light on
and watch the potatoes
closely toward the end of
the cooking time. Pull them
out right away if it looks like
they're starting to burn.

- **Preheat oven to 400°F (200°C)**
- **Large rimmed baking sheet**

2 tsp	olive oil, divided	10 mL
1	baking potato, such as russet, thinly sliced	1
2 tsp	dried oregano	10 mL
	Salt and freshly ground black pepper (optional)	

1. Lightly grease baking sheet with half the oil. Arrange potato slices in a single layer on prepared baking sheet. Brush each slice with some of the remaining oil. Sprinkle with oregano. If desired, season to taste with salt and pepper.

2. Bake in preheated oven for 10 minutes. Carefully run a metal spatula under potatoes and flip over. Bake for about 10 minutes or until potatoes are browned and tender, being careful to not let them burn.

Variation

Substitute $\frac{1}{2}$ sweet potato, thinly sliced, for the potato.

Nutrients
PER SERVING

Calories	43
Fat	0.7 g
Sodium	2 mg
Carbohydrate	8.5 g
Fiber	0.7 g
Sugar	0.3 g
Protein	1.0 g
Calcium	10 mg
Iron	0.5 mg

Protein Potato Topping

*Add this topping to cooked
potatoes to enhance the
flavor and increase the
protein. It's also delicious
with grilled chicken or
pork, and makes a terrific
spread for Melba toast,
flatbread or crackers.*

Kitchen Tips

To save time chopping, add
all of the ingredients to a
blender or food processor
and process until smooth.

Store leftovers in an airtight
container in the refrigerator
for up to 3 days.

I	shallot, minced	I
I	clove garlic, minced	I
2 tbsp	chopped fresh parsley	30 mL
I tbsp	chopped fresh chives	15 mL
I cup	low-fat cottage cheese, puréed	250 mL
¼ cup	Greek-style low-fat plain yogurt	60 mL
I tbsp	white vinegar	15 mL
2 tsp	olive oil	10 mL
⅛ tsp	salt (or to taste)	0.5 mL
	Freshly ground black pepper	

1. In a small bowl, combine shallot, garlic, parsley, chives,
cottage cheese, yogurt, vinegar and oil. Season with up to
⅛ tsp (0.5 mL) salt and pepper to taste.

Nutrients PER SERVING	
Calories	31
Fat	1.0 g
Sodium	126 mg
Carbohydrate	2.7 g
Fiber	0.1 g
Sugar	1.7 g
Protein	2.8 g
Calcium	52 mg
Iron	0.1 mg

Snacks

Snacks sustain you and give you energy if you are not able to eat enough at meals or if you have a long wait between meals. Making healthier snack choices will help you achieve your weight-loss or weight-maintenance goals. If you want your snack to keep you full a little longer, opt for foods that include protein and/or fiber. When choosing your snack, you should also try to include food groups you may have missed at mealtimes, to ensure you are getting balanced nutrition on a daily basis.

The recipes in this chapter provide some delicious homemade snack options. Some of them can also serve as wonderful appetizers or desserts when you're entertaining. For example, Low-Fat Tzatziki (page 301), Black Bean Dip (page 303) and Hummus (page 304) make delectable dips and spreads, and the Fruit Kebabs (page 310) and Egg and Ham Pinwheels (page 308) look and taste sensational on an hors d'oeuvres tray.

Applesauce

*Applesauce is a classic
snack that can double as a
fat substitute in baking. It
couldn't be easier to make.*

Kitchen Tips

This recipe can easily be
doubled.

Store leftovers in an airtight
container in the refrigerator
for up to 1 week. Or store
individual portions in airtight
containers for up to 1 year.
Thaw in the microwave, on
the stovetop or overnight in
the refrigerator.

• Blender or food processor

1/2 cup	water	125 mL
2	cooking apples that soften (such as Empire, McIntosh or Idared), peeled and chopped	2
	Ground cinnamon (optional)	
	Ground nutmeg (optional)	

1. In a small saucepan, bring water to a boil over high heat. Add apples, reduce heat to medium-low, cover and boil gently, stirring occasionally, for about 25 minutes or until apples are very soft.

2. Using a slotted spoon, transfer apples to blender, reserving cooking water. Purée apples until smooth. If necessary for a smooth texture, add cooking water 1 tbsp (15 mL) at a time and purée until the desired texture is achieved.

3. Transfer to a bowl and season to taste with cinnamon and nutmeg (if using).

Variations

Omit 1 apple and add 1 small chopped carrot.

Use 2 peeled and chopped pears in place of the apple, or use 1 apple and 1 pear.

Place whole, unpeeled apples in a roasting pan and add 1/4 to 1/2 inch (0.5 to 1 cm) water. Roast in a 400°F (200°C) oven for 30 minutes. Let cool for 20 minutes. Slip off skins and purée apples as described in step 2.

Nutrients
PER SERVING

Calories	39
Fat	0.1 g
Sodium	1 mg
Carbohydrate	10.3 g
Fiber	1.1 g
Sugar	8.1 g
Protein	0.2 g
Calcium	5 mg
Iron	0.1 mg

Low-Fat Tzatziki

*Enjoy tzatziki as a dip for
vegetables or pita chips,
as a sauce to help moisten
chicken when you are
introducing solid textures,
or simply to add flavor to
your food in a low-fat way.*

Kitchen Tips

Salt pulls the water out of
the cucumber, making it
easier to drain.

If you tolerate garlic and
like the way it tastes, add as
much as you like.

I	small cucumber, peeled, seeded and coarsely grated	I
⅛ tsp	salt	0.5 mL
¾ cup	Greek-style low-fat plain yogurt	175 mL
I	clove garlic, minced (optional)	I
I tsp	chopped fresh mint	5 mL
I tsp	olive oil	5 mL
	Freshly ground black pepper (optional)	

1. Place cucumber in a fine-mesh sieve set over a bowl
   and sprinkle evenly with salt. Let drain for 1 hour,
   occasionally pushing cucumber along the edges of the
   sieve with the back of a spoon. Discard drained liquid.

2. In a bowl, combine drained cucumber, yogurt, garlic (if
   using), mint and oil. Season to taste with pepper (if using).

Variations

If you cannot find Greek-style yogurt, use 1⅓ cups
(325 mL) Balkan-style low-fat plain yogurt and drain
it by pouring yogurt into a fine-mesh sieve set over a
bowl; let drain for 1 hour. Discard drained liquid.

Nutrients
PER SERVING

Calories	25
Fat	0.8 g
Sodium	70 mg
Carbohydrate	2.5 g
Fiber	0.2 g
Sugar	2.3 g
Protein	1.5 g
Calcium	53 mg
Iron	0.1 mg

Vegetable Dip

The blend of cottage cheese and yogurt makes this dip higher in protein than the usual store-bought dip.

Kitchen Tip

You can also use this dip for chicken or pork, or as a spread on crackers.

Weight-Loss Surgery Tip

On its own, this dip is safe to eat during diet stages 2 to 4. If you are using it as a vegetable dip during diet stage 3, steam the vegetables first, so they're soft enough to tolerate. Otherwise, enjoy this recipe during diet stage 4, once you have introduced raw vegetables.

Nutrients
PER SERVING

Calories	54
Fat	0.7 g
Sodium	364 mg
Carbohydrate	3.3 g
Fiber	0 g
Sugar	2.2 g
Protein	8.0 g
Calcium	50 mg
Iron	0.1 mg

- **Blender, food processor or immersion blender**

1 cup	low-fat cottage cheese	250 mL
⅓ cup	Greek-style low-fat plain yogurt	75 mL
2 tbsp	dry ranch salad dressing mix	30 mL
½ tsp	freshly squeezed lemon juice	2 mL

1. In blender (or using an immersion blender in a bowl), combine cottage cheese, yogurt, salad dressing mix and lemon juice; purée until smooth.

Black Bean Dip

*Enjoy this dip with whole-
grain Melba rounds or
crackers. It also makes a
fabulous, guest-worthy
appetizer.*

Kitchen Tips

One 19-oz (540 mL)
can of black beans yields
about 2 cups (500 mL). If
you use 2 smaller cans or
1 larger can, measure 2 cups
(500 mL), then refrigerate
any extras in an airtight
container for up to 3 days or
freeze for up to 3 months.

For a smooth dip, purée all
of the ingredients except
the cheese in a blender or
food processor. Transfer to
a serving bowl and sprinkle
with cheese.

Nutrients PER SERVING	
Calories	47
Fat	1.0 g
Sodium	191 mg
Carbohydrate	6.8 g
Fiber	1.7 g
Sugar	0.4 g
Protein	2.6 g
Calcium	31 mg
Iron	0.5 mg

2 cups	drained rinsed canned black beans	500 mL
1	clove garlic, minced	1
2 tbsp	finely chopped fresh cilantro	30 mL
½ cup	mild salsa	125 mL
1 tsp	freshly squeezed lime juice	5 mL
¼ cup	shredded light Cheddar cheese	60 mL

1. In a bowl, mash beans with a potato masher. Stir in garlic, cilantro, salsa and lime juice.
2. Transfer to a serving bowl and sprinkle with cheese.

Variation

Substitute white pea (navy) beans for the black beans.

Hummus

*Use hummus as a spread
or as a dip for vegetables or
pita bread.*

Kitchen Tips

One 28-oz (796 mL) can
of chickpeas yields about
3 cups (750 mL). If you use
2 smaller cans or 1 larger
can, measure 3 cups
(750 mL), then refrigerate
any extras in an airtight
container for up to 3 days or
freeze for up to 3 months.

Leftovers can be stored in
an airtight container in the
refrigerator for up to 1 week.

• **Food processor**

2	cloves garlic, minced	2
3 cups	drained rinsed canned chickpeas	750 mL
1/3 cup	water	75 mL
1/4 cup	freshly squeezed lemon juice	60 mL
2 tbsp	tahini (sesame seed paste)	30 mL
2 tbsp	olive oil	30 mL
1/2 tsp	ground cumin	2 mL
1/4 tsp	salt (or to taste)	1 mL

1. In food processor, combine garlic, chickpeas, water, lemon juice, tahini, oil and cumin; purée until smooth.
2. Transfer to an airtight container and season with up to 1/4 tsp (1 mL) salt. Refrigerate for at least 2 hours or overnight to blend the flavors.

Variations

For a different flavor, substitute white pea (navy) beans for the chickpeas.

Substitute smooth peanut butter for the tahini.

Nutrients
PER SERVING

Calories	62
Fat	3.1 g
Sodium	155 mg
Carbohydrate	6.5 g
Fiber	1.5 g
Sugar	1.2 g
Protein	2.5 g
Calcium	18 mg
Iron	0.6 mg

Green Salsa Mini Pita Pizza

Green salsa gives a different look and flavor to a familiar snack option. Make extra and serve as a neat little appetizer for guests or as a snack for the whole family.

● **Preheat broiler or toaster oven**

1 tsp	green salsa (salsa verde)	5 mL
2	2-inch (5 cm) mini whole wheat pita pockets	2
1 tsp	shredded light sharp (old) Cheddar cheese	5 mL
½ tsp	chopped fresh cilantro	2 mL

1. Spoon salsa evenly on top of each pita, then top with cheese and cilantro.

2. Broil or toast for about 1 minute or until cheese is melted.

Variations

Use regular red salsa instead of green salsa.

Replace the pitas with crisp, cracker-like flatbreads, such as lavash, or Melba toasts or rounds.

Substitute different types of light cheese, such as light Havarti or part-skim mozzarella.

Add 1 tbsp (15 mL) chopped cooked vegetables, such as zucchini, bell peppers, onions and/or mushrooms with the salsa.

Nutrients
PER SERVING

Calories	43
Fat	0.6 g
Sodium	118 mg
Carbohydrate	8.4 g
Fiber	1.1 g
Sugar	0.4 g
Protein	2.0 g
Calcium	12 mg
Iron	0.5 mg

Pita Pocket Chips

Nutrients PER SERVING	
Calories	79
Fat	2.9 g
Sodium	186 mg
Carbohydrate	12.1 g
Fiber	1.7 g
Sugar	0.2 g
Protein	2.2 g
Calcium	4 mg
Iron	0.7 mg

- **Preheat oven to 400°F (200°C)**

6	2-inch (5 cm) mini whole wheat pita pockets	6
½ tsp	dried oregano	2 mL
½ tsp	garlic powder	2 mL
¼ tsp	onion powder	1 mL
2 tsp	olive oil	10 mL
⅛ tsp	salt (or to taste)	0.5 mL

1. Cut each pita into quarters, making small triangle wedges.

2. In a small bowl, combine oregano, garlic powder, onion powder and oil. Brush onto both sides of pita wedges. Season with up to ⅛ tsp (0.5 mL) salt. Spread pita wedges out on a small baking sheet.

3. Bake in preheated oven for 4 minutes. Turn pitas over and bake for 4 minutes or until crisp and lightly browned.

Pearl Bocconcini with Tomato

Nutrients PER SERVING	
Calories	46
Fat	4.0 g
Sodium	16 mg
Carbohydrate	1.2 g
Fiber	0.3 g
Sugar	0.6 g
Protein	1.6 g
Calcium	26 mg
Iron	0.2 mg

1	clove garlic, minced	1
½ cup	diced tomato	125 mL
½ cup	drained light pearl bocconcini cheese	125 mL
1 tbsp	finely chopped fresh basil	15 mL
1 tbsp	finely chopped fresh parsley	15 mL
2 tsp	olive oil	10 mL
	Salt and freshly ground black pepper (optional)	

1. In a small bowl, combine garlic, tomato, bocconcini, basil, parsley and oil. Season to taste with salt and pepper (if using).

Oven-Roasted Chickpeas

Makes about 2¼ cups (550 mL)

Serving size: ¼ cup (60 mL)

Diet Stage 4

Nutrients
PER SERVING

Calories	55
Fat	1.7 g
Sodium	151 mg
Carbohydrate	7.3 g
Fiber	1.9 g
Sugar	1.3 g
Protein	2.7 g
Calcium	19 mg
Iron	0.7 mg

- **Preheat oven to 400°F (200°C)**
- **Rimmed baking sheet, lightly sprayed with light nonstick cooking spray**

½ tsp	ground cumin	2 mL
½ tsp	ground coriander	2 mL
½ tsp	ground turmeric	2 mL
⅛ tsp	freshly ground black pepper	0.5 mL
2 tsp	olive oil	10 mL
2 cups	drained rinsed canned chickpeas	500 mL

1. In a medium bowl, combine cumin, coriander, turmeric, pepper and oil. Add chickpeas and toss to coat. Spread chickpeas out on prepared baking sheet.
2. Bake in preheated oven for 35 to 45 minutes, turning halfway through, until golden brown and crisp. Let cool on baking sheet on a wire rack. Store loosely covered with foil at room temperature for up to 3 days.

Ricotta Cheese with Pear

Makes 2 servings

Diet Stages 3 to 4

Nutrients
PER SERVING

Calories	92
Fat	3.1 g
Sodium	150 mg
Carbohydrate	11.4 g
Fiber	1.4 g
Sugar	6.4 g
Protein	7.2 g
Calcium	105 mg
Iron	0.1 mg

½	pear, grated	½
½ cup	low-fat ricotta cheese	125 mL
2 tbsp	granulated sucralose artificial sweetener, such as Splenda	30 mL

1. In a bowl, combine pear, ricotta and sweetener. Serve immediately.

Variation

Use grated apple instead of pear and sprinkle the mixture with some ground cinnamon and/or nutmeg.

Egg and Ham Pinwheels

Makes 4 servings

Serving size: 2 pinwheels

Diet Stages 3 to 4

Serve these eye-catching rolls as a party appetizer or enjoy them as an afternoon snack.

Kitchen Tips

Cut the parchment paper to fit evenly into the baking sheet and dab a little margarine along the bottom edges of the paper to stick it to the pan.

Insert a decorative wooden skewer through each pinwheel to hold it together.

Wrap and refrigerate any leftovers to enjoy for breakfast the next day.

- **Preheat oven to 325°F (160°C)**
- **15- by 10-inch (40 by 25 cm) rimmed baking sheet, lined with parchment paper**

2 tbsp	all-purpose flour	30 mL
2 tbsp	skim milk	30 mL
3	eggs	3
2	egg whites	2
2 tbsp	light cream cheese, softened	30 mL
5 oz	thinly sliced low-fat deli ham	150 g

1. Place flour in a small bowl and slowly whisk in milk until a smooth paste forms.

2. In a medium bowl, lightly beat eggs and egg whites. Whisk in flour paste. Pour onto prepared baking sheet.

3. Bake in preheated oven for 10 minutes or until set. Remove from heat and let cool for 10 minutes. Cover with plastic wrap and refrigerate for 1 hour.

4. Remove plastic wrap and spread an even layer of cream cheese over set eggs. Top evenly with ham. Tightly roll up lengthwise, using the parchment paper as a guide. Cut the roll into 8 pinwheels.

Variations

Use any type of low-fat deli meat, such as turkey, lean mortadella and/or smoked chicken breast.

Replace the cream cheese with a mixture of $1\frac{1}{2}$ tbsp (22 mL) light mayonnaise and $1\frac{1}{2}$ tsp (7 mL) Dijon mustard.

Add a layer of red leaf lettuce between the cream cheese and the ham.

Nutrients
PER SERVING

Calories	130
Fat	5.8 g
Sodium	492 mg
Carbohydrate	5.2 g
Fiber	0.1 g
Sugar	1.2 g
Protein	14.2 g
Calcium	52 mg
Iron	1.3 mg

Mini Banana Bread Muffins

These moist mini muffins make a delicious snack just as they are, but for an extra-special treat, top each muffin with 3 or 4 mini chocolate chips before baking.

Kitchen Tips

Make sure to use granulated sucralose artificial sweetener that measures like sugar, not the packets.

You may store these muffins at room temperature for a few days, but it is better to keep them refrigerated, as they do not contain enough sugar to preserve them. For longer storage, freeze in an airtight container for up to 3 months.

Nutrients
PER SERVING

Calories	56
Fat	0.6 g
Sodium	45 mg
Carbohydrate	11.2 g
Fiber	1.1 g
Sugar	2.1 g
Protein	2.0 g
Calcium	11 mg
Iron	0.4 mg

- **Preheat oven to 350°F (180°C)**
- **12-cup mini muffin pan, lightly sprayed with light nonstick cooking spray or lined with paper liners**

1/2 cup	whole wheat flour	125 mL
1/2 cup	spelt flour	125 mL
3/4 tsp	baking powder	3 mL
1/4 tsp	baking soda	1 mL
1/2 cup	granulated sucralose artificial sweetener, such as Splenda	125 mL
1	egg	1
1/2 cup	mashed ripe banana (about 1 large)	125 mL
1/4 cup	unsweetened applesauce	60 mL
2 tbsp	low-fat plain yogurt	30 mL
1/2 tsp	vanilla extract	2 mL

1. In a small bowl, whisk together whole wheat flour, spelt flour, baking powder and baking soda.

2. In a medium bowl, whisk together sweetener, egg, banana, applesauce, yogurt and vanilla until well blended. Whisk in flour mixture until just blended.

3. Divide batter equally among prepared muffin cups. Bake in preheated oven for 16 to 18 minutes or until a tester inserted in the center comes out clean. Let cool in pan on a wire rack for 10 minutes, then transfer to the rack to cool completely.

Variations

Mini Pumpkin Muffins: Substitute 1/2 cup (125 mL) canned pumpkin purée (not pie filling) for the banana. Add 1/4 tsp (1 mL) ground cinnamon and 1/8 tsp (0.5 mL) ground nutmeg to the flour mixture.

Replace the spelt flour with ground millet flour, which is also rich in protein.

Fruit Kebabs

* **Eight 6-inch (15 cm) wooden skewers**

2 cups	hulled strawberries	500 mL
2 cups	honeydew melon chunks	500 mL

1. Thread fruit evenly onto skewers, alternating strawberries and melon chunks.

Nutrients
PER SERVING

Calories	29
Fat	0.2 g
Sodium	8 mg
Carbohydrate	7.1 g
Fiber	1.2 g
Sugar	5.5 g
Protein	0.5 g
Calcium	9 mg
Iron	0.2 mg

Trail Mix Treat

5	almonds	5
1 tbsp	low-sugar cereal (such as Cheerios)	15 mL
1 tsp	semisweet chocolate chips	5 mL
1 tsp	raisins (optional)	5 mL

1. In a sealable food storage bag or airtight container, combine almonds, cereal, chocolate chips and raisins (if using).

Nutrients
PER SERVING

Calories	70
Fat	4.4 g
Sodium	16 mg
Carbohydrate	6.4 g
Fiber	0.9 g
Sugar	1.0 g
Protein	1.9 g
Calcium	24 mg
Iron	0.6 mg

Desserts

Although you've had weight-loss surgery, that doesn't mean you can never enjoy desserts again. The recipes in this chapter provide just enough sweetness to enjoy as part of a healthy, well-balanced diet. Prepare these desserts for holidays and special occasions. Serve them to guests or bring them along to a potluck. Keep your portions to a minimum and include the amount of dessert you are having in the total portion size of your meal if you are having your treat right after a meal.

On special occasions or holidays, or at dinner party gatherings, consider going out for a walk with your family or friends and then coming home to a small portion of dessert. Take the focus off food and enjoy socializing, playing games and spending time together.

Blueberry Crumble

Warm and vibrant blue, this dessert can be enjoyed warm or cold.

Kitchen Tip

Just before serving, top each custard cup with 1 tbsp (15 mL) low-fat plain yogurt and sprinkle with ground cinnamon.

- **Preheat oven to 400°F (200°C)**
- **Four ³⁄₄-cup (175 mL) custard cups or ramekins, lightly sprayed with light nonstick cooking spray**

2 cups	blueberries	500 mL
1 tbsp	cornstarch	15 mL
¼ cup	quick-cooking rolled oats	60 mL
1½ tbsp	sucralose artificial sweetener mixed with brown sugar, such as Splenda Brown Sugar Blend	22 mL
½ tsp	ground cinnamon	2 mL
2 tsp	margarine	10 mL
3 tbsp	water	45 mL

1. In a bowl, combine blueberries and cornstarch. Spoon ½ cup (125 mL) coated blueberries into each prepared custard cup.

2. In a small bowl, combine oats, sweetener, cinnamon and margarine. Stir in water. Spoon evenly over blueberries.

3. Bake in preheated oven for 15 minutes or until berries are bubbling. Let cool for 10 minutes before serving.

Variation

Substitute whole cranberries or chopped peeled apples for the blueberries. Or come up with your own creation, using a variety of fruit.

Nutrients
PER SERVING

Calories	113
Fat	2.5 g
Sodium	2 mg
Carbohydrate	21.5 g
Fiber	2.5 g
Sugar	12.0 g
Protein	1.3 g
Calcium	12 mg
Iron	0.6 mg

Crustless No-Bake Pumpkin Pie

This version of pumpkin pie does not require a crust or baking, but does need a night to set.

Kitchen Tips

Be sure to use unsweetened pumpkin purée, not the sweetened, spiced pie filling.

Make sure to use granulated sucralose artificial sweetener that measures like sugar, not the packets.

Serve with a dollop of low-fat whipped topping and sprinkle ground cinnamon over top.

Nutrients
PER SERVING

Calories	79
Fat	0.4 g
Sodium	127 mg
Carbohydrate	15.6 g
Fiber	1.4 g
Sugar	13.0 g
Protein	2.9 g
Calcium	54 mg
Iron	0.3 mg

• **9-inch (23 cm) pie plate, lightly sprayed with light nonstick cooking spray**

1	can (28 oz/796 mL) pumpkin purée (not pie filling)	1
1/2 cup	sucralose artificial sweetener mixed with brown sugar, such as Splenda Brown Sugar Blend	125 mL
1/4 cup	granulated sucralose artificial sweetener, such as Splenda	60 mL
1 1/2 tsp	ground cinnamon	7 mL
1/2 tsp	ground nutmeg	2 mL
1/4 tsp	ground ginger	1 mL
1/4 tsp	salt	1 mL
1 tsp	vanilla extract	5 mL
1 cup	skim milk	250 mL
3/4 cup	evaporated skim milk	175 mL
2	envelopes (each 1/4 oz/7 g) unflavored gelatin powder	2
1/4 cup	water	60 mL

1. In a large bowl, combine pumpkin, brown sugar sweetener, sweetener, cinnamon, nutmeg, ginger, salt and vanilla until well blended.

2. In a small saucepan, warm milk and evaporated milk over medium heat, stirring often.

3. In a small bowl, combine gelatin and water, stirring until gelatin is softened. Stir into warmed milk and heat, stirring constantly, for 1 minute or until gelatin is dissolved. Remove from heat and let cool for 2 minutes. Stir into pumpkin mixture.

4. Pour pumpkin mixture into prepared pie plate, cover and refrigerate overnight or until set. Cut into 16 even wedges.

Petite Ricotta Cream Tarts

Why not make these little tarts for your next birthday party? Arrange them on a serving platter lined with a paper doily and insert a colorful or fun candle into each tart.

Kitchen Tips

To finely crush graham crackers, place them in a sealable plastic bag, seal and pound with a rolling pin.

If you can't find small eggs, whisk 1 large egg until blended, then measure 2 tbsp + 1 tsp (35 mL) to equal the volume of 1 small egg, reserving any remaining egg for another use.

Leftover tarts can be stored in the refrigerator for up to 3 days.

Nutrients PER SERVING	
Calories	91
Fat	5.3 g
Sodium	155 mg
Carbohydrate	8.5 g
Fiber	0.2 g
Sugar	2.4 g
Protein	5.1 g
Calcium	62 mg
Iron	0.2 mg

- **Preheat oven to 325°F (160°C)**
- **12-cup mini muffin pan, lightly sprayed with light nonstick cooking spray**

Crust

4	low-fat graham crackers, finely crushed (about $1/3$ cup/75 mL)	4
$2^1/_2$ tsp	seedless no-sugar-added fruit spread (any flavor)	12 mL

Filling

1	small egg (see tip, at left)	1
4 oz	light cream cheese, softened	125 g
$1/_2$ cup	low-fat ricotta cheese	125 mL
2 tbsp	granulated sucralose artificial sweetener, such as Splenda	30 mL
1 tbsp	grated lemon zest	15 mL
$1^1/_2$ tsp	freshly squeezed lemon juice	7 mL

Topping

$1/_4$ cup	no-sugar-added fruit spread (any flavor), preferably seedless	60 mL

1. *Crust:* Divide graham cracker crumbs equally among prepared muffin cups. Spoon fruit spread on top, dividing equally.

2. *Filling:* In a medium bowl, using a wooden spoon, combine egg, cream cheese, ricotta cheese, sweetener, lemon zest and lemon juice until well blended. Spoon evenly on top of fruit spread.

3. Bake in preheated oven for 18 to 20 minutes or until a tester inserted in the center of a tart comes out clean. Let cool for 10 minutes.

4. Carefully slide a knife around the edge of each tart and remove from pan. Transfer to a serving platter. Cover with plastic wrap and refrigerate for 1 hour.

5. *Topping:* Just before serving, top each tart with 1 tsp (5 mL) fruit spread.

Almond Orange Panna Cotta

Panna cotta *means "cooked cream." I've transformed this classic Italian dessert into a low-fat, low-sugar treat that is easy to make yet elegant enough to serve to guests.*

Kitchen Tips

Save some time and make this simple dessert a day or two before entertaining.

Make sure to use granulated sucralose artificial sweetener that measures like sugar, not the packets.

Weight-Loss Surgery Tip

If you have difficulty tolerating lactose, use lactose-free skim milk.

- **Four ³/₄-cup (175 mL) custard cups or ramekins**

2 cups	skim milk, divided	500 mL
1	envelope (¹/₄ oz/7 g) unflavored gelatin powder	1
¹/₄ cup	granulated sucralose artificial sweetener, such as Splenda	60 mL
¹/₈ tsp	almond extract	1 mL
¹/₈ tsp	orange extract	1 mL

1. In a small saucepan, warm 1¹/₂ cups (375 mL) of the skim milk over medium heat, stirring occasionally.

2. Meanwhile, in a small bowl, combine gelatin and the remaining ¹/₂ cup (125 mL) milk, stirring until gelatin is softened.

3. Add sweetener, almond extract and orange extract to the warm milk. Stir in gelatin mixture and heat, stirring constantly, for 1 minute or until gelatin is dissolved.

4. Pour milk mixture into custard cups, dividing equally. Cover and refrigerate for at least 2 hours, until completely set, or for up to 2 days.

Variation

Change the flavor of this versatile dessert by experimenting with different extracts. Try peppermint, amaretto, maple, lemon, banana, rum and/or coconut extract. Combine flavors such as banana and coconut, then top with fresh banana.

Nutrients
PER SERVING

Calories	57
Fat	0 g
Sodium	68 mg
Carbohydrate	8.0 g
Fiber	0 g
Sugar	6.0 g
Protein	6.0 g
Calcium	126 mg
Iron	0 mg

Amaretto Espresso Cups

These little espresso cups make an elegant, low-fat dessert that is ideal for entertaining.

Kitchen Tips

If you do not have decaffeinated espresso, use 3 tbsp (45 mL) decaffeinated instant coffee granules instead.

If you cannot find chocolate-covered espresso beans, use mini chocolate chips.

Weight-Loss Surgery Tips

In diet stages 2 and 3, omit the chocolate-covered espresso bean on your serving.

If you have difficulty tolerating lactose, use lactose-free skim milk.

Nutrients
PER SERVING

Calories	44
Fat	1.1 g
Sodium	35 mg
Carbohydrate	5.7 g
Fiber	0 g
Sugar	4.2 g
Protein	2.9 g
Calcium	59 mg
Iron	0.1 mg

- **Eight $\frac{1}{2}$-cup (125 mL) espresso cups or ramekins**

1$\frac{3}{4}$ cups	skim milk, divided	425 mL
1	envelope ($\frac{1}{4}$ oz/7 g) unflavored gelatin powder	1
$\frac{1}{4}$ cup	granulated sucralose artificial sweetener, such as Splenda (see tip, page 315)	60 mL
$\frac{1}{4}$ cup	brewed decaffeinated espresso	60 mL
$\frac{1}{8}$ tsp	amaretto or almond extract	1 mL
$\frac{1}{2}$ cup	frozen low-fat whipped topping, thawed (optional)	125 mL
8	chocolate-covered espresso beans (optional)	8

1. In a small saucepan, warm 1$\frac{1}{4}$ cups (300 mL) of the milk over medium heat, stirring occasionally, just until steaming.

2. Meanwhile, in a small bowl, combine gelatin and the remaining $\frac{1}{2}$ cup (125 mL) milk, stirring until gelatin is softened.

3. Add sweetener, espresso and amaretto extract to the warm milk. Stir in gelatin mixture and heat, stirring constantly, for 1 minute or until gelatin is dissolved.

4. Pour milk mixture into espresso cups, dividing equally. Cover and refrigerate for at least 2 hours, until completely set, or for up to 2 days.

5. If desired, dollop about 1 tbsp (15 mL) whipped topping on each espresso cup and top with a chocolate-covered espresso bean.

Wheat Berry Fruit Salad

Makes 4 servings

Diet Stage 4

Wheat berries are whole, unprocessed wheat kernels — wheat in its natural form. Here, they add extra appeal to this healthy dessert.

Kitchen Tip

Prepare the wheat berries ahead of time, as they take a while to cook. Store in an airtight container in the refrigerator for up to 3 days.

½ cup	wheat berries	125 mL
1 ½ cups	water	375 mL
½ cup	blueberries	125 mL
¼ cup	chopped strawberries	60 mL
¼ cup	raspberries	60 mL
	Artificial sweetener equivalent to 1 tbsp (15 mL) granulated sugar	
¼ cup	low-fat plain yogurt	60 mL
	Ground cinnamon	

1. In a medium saucepan, combine wheat berries and water. Bring to a boil over high heat. Reduce heat and simmer, stirring occasionally, for about 90 minutes or until wheat berries are tender. Drain and rinse under cold water. Transfer to a bowl.

2. Stir in blueberries, strawberries, raspberries and sweetener. Divide equally among 4 serving bowls. Top each with 1 tbsp (15 mL) yogurt and sprinkle with cinnamon.

Variations

Use any variety of fresh fruit.

Substitute a low-fat, no-sugar-added flavored yogurt of your choice for the plain yogurt.

Nutrients
PER SERVING

Calories	107
Fat	0.8 g
Sodium	11 mg
Carbohydrate	22.5 g
Fiber	3.7 g
Sugar	3.0 g
Protein	4.4 g
Calcium	36 mg
Iron	1.0 mg

Fruit Salad with Pecans

Diet Stage 4

You don't need to wait for a holiday or special occasion to enjoy this delicious dessert. Enjoy it as a snack, at breakfast or as a filling in a homemade crêpe (see recipe, page 322).

- **Four ³/₄-cup (175 mL) custard cups or ramekins**

	Artificial sweetener equivalent to 1 tbsp (15 mL) granulated sugar	
1	can (4 oz/125 mL) no-sugar-added diced peaches, drained and juice reserved	1
2 tbsp	freshly squeezed lemon juice	30 mL
1	small banana, sliced	1
½ cup	sliced strawberries	125 mL
½ cup	blueberries	125 mL
¼ cup	vanilla-flavored low-fat no-sugar-added yogurt	60 mL
2 tbsp	chopped pecans	30 mL
	Ground cinnamon	

1. In a bowl, combine sweetener, peach juice and lemon juice. Stir in peaches, banana, strawberries and blueberries.
2. Divide equally among 4 serving bowls. Top with yogurt, then sprinkle with pecans and cinnamon to taste.

Variations

Substitute 2 cups (500 mL) of any combination of seasonal fruits.

Use any flavored low-fat yogurt to top this fruit salad.

Nutrients
PER SERVING

Calories	82
Fat	2.9 g
Sodium	12 mg
Carbohydrate	14.1 g
Fiber	2.3 g
Sugar	8.7 g
Protein	1.7 g
Calcium	35 mg
Iron	0.4 mg

Melon Ball Fruit Cup

Mid Diet Stage 3 to Diet Stage 4

These fruit cups are sure to impress your guests at your next dinner party. Use clear glass, stemmed serving bowls or wine glasses for a cool look.

Kitchen Tips

If you do not have a melon baller, chopping the melons into equal size pieces is just fine.

Rose water, a flavoring used in Middle Eastern, Indian and Asian cuisines, tastes and smells like roses. It is commonly used to flavor desserts. If you cannot find rose water in your grocery store, try specialty food stores. If you cannot find rose water, substitute 1/8 tsp (0.5 mL) almond or orange extract.

Nutrients
PER SERVING

Calories	32
Fat	0.1 g
Sodium	10 mg
Carbohydrate	8.0 g
Fiber	0.6 g
Sugar	6.3 g
Protein	0.6 g
Calcium	7 mg
Iron	0.2 mg

- **Six 1/2-cup (125 mL) glass bowls or custard cups**

2 tbsp	sucralose artificial sweetener	30 mL
2 tbsp	freshly squeezed lemon juice	30 mL
1 tsp	rose water	5 mL
1 cup	honeydew melon balls	250 mL
1 cup	cantaloupe melon balls	250 mL
1 cup	watermelon melon balls	250 mL
6	fresh mint leaves	6

1. In a large bowl, combine sweetener, lemon juice and rose water. Gently stir in honeydew, cantaloupe and watermelon.
2. Divide equally among 6 serving bowls. Garnish each with a mint leaf.

Variations

Use any other fruit, such as sliced strawberries, sliced peaches or grapes.

For a frozen treat, after step 1, lay melon balls in a single layer on a baking sheet lined with parchment paper and freeze for about 2 hours. Proceed with step 2.

Frozen Berry Yogurt Cubes

These flavorful little treats are just like ice cream, minus the fat and sugar.

Kitchen Tips

You can also use a mini muffin pan or an ice pop mold instead of an ice cube tray.

Once solid, transfer cubes to an airtight container or freezer bag and store in the freezer for up to 3 months.

- **Blender or food processor**
- **Ice cube tray with at least 10 compartments**
- **10 small ice pop sticks**

1 cup	frozen mixed berries, partially thawed	250 mL
1 cup	low-fat plain yogurt	250 mL
	Artificial sweetener equivalent to 2 tsp (10 mL) granulated sugar	

1. In blender, combine berries, yogurt and sweetener (if using); purée until smooth.
2. Pour about 2 tbsp (30 mL) berry mixture into each of 10 ice cube tray compartments. Insert an ice pop stick into each. Freeze for 30 minutes, then check on the ice pop sticks to see if they need straightening out. Freeze for about 30 minutes or until solid. Let stand at room temperature for 2 to 3 minutes before trying to remove the ice pops from the molds.

Variation

Any frozen fruit will work. Try chopped peaches, strawberries or mangos.

Nutrients
PER SERVING

Calories	43
Fat	0.7 g
Sodium	34 mg
Carbohydrate	6.8 g
Fiber	0.8 g
Sugar	5.4 g
Protein	2.4 g
Calcium	84 mg
Iron	0.1 mg

Sautéed Apple Slices

These sautéed apples taste wonderful rolled in a crêpe (see recipe, page 322) or served on top of low-fat ricotta cheese or yogurt.

Kitchen Tips

The cooking time will vary depending on the apple variety you use and how thinly you slice it.

If desired, top each serving with flavored or plain low-fat yogurt.

Choose a variety of apple that will hold its shape and flavor when cooked.

Adjust the amount of sweetener to your liking.

½ tsp	margarine	2 mL
I	large cooking apple, such as Honey Crisp, Golden Delicious, Empire or Cortland, peeled and thinly sliced	I
	Ground cinnamon	
	Ground nutmeg	
2 tbsp	freshly squeezed lemon juice	30 mL
I tsp	granulated sucralose artificial sweetener, such as Splenda	5 mL
I to 2 tbsp	water	I5 to 30 mL
I tbsp	no-added-sugar maple-flavored syrup	I5 mL

I. In a medium nonstick skillet, melt margarine over medium heat. Add apple, cinnamon to taste, nutmeg to taste and lemon juice; sauté for 5 minutes or until apple is partially softened.

2. Stir in sweetener, 1 tbsp (15 mL) water and syrup; cook, stirring, for 1 minute. (If necessary, add another 1 tbsp/ 15 mL water to prevent apple from sticking.) Turn heat off and let cook over residual heat (if using a gas burner, reduce heat to low), stirring, for 1 to 2 minutes or until apple is tender.

Variation

Use 2 small pears or peaches, peeled and thinly sliced, instead of the apple. Adjust the cooking time to the fruit you use, cooking until tender.

Nutrients
PER SERVING

Calories	60
Fat	0.8 g
Sodium	II mg
Carbohydrate	I5.5 g
Fiber	1.9 g
Sugar	8.0 g
Protein	0.2 g
Calcium	7 mg
Iron	0.I mg

Fruit-Filled Crêpes

Serving size: 1 fruit-filled crêpe

Diet Stage 4

Here's a yummy treat for your next birthday. Drizzle each crêpe with a little no-sugar-added chocolate sauce for an extra-special treat. Insert a sparkler and sing "Happy Birthday"!

Kitchen Tips

The key to making perfect crêpes is using the right pan and the right amount of batter. A nonstick pan is important, as is spraying it with light nonstick cooking spray between crêpes.

Specialty equipment, such as crêpe pans and spatulas, can be purchased at kitchen stores if you enjoy making crêpes. You may need to try this recipe a few times before you get the hang of it.

Nutrients
PER SERVING

Calories	101
Fat	2.5 g
Sodium	109 mg
Carbohydrate	16.2 g
Fiber	2.6 g
Sugar	7.2 g
Protein	4.1 g
Calcium	59 mg
Iron	0.8 mg

- **Blender, food processor or immersion blender**
- **9 $\frac{1}{2}$-inch (24 cm) nonstick skillet or crêpe pan**

Crêpes

2 tbsp	all-purpose flour	30 mL
2 tbsp	spelt flour	30 mL
2 tsp	granulated sucralose artificial sweetener, such as Splenda (optional)	10 mL
$\frac{1}{8}$ tsp	salt	0.5 mL
1	egg	1
$\frac{1}{2}$ cup	skim milk	125 mL
	Light nonstick cooking spray	

Filling

1 tsp	margarine	5 mL
1	cooking apple, such as Honey Crisp, Golden Delicious, Empire or Cortland, peeled and thinly sliced	1
$\frac{1}{4}$ tsp	ground cinnamon	1 mL
$\frac{3}{4}$ cup	blackberries	175 mL
2 tsp	granulated sucralose artificial sweetener, such as Splenda	10 mL
$\frac{1}{4}$ cup	water	60 mL

Topping

4 tsp	low-fat plain or no-sugar-added flavored yogurt	20 mL
	Ground cinnamon	

1. *Crêpes:* In blender (or using an immersion blender in a bowl), combine all-purpose flour, spelt flour, sweetener (if using), salt, egg and milk; process until smooth. Transfer to a bowl if necessary, cover and refrigerate for 1 hour.

2. Spray nonstick skillet with light nonstick cooking spray and heat over medium heat. Pour a little more than 3 tbsp (45 mL) batter into skillet, tilting and swirling the pan to coat it evenly. Cook for 1 to 2 minutes or until set on the bottom. Using a thin spatula, carefully flip crêpe over and cook for 30 to 60 seconds or until light golden. Transfer crêpe to a serving plate. Repeat with the remaining batter, spraying pan with cooking spray between each crêpe. Wrap crêpes in foil to keep them warm, and set aside.

Weight-Loss Surgery Tip

One filled crêpe may be too much for you to eat right after a meal. Enjoy this dessert once in a while after a lighter meal, make your crêpe a little smaller than others or wait to serve dessert to your guests until later in the evening. These crêpes are also great for brunch!

3. *Filling*: In the same skillet, melt margarine over medium heat. Sauté apples and cinnamon for 3 minutes. Turn off heat and stir in blackberries, sweetener and water; let cook over residual heat (if using a gas burner, reduce heat to low), stirring constantly, for 2 minutes. Remove from heat and let cool for 2 minutes.

4. *Topping*: Spoon one-quarter of the filling evenly along the center of each crêpe and roll crêpes up. Top each with 1 tsp (5 mL) of yogurt and sprinkle with cinnamon.

Variations

In place of the spelt flour, you can use any type of specialty flour, such as buckwheat, quinoa or millet flour.

The possible fillings for crêpes are endless. Try spreading them with no-sugar-added fruit spread and/or filling them with any type of fruit, such as sliced bananas, raspberries, blueberries or sliced strawberries. Or use Sautéed Apple Slices (page 321) as a filling.

To make savory crêpes, omit the sweetener in the batter. Fill each crêpe with 2 oz (60 g) lean deli meat and $\frac{1}{4}$ cup (60 mL) shredded light cheese.

Blueberry Lemon Parfait

Makes 4 servings

Diet Stage 4

This easy parfait makes an economical, elegant dessert that is sure to entice you and your guests.

Kitchen Tip

For outstanding visual appeal, serve in tall, clear wine glasses instead of custard cups. Sprinkle some grated lemon zest on top.

- **Four ¾-cup (175 mL) custard cups or ramekins**

1	envelope (⅓ oz/10 g) lemon-flavored no-sugar-added gelatin powder	1
1 cup	boiling water	250 mL
2 tsp	granulated sucralose artificial sweetener, such as Splenda	10 mL
¾ cup	Greek-style low-fat plain yogurt	175 mL
4 tsp	frozen low-fat whipped topping, thawed	20 mL
¼ cup	blueberries	60 mL

1. In a medium bowl, combine gelatin and boiling water, stirring until gelatin is dissolved. Let cool to room temperature.

2. Whisk sweetener and yogurt into gelatin mixture. Pour into custard cups, dividing equally. Refrigerate for 2 to 3 hours or until set.

3. Top each custard cup with 1 tsp (5 mL) whipped topping and 1 tbsp (15 mL) blueberries.

Variation

Try using gelatin powder and low-fat yogurt in different flavors. Raspberry-flavored gelatin works well with banana-flavored yogurt, as does orange-flavored gelatin with vanilla-flavored yogurt. Be sure to use no-sugar-added products.

Nutrients
PER SERVING

Calories	45
Fat	0.8 g
Sodium	35 mg
Carbohydrate	5.0 g
Fiber	0.2 g
Sugar	4.3 g
Protein	5.0 g
Calcium	78 mg
Iron	0 mg

Berry Gelatin Dessert

Makes 4 servings

Diet Stage 4

Not just your ordinary gelatin dessert — with added fiber from the berries and protein from the yogurt, this one is especially good for you.

Kitchen Tip

For the mixed berries, try raspberries, blackberries and chopped strawberries. Or experiment with any berry combination you like!

Weight-Loss Surgery Tip

Use Greek-style low-fat plain yogurt for extra protein.

- **Four ³⁄₄-cup (175 mL) custard cups or ramekins**

1	envelope (¹⁄₃ oz/10 g) strawberry-flavored no-sugar-added gelatin powder	1
1 cup	boiling water	250 mL
¹⁄₃ cup	cold water	75 mL
¹⁄₃ cup	low-fat plain yogurt	75 mL
1 cup	mixed berries	250 mL

1. In a medium bowl, combine gelatin and boiling water, stirring until gelatin is dissolved. Let cool to room temperature.

2. Whisk cold water into gelatin mixture. Whisk in yogurt. Stir in berries. Pour into custard cups, dividing equally. Refrigerate for 2 to 3 hours or until set.

Nutrients
PER SERVING

Calories	34
Fat	0.4 g
Sodium	22 mg
Carbohydrate	4.5 g
Fiber	0.8 g
Sugar	3.4 g
Protein	3.4 g
Calcium	44 mg
Iron	0.2 mg

Grapey Green Gelatin

This beautifully delicious gelatin dessert is easy to prepare.

- **Four ³/₄-cup (175 mL) custard cups or ramekins**

1	envelope (¹/₃ oz/10 g) lime-flavored no-sugar-added gelatin powder	1
1 cup	boiling water	250 mL
²/₃ cup	cold water	150 mL
²/₃ cup	quartered green seedless grapes	150 mL

1. In a medium bowl, combine gelatin and boiling water, stirring until gelatin is dissolved. Let cool to room temperature.
2. Whisk in cold water. Stir in grapes. Pour into custard cups, dividing equally. Refrigerate for 2 to 3 hours or until set.

Nutrients
PER SERVING

Calories	26
Fat	0 g
Sodium	8 mg
Carbohydrate	4.6 g
Fiber	0.2 g
Sugar	3.9 g
Protein	2.4 g
Calcium	6 mg
Iron	0.1 mg

Beverages

This chapter provides recipes that will enhance your fluid intake. It is very important to stay hydrated after weight-loss surgery, but that can sometimes be difficult because of the limited amount you can drink at once and the need to sip fluids rather than gulp them quickly. Inadequate fluid consumption may lead to mild, moderate or even severe dehydration. Water is your best hydrator, so sip it throughout the day. Remember to choose decaffeinated beverages more often than caffeinated beverages, as caffeine has a dehydrating effect on the body.

Protein is a key component of your menu after weight-loss surgery. Protein drinks can provide you with supplemental protein when you are having difficulty getting adequate protein from food. Protein powders come in a variety of flavors and can simply be mixed with water or low-fat milk. But you'll enjoy protein drinks even more when you change up the taste with the help of the creative recipes in this chapter, which are both tasty and high in nutrition. I've provided a bunch of variations for a wide variety of drinks, and by all means be creative and create your own tasty concoctions!

Fruit Smoothie

Build your bones with this berry beverage!

Weight-Loss Surgery Tips

If you have difficulty tolerating lactose, use lactose-free skim milk.

For more protein, use Greek-style yogurt and/or add 1 scoop of the protein powder of your choice, such as vanilla-flavored or unflavored.

Once you're in diet stage 4, you can skip straining out the seeds.

• **Blender or immersion blender**

¾ cup	skim milk	175 mL
½ cup	frozen mixed berries	125 mL
3 tbsp	smooth tofu	45 mL
2 tbsp	low-fat plain yogurt	30 mL
	Artificial sweetener equivalent to 1 tsp (5 mL) granulated sugar (optional)	

1. In a blender (or using an immersion blender in a tall cup), combine milk, berries, tofu and yogurt; blend for 30 to 45 seconds or until smooth.

2. Strain through a fine-mesh sieve to remove seeds. If desired, stir in sweetener.

Variations

Substitute frozen chopped peaches or mangos, or any frozen fruit you like, for the mixed berries.

Omit the tofu and add 3 tbsp (45 mL) more yogurt.

Replace the sweetener with 1 to 2 tsp (5 to 10 mL) sugar-free flavoring syrup, such as vanilla-flavored syrup (or add as directed on the label).

Nutrients
PER SERVING

Calories	74
Fat	1.3 g
Sodium	49 mg
Carbohydrate	10.2 g
Fiber	1.1 g
Sugar	8.5 g
Protein	5.8 g
Calcium	175 mg
Iron	0.4 mg

Strawberry Banana Protein Smoothie

Makes 2 servings

Diet Stages 2 to 4

Your body needs extra nutrition after a workout. Enjoy this high-protein, flavorful smoothie after hitting the gym.

Weight-Loss Surgery Tip

If you have difficulty tolerating lactose, use lactose-free skim milk.

- **Blender or immersion blender**

3	ice cubes	3
1	scoop strawberry-flavored protein powder	1
¼	banana	¼
¾ cup	skim milk	175 mL
3 tbsp	low-fat plain yogurt	45 mL

1. In a blender (or using an immersion blender in a tall cup), combine ice cubes, protein powder, banana, milk and yogurt; blend for 45 to 60 seconds or until ice cubes are crushed.

Variation

Use vanilla-flavored or unflavored protein powder and add 3 frozen strawberries. For diet stages 2 and 3, you will need strain the strawberry seeds out with a fine-mesh sieve after blending.

Nutrients
PER SERVING

Calories	108
Fat	0.4 g
Sodium	54 mg
Carbohydrate	10.4 g
Fiber	0.4 g
Sugar	7.9 g
Protein	15.8 g
Calcium	155 mg
Iron	0.1 mg

Almond Coffee Protein Shake

Makes 1 serving

Diet Stages 2 to 4

Trick your taste buds with this nutty java-flavored protein drink.

Weight-Loss Surgery Tip

If you have difficulty tolerating lactose, use lactose-free skim milk.

- **Blender or immersion blender**

3	ice cubes	3
1	scoop vanilla-flavored protein powder	1
¾ cup	skim milk	175 mL
2 tsp	decaffeinated instant coffee granules	10 mL
⅛ tsp	almond extract	0.5 mL
	Artificial sweetener equivalent to 1 tsp (5 mL) granulated sugar (optional)	

1. In a blender (or using an immersion blender in a tall cup), combine ice cubes, protein powder, milk, coffee, almond extract and sweetener (if using); blend for 45 to 60 seconds or until ice cubes are crushed.

Variations

If you don't have vanilla-flavored protein powder, use unflavored protein powder and add a few drops of vanilla extract.

Omit the sweetener and almond extract, and add 1 tsp (5 mL) sugar-free flavoring syrup, such as almond-flavored syrup (or add as directed on the label).

Nutrients
PER SERVING

Calories	171
Fat	0.2 g
Sodium	77 mg
Carbohydrate	12.5 g
Fiber	0 g
Sugar	9.2 g
Protein	29.5 g
Calcium	238 mg
Iron	0.2 mg

Chocolate Mint Protein Drink

Makes 1 to 2 servings

Diet Stages 2 to 4

Nutrients
PER SERVING

Calories	81
Fat	0.1 g
Sodium	38 mg
Carbohydrate	5.5 g
Fiber	0 g
Sugar	4.6 g
Protein	14.6 g
Calcium	116 mg
Iron	0 mg

- **Blender or immersion blender**

2	ice cubes	2
1	scoop chocolate-flavored protein powder	1
¾ cup	skim milk	175 mL
⅛ tsp	peppermint extract	0.5 mL

1. In a blender (or using an immersion blender in a tall cup), combine ice cubes, protein powder, milk and peppermint extract; blend for 45 to 60 seconds or until ice cubes are crushed.

Variations

To give this drink a mocha flavor, add 2 tsp (10 mL) decaffeinated instant coffee granules.

Omit the peppermint extract and add ¼ banana.

Lemonade

Makes 2 servings

Diet Stages 1 to 4

Nutrients
PER SERVING

Calories	5
Fat	0 g
Sodium	4 mg
Carbohydrate	1.5 g
Fiber	0.1 g
Sugar	0.6 g
Protein	0.1 g
Calcium	5 mg
Iron	0 mg

1½ cups	cold water	375 mL
2 tbsp	freshly squeezed lemon juice	30 mL
⅛ tsp	rose water (optional)	0.5 mL
	Artificial sweetener equivalent to 2 tsp (10 mL) granulated sugar	

1. In a small pitcher, combine cold water, lemon juice, rose water (if using) and sweetener. Refrigerate for 1 to 2 hours or until chilled.

Variation

Instead of water, use steeped decaffeinated green tea.

Homemade Iced Tea

Enjoy this cool drink on a warm summer day. Make a jug to keep in your refrigerator for a refreshing beverage any time.

Kitchen Tips

You can also enjoy this homemade tea warm.

Use the cooked apple to make applesauce, or enjoy it as a snack topped with yogurt. Just make sure to discard the cloves and cinnamon stick!

2 cups	water	500 mL
1	small apple, cored, peeled and quartered	1
5	whole cloves	5
1	2-inch (5 cm) cinnamon stick	1
1	decaffeinated orange pekoe tea bag	1
	Artificial sweetener equivalent to 2 tsp (10 mL) granulated sugar	

1. In a small pot, bring water to a boil over high heat. Add apple, cloves and cinnamon stick. Reduce heat to low and simmer for 10 minutes. Add tea bag and simmer for 2 minutes. Remove from heat and let cool for 10 minutes.

2. Strain through a fine-mesh sieve into a pitcher, discarding solids (or save the apple for another use). Stir in sweetener. Refrigerate for 2 to 4 hours or until chilled.

Variations

Use any fruit in place of the apple, such as a quartered pear or orange wedges.

Omit the tea bag for an iced spiced fruit drink.

Replace the sweetener with 1 tbsp (15 mL) sugar-free flavoring syrup, such as apple-flavored syrup (or add as directed on the label).

Nutrients
PER SERVING

Calories	17
Fat	0.1 g
Sodium	0 mg
Carbohydrate	4.5 g
Fiber	0.6 g
Sugar	3.4 g
Protein	0.1 g
Calcium	4 mg
Iron	0.1 mg

Chai

*This spicy taste of India will
warm your senses.*

Kitchen Tip

If you do not have loose
decaffeinated black tea
leaves, use a decaffeinated
tea bag instead.

Weight-Loss
Surgery Tip

If you have difficulty
tolerating lactose, use
lactose-free skim milk.

⅓ cup	water	75 mL
4	cardamom pods	4
4	whole cloves	4
1	1-inch (2.5 cm) cinnamon stick	1
1	¼-inch (0.5 cm) slice gingerroot	1
¾ cup	skim milk	175 mL
1½ tsp	loose decaffeinated black tea leaves	7 mL
	Artificial sweetener equivalent to 1 tsp (5 mL) granulated sugar	

1. In a small saucepan, combine water, cardamom, cloves, cinnamon and ginger. Bring to a boil over high heat. Reduce heat to low, cover and simmer for 10 minutes. Add milk and return to a simmer, uncovered; simmer, stirring often, for 1 minute.

2. Add tea leaves, remove from heat, cover and let steep for 3 minutes. Strain through a fine-mesh sieve into serving mug(s), discarding solids. Stir in sweetener.

Variation

Experiment with different tea leaves for a variety of flavors.

Nutrients
PER SERVING

Calories	34
Fat	0.1 g
Sodium	39 mg
Carbohydrate	5.2 g
Fiber	0.3 g
Sugar	4.9 g
Protein	3.2 g
Calcium	120 mg
Iron	0.2 mg

Orange Cinnamon Decaf Coffee

Makes 4 servings

Diet Stages 1 to 4

Nutrients PER SERVING	
Calories	7
Fat	0 g
Sodium	1 mg
Carbohydrate	1.5 g
Fiber	0.2 g
Sugar	0 g
Protein	0.3 g
Calcium	7 mg
Iron	0.2 mg

- **Paper coffee filter**
- **Coffee pot**

2 tbsp	ground decaffeinated coffee	30 mL
2	1-inch (2.5 cm) cinnamon sticks	2
2 tsp	grated orange zest	10 mL
2 cups	boiling water	500 mL

1. Place paper filter over coffee pot and add coffee, cinnamon sticks and orange zest. Pour boiling water over coffee mixture. Discard solids.

Decaf Caffè Latte

Makes 1 serving

Diet Stages 2 to 4

Nutrients PER SERVING	
Calories	67
Fat	0.2 g
Sodium	78 mg
Carbohydrate	10.1 g
Fiber	0 g
Sugar	9.6 g
Protein	6.4 g
Calcium	232 mg
Iron	0.1 mg

¾ cup	skim milk	175 mL
1 tsp	decaffeinated instant coffee granules	5 mL
	Artificial sweetener equivalent to 1 tsp (5 mL) granulated sugar	

1. In a small saucepan, warm milk over medium heat, stirring often. Add coffee and stir well. Stir in sweetener.

Variation

Replace the sweetener with 1 tsp (5 mL) sugar-free flavoring syrup, such as almond-flavored syrup (or add as directed on the label).

Skinny High-Protein Cappuccino

Who needs expensive coffee shops when you can make cappuccino right in your own kitchen?

Kitchen Tip

If you do not own an espresso maker, make the espresso Turkish-style. Use either decaffeinated Turkish ground coffee or decaffeinated finely ground espresso. In a saucepan, bring 1 cup (250 mL) cold water to a boil over high heat. Add 1 tsp (5 mL) coffee and return to a boil, then quickly remove from heat. Stir and let the grinds settle before pouring. Slowly pour the amount you need.

¾ cup	skim milk	175 mL
1	scoop unflavored protein powder	1
2 tbsp	hot brewed decaffeinated espresso	30 mL
	Artificial sweetener equivalent to 1 tsp (5 mL) granulated sugar	
	Ground cinnamon	

1. In a small saucepan, warm milk over medium heat, stirring often. Remove from heat and froth milk using a frother or a wire whisk. Stir in protein powder.

2. Pour espresso into a mug and stir in sweetener. Pour in warm milk mixture, using the back of a spoon to hold back the froth. Scoop froth on top. Sprinkle with cinnamon.

Variation

Replace the sweetener with 1 tsp (5 mL) sugar-free flavoring syrup, such as Irish cream–, hazelnut- or almond-flavored syrup (or add as directed on the label).

Nutrients
PER SERVING

Calories	164
Fat	0.2 g
Sodium	81 mg
Carbohydrate	11.6 g
Fiber	0.2 g
Sugar	9.6 g
Protein	29.2 g
Calcium	240 mg
Iron	0.2 mg

Light Hot Chocolate

This homemade hot chocolate is easy and delicious, and cocoa powder offers beneficial antioxidants.

Weight-Loss Surgery Tips

Warming the milk helps to break down some of the lactose, but if you have lactose intolerance, use lactose-free skim milk or unsweetened soy milk.

For extra protein, add 1 scoop unflavored protein powder with the sweetener.

¾ cup	skim milk	175 mL
1 tbsp	unsweetened cocoa powder	15 mL
⅛ tsp	vanilla extract	0.5 mL
	Artificial sweetener equivalent to 1 tsp (5 mL) granulated sugar	

1. In a small saucepan, warm milk over medium heat, stirring often.
2. Place cocoa in a small cup and add 2 tbsp (30 mL) of the warm milk. Stir quickly with a metal spoon until dissolved. Stir into the saucepan. Stir in vanilla and sweetener.

Variation

Omit the vanilla and sweetener, and add 1 tsp (5 mL) sugar-free flavoring syrup, such as Irish cream–, vanilla-, hazelnut- or almond-flavored syrup (or add as directed on the label).

Nutrients
PER SERVING

Calories	77
Fat	0.9 g
Sodium	78 mg
Carbohydrate	12.5 g
Fiber	1.8 g
Sugar	9.7 g
Protein	7.3 g
Calcium	237 mg
Iron	0.8 mg

Acknowledgments

I would like to thank the Bariatric Team at Humber River Regional Hospital (HRRH) and St. Joseph's Health Centre, Toronto, including but not limited to the surgeons, the medical team, the interdisciplinary team and the girls at the front. With special thanks to Jackie, Jennifer, Melice, Denise, Diana (and your mom!), Michelle, Lori, Janet, Jhanvi and Dr. Glazer. Dr. Klein, thank for your encouragement, support and kindness and, most important, for agreeing to write with me; your enthusiasm and devotion to bariatrics are incredible. Thanks to all my other friends and colleagues at HRRH, who inspire me each and every day. A special thank you to the physiotherapists on 5CD, Ronald Wu and Anthony Partipilo, for their expertise and assistance in the writing of the active lifestyle section.

Thank you to Karen Coulman, a bariatric dietitian from the United Kingdom, for your knowledge and expertise and prompt feedback, and to all the Ontario bariatric dietitians for your devotion to this area of dietetics and making a difference in every patient's life. Thank you to the Ontario Bariatric Network and the University of Toronto's Collaborative Bariatric Surgery Program.

Thank you to the staff of Robert Rose Inc., and in particular to Bob Dees for believing in this idea and in me. Thank you to the editing team, Bob Hilderley, Sue Sumeraj and Jennifer MacKenzie, for all your tremendous work from start to finish. To the staff at PageWave Graphics, thank you for your work on the design of the book. Thank you also to Dr. Len Piché and his team for nutrient analysis of the recipes.

A great big thank you to all my friends and relatives for your everlasting love and support, especially Rita, Diana, Vina, Cheryl and Renée, Kristine, Anthony and Rina, Prat and Wayne, Rami and Sonja, and Paola and Claudia. And to anyone I may have inadvertently missed.

Thank you also to my family, who instilled a love of cooking and helping others. I put these two ingredients together to create this book. Mom, Dad, Dan, Rina and Angelina, Medz Mama, Dede, Amo and Tantig, Nonno and Luna and everyone else in my family of three hundred! Mom, thank you for the Italian-themed recipes, and Medz Mama, thank you for the Armenian recipes.

And last, to the one and only Ekserci family, Garo, Alex and Lily — you are the world to me. Thank you for believing in me and for tasting and eating the good (and the not-so-good). Alex, for your words of encouragement — "Mommy, you're a super-duper cooker." Lily, for lapping up the food with no hesitation! And finally Garo, for getting in the kitchen with me and whipping up a storm, for going out to get flour or eggs because I ran out, not once but a few times, and then going back again because the cupcake liners were too big, and then again because they were too small. You helped me set my goals and timelines. Thank you for introducing me to the wonderful variety of flavors that cultural foods have to offer, for making me taste something even just once, and for all your love, patience and kindness to see this through to the end.

The intention of this book is to help all people who are considering or have undergone weight-loss surgery. I dedicate this book to all my patients past, present and future. You inspire me to be all that I can be.

Thank you to God for giving me the power to believe in myself and pursue this dream, and for giving me such wonderful family, friends and colleagues, whose love and support never fail.

— Sue Ekserci

References

Aills L, Blankenship J, Buffington C, et al. ASMBS Allied Health nutritional guidelines for the surgical weight loss patient. *Surgery for Obesity and Related Diseases*, 2008;4(5S):S73–S108.

Alvarado R, Alami RS, Hsu G, et al. The impact of preoperative weight loss in patients undergoing laparoscopic Roux-en-Y gastric bypass. *Obesity Surgery*, 2005;15(9):1282–86.

Alverdy JC, Prachand V, Flanagan B, et al. Bariatric surgery: A history of empiricism, a future in science. *Journal of Gastrointestinal Surgery*, 2009;13(3):465–77.

American Association of Clinical Endocrinologists website. Available at: www.aace.com. Accessed October 2010.

American Dietetic Association website. Available at: www.eatright.org. Accessed September 2010.

American Heart Association website. Available at: www.heart.org. Accessed September 2010.

American Society for Metabolic and Bariatric Surgery website. Available at: www.asmbs.org. Accessed October 2010.

Apovian CM, Cummings S, Anderson W, et al. Best practice updates for multidisciplinary care in weight loss surgery. *Obesity*, 2009;17(5):871–79.

Arkinson J, Ji H, Fallah S, et al. Bariatric surgery in Canada: A focus on day surgery procedures. *Healthcare Quarterly*, 2010;13(3):15–18.

Ashley MJ, Ferrence R, Room R, et al. Moderate drinking and health: Implications of recent evidence. *Canadian Family Physician*, 1997;43:687–94.

Beckman LM, Beckman TR, Earthman CP. Changes in gastrointestinal hormones and leptin after Roux-en-Y gastric bypass procedure: A review. *Journal of the American Dietetic Association*, 2010;110(4):571–84.

Biesemeir CK, Garland J. Weight Management Dietetic Practice Group. *ADA Pocket Guide to Bariatric Surgery*. Chicago: American Dietetic Association, 2009.

Bond DS, Phelan S, Wolfe LG, et al. Becoming physically active after bariatric surgery is associated with improved weight loss and health-related quality of life. *Obesity*, 2008;17(1):78–83.

Bondy SJ, Rehm J, Ashley MJ, et al. Low-risk drinking guidelines: The scientific evidence. *Canadian Journal of Public Health*, 1999;90(4):264–70.

Bonelli S. Spotlight: How fitness professionals can help gastric bypass patients make the transition to healthier lifestyles. *ACE Certified News*, August/September 2005;3–15.

Brethauer S, Hammel JP, Schauer PR. Systematic review of sleeve gastrectomy as staging and primary bariatric procedure. *Surgery for Obesity and Related Diseases*, 2009;5(4):469–75.

The British Dietetic Association website. Available at: www.bda.uk.com. Accessed December 2010.

British Obesity and Metabolic Surgery Society website. Available at: www.british-obesity-surgery.org. Accessed November 2010.

Buchwald H, Avidor Y, Braunwald E, et al. Bariatric surgery: A systematic review and meta-analysis. *Journal of the American Medical Association*, 2004;292(14):1724–37.

Budak AR, Thomas SE. Food craving as a predictor of "relapse" in the bariatric surgery population: A review with suggestions. *Bariatric Nursing and Surgical Patient Care*, 2009;4(2):115–21.

Burns EM, Naseem H, Bottle A, et al. Introduction of laparoscopic bariatric surgery in England: Observational population cohort study. *British Medical Journal*, 2010;341:c4296.

Canadian Association of Bariatric Physicians and Surgeons website. Available at: www.cabps.ca. Accessed November 2010.

Canadian Diabetes Association website. Available at: www.diabetes.ca. Accessed September 2010.

Canadian Diabetes Association. *Alcohol + Diabetes*. Available at: www.diabetes.ca/files/CDAAlcoholFinal.pdf. Accessed September 2010.

Canadian Diabetes Association. *The Glycemic Index*. Available at: www.diabetes.ca/files/glycemicindex_08.pdf. Accessed September 2010.

Canadian Diabetes Association. Guidelines for the nutritional management of diabetes mellitus in the new millennium: A position statement by the Canadian Diabetes Association. *Canadian Journal of Diabetes Care*, 1999;23:56–69.

Canadian Diabetes Association. *Sugar Alcohols: Sugars & Sweeteners*. Available at: www.diabetes.ca/files/for-professionals/sugar-alcohol.pdf. Accessed September 2010.

Canadian Obesity Network website. Available at: www.obesitynetwork.ca. Accessed September 2010.

Canadian Partnership for Consumer Food Safety Education. *Mrs. Cookwell Handy Charts*. Available at: www.canfightbac.org/cpcfse/en/cookwell/charts/. Accessed October 2010.

Centers for Disease Control and Prevention. Physical activity trends — United States, 1990–1998. *Morbidity and Mortality Weekly Report*, 2001;50(9):166–69.

Centers for Disease Control and Prevention. *Key Statistics from NHANES*. Available at: wwwn.cdc.gov/nchs/nhanes/bibliography/key_statistics.aspx. Accessed November 2010.

Centre for Addiction and Mental Health website. Available at: www.camh.net. Accessed November 2010.

Centre for Addiction and Mental Health. *Low-Risk Drinking Guidelines: Maximize Life, Minimize Risk*. Available at: www.camh.net/About_Addiction_Mental_Health/Drug_and_Addiction_Information/low_risk_drinking_guidelines.html. Accessed November 2010.

Christou NV. Impact of obesity and bariatric surgery on survival. *World Journal of Surgery*, 2009;33(10):2022–27.

Christou NV, MacLean LD. Effect of bariatric surgery on long-term mortality. *Advances in Surgery*, 2005;39:165–79.

Christou NV, Sampalis JS, Liberman M, et al. Surgery decreases long-term mortality, morbidity, and health care use in morbidly obese patients. *Annals of Surgery*, 2004;240(3):416–23.

The Cleveland Clinic Bariatric and Metabolic Institute website. Available at: weightloss.clevelandclinic.org/index.aspx. Accessed December 2010.

The Coca-Cola Company. *Soft Drink Nutrition Information for Carbonated Beverages*. Available at: web.archive.org/web/20070928010037/http://www.thecoca-colacompany.com/mail/goodanswer/soft_drink_nutrition.pdf. Accessed September 2010.

Committee to Develop Criteria for Evaluating the Outcomes of Approaches to Prevent and Treat Obesity, Food and Nutrition Board, Institute of Medicine, National Academy of Sciences. Summary: Weighing the options — Criteria for evaluating weight-management programs. *Journal of the American Dietetic Association*, 1995;95(1):96–105.

Deitel M, Gagner M, Dixon JB, et al. *Handbook of Obesity Surgery: Current Concepts and Therapy of Morbid Obesity and Related Disease*. Toronto: FD Communications Inc., 2010.

DeMaria EJ. Bariatric surgery for morbid obesity. *The New England Journal of Medicine*, 2007;356(21):2176–83.

Deusinger SS, Deusinger RH, Racette SB. The obesity epidemic: Health consequences and implications for physical therapy. *Physical Therapy*, 2003;83:276–88.

Dietitians of Canada website. Available at: www.dietitians.ca. Accessed September 2010.

Dietitians of Canada. *Eating Guidelines for Lacto-Ovo Vegetarians*. Available at: www.dietitians.ca/Nutrition-Resources-A-Z/Fact-Sheet-Pages(HTML)/Vegetarian/Eating-Guidelines-for-Lacto-Ovo-Vegetarians.aspx. Accessed September 2010.

EBariatricSurgery.com website. Available at: www.ebariatricsurgery.com. Accessed December 2010.

Elte JWF, Castro Cabeza M, Vrijland WW, et al. Proposal for a multidisciplinary approach to the patient with morbid obesity: The St. Franciscus Hospital morbid obesity program. *European Journal of Internal Medicine*, 2008;19 (2):92–98.

Field AE, Austin SB, Taylor CB, et al. Relation between dieting and weight change among preadolescents and adolescents. *Pediatrics*, 2003;112(4):900–906.

Flancbaum L, Belsley S, Drake V, et al. Preoperative nutritional status of patients undergoing Roux-en-Y gastric bypass for morbid obesity. *Journal of Gastrointestinal Surgery*, 2006;10(7):1033–37.

FoodSafety.gov. *Charts: Food Safety at a Glance*. Available at: www.foodsafety.gov/keep/charts/index.html. Accessed October 2010.

Food Standards Agency website. Available at: www.eatwell.gov.uk. Accessed October 2010.

Food Standards Agency. *Traffic Light Labelling*. Available at: www.eatwell.gov.uk/foodlabels/trafficlights/. Accessed October 2010.

Forti E, Ike D, Barbalho-Moulim M, et al. Effects of chest physiotherapy on the respiratory function of postoperative gastroplasty patients. *Clinics* (Sao Paulo, Brazil), 2009;64(7):683–89.

Guthrie HA, Picciano MF. *Human Nutrition*. Boston: McGraw-Hill, 1995.

Health Canada website. Available at: www.hc-sc.gc.ca. Accessed September 2010.

Health Canada. *Canadian Guidelines for Body Weight Classification in Adults*. Available at www.hc-sc.gc.ca/fn-an/nutrition/weights-poids/guide-ld-adult/cg_quick_ref-ldc_rapide_ref-eng.php. Accessed September 2010.

Health Canada. *The Canadian Nutrient File*. Available at: www.hc-sc.gc.ca/fn-an/nutrition/fiche-nutri-data/index-eng.php. Accessed September 2010.

Health Canada. *Fish Oil*. Available at www.hc-sc.gc.ca/dhp-mps/prodnatur/applications/licen-prod/monograph/mono_fish_oil_huile_poisson-eng.php. Accessed November 2010.

Health Canada. *Nutrition Labelling*. Available at: www.hc-sc.gc.ca/fn-an/label-etiquet/nutrition/index-eng.php. Accessed September 2010.

Health risks and benefits of alcohol consumption. *Alcohol Research and Health*. 2000;24(1):5–11.

Heber D, Greenway FL, Kaplan LM, et al. Endocrine and nutritional management of the post-bariatric surgery patient: An Endocrine Society clinical practice guideline. *Journal of Clinical Endocrinology and Metabolism*, 2010;95(11):4823–43.

Heinlein CR. Dumping syndrome in Roux-en-Y bariatric surgery patients: Are they prepared? *Bariatric Nursing and Surgical Patient Care*, 2009;4(1):39–47.

Herbst ST, Herbst R. *The Deluxe Food Lover's Companion*. Hauppauge, NY: Barron's Educational Series, Inc., 2009.

Howard AA, Arnsten JH, Gourevitch MN. Effect of alcohol consumption on diabetes mellitus: A systematic review. *Annals of Internal Medicine*, 2004;140(3):211–19.

Hrabosky JI, Masheb RM, White MA, et al. A prospective study of body dissatisfaction and concerns in extremely obese gastric bypass patients: 6- and 12-month postoperative outcomes. *Obesity Surgery*, 2006; 16(12):1615–21.

Hsu LK, Benotti PN, Dwyer J, et al. Nonsurgical factors that influence the outcome of bariatric surgery: A review. *Psychosomatic Medicine*, 1998;60(3):338–46.

International Federation for the Surgery of Obesity and Metabolic Disorders (IFSO) website. Available at: www.ifso.com. Accessed November 2010.

Josbeno DA, Jakicic JM, Hergenroeder A, Eid GM. Physical activity and physical function changes in obese individuals after gastric bypass surgery. *Surgery for Obesity and Related Diseases*, 2010;6(4):361–66.

Kanadys WM, Leszczy_ska-Gorzelak B, Oleszczuk J. Obesity among women: Pregnancy after bariatric surgery — A qualitative review [Article in Polish]. *Ginekologia Polska*, 2010;81(3):215–23.

Kris-Etherton PM, Innis S, American Dietetic Association, Dietitians of Canada. Position of the American Dietetic Association and Dietitians of Canada: Dietary fatty acids. *Journal of the American Dietetic Association*, 2007;107(9):1599–1611.

Kulick D, Hark L, Deen D. The bariatric surgery patient: A growing role for registered dietitians. *Journal of the American Dietetic Association*, 2010;110(4):593–99.

Lau DC, Douketis JD, Morrison KM, et al. 2006 Canadian clinical practice guidelines on the management and prevention of obesity in adults and children [summary]. *Canadian Medical Association Journal*, 2007;176(8):S1–S13.

Lee YS. The role of genes in the current obesity epidemic. *Annals, Academy of Medicine, Singapore*, 2009;38(1):45–47.

Le Grange D, Loeb KL. Early identification and treatment of eating disorders: Prodrome to syndrome. *Early Intervention in Psychiatry*, 2007;1(1):27–39.

LePage CT. The lived experience of individuals following Roux-en-Y gastric bypass surgery: A phenomenological study. *Bariatric Nursing and Surgical Patient Care*, 2010;5(1):57–64.

Levy L. *Conquering Obesity: Your Guide to Healthy and Successful Weight Management*. Toronto: Key Porter Books, 2002.

Livhits M, Mercado C, Yermilov I, et al. Does weight loss immediately before bariatric surgery improve outcomes? A systematic review. *Surgery for Obesity and Related Diseases*, 2009;5(6):713–21.

Livhits M, Mercado C, Yermilov I, et al. Exercise following bariatric surgery: A systematic review. *Obesity Surgery*, 2010;20(5):657–65.

Longitudinal Assessment of Bariatric Surgery (LABS) Consortium. Perioperative safety in the longitudinal assessment of bariatric surgery. *New England Journal of Medicine*, 2009;361(5):445–54.

Lutfi R, Torquati A, Sekhar N, Richards WO. Predictors of success after laparoscopic gastric bypass: A multivariate analysis of socioeconomic factors. *Surgical Endoscopy*, 2006;20(6):864–67.

Maggard MA, Yermilov I, Li Z, et al. Pregnancy and fertility following bariatric surgery: A systematic review. *Journal of the American Medical Association*, 2008;300(19):2286–96.

Mahan LK, Escott-Stump S. *Krause's Food, Nutrition, & Diet Therapy*, 10th ed. Philadelphia: W.B. Saunders Company, 2000.

Mayo Clinic website. Available at: www.mayoclinic.com. Accessed October 2010.

McCullough PA, Gallagher MJ, deJong AT, et al. Cardiorespiratory fitness and short-term complications after bariatric surgery. *Chest*, 2006;130(2):517–25.

McGill First Canadian Summit on Metabolic Surgery for Type II Diabetes website. *An Ecomonic Tsunami: The Cost of Diabetes in Canada*. Available at: www.t2dmcanadasummit.com/FINAL_Economic_Report.pdf. Accessed November, 2010.

McMahon MM, Sarr MG, Clark MM, et al. Clinical management after bariatric surgery: Value of a multidisciplinary approach. *Mayo Clinic Proceedings*, 2006;81(10 Suppl):S35–S45.

Mechanick JI, Kushner RF, Sugerman HJ et al. American Association of Clinical Endocrinologists, the Obesity Society, and American Society for Metabolic and Bariatric Surgery Medical guidelines for clinical practice for the perioperative nutritional, metabolic, and nonsurgical support of the bariatric surgery patient. *Obesity*, 2009;17(S1):S1–S70.

Messina V, Melina V, Mangels AR. A new food guide for North American vegetarians. *Journal of the American Dietetic Association*, 2003;103(6):771–75.

Miller GD, Nicklas BJ, You T, Fernandez A. Physical function improvements after laparoscopic Roux-en-Y gastric bypass surgery. *Surgery for Obesity and Related Diseases*, 2009;5(5):530–37.

Ministry of Health and Long-Term Care. 2004 *Chief Medical Officer of Health Report: Healthy Weights, Healthy Lives*. Available at: www.health.gov.on.ca/english/public/pub/ministry_reports/cmoh04_report/healthy_weights_112404.pdf. Accessed October 2010.

Modest Meanings. *Stages of Change*. Available at: www.modestmeanings.com/2009/07/change-is-addictive/stages-of-change-2/. Accessed December 2010.

Moizé VL, Pi-Sunyer X, Mochari H, Vidal J. Nutritional pyramid for post-gastric bypass patients. *Obesity Surgery*, 2010;20(8):1133–41.

Murphy KG, Dhillo WS, Bloom SR. Gut peptides in the regulation of food intake and energy homeostasis. *Endocrine Reviews*, 2006;27(7):719–27.

NHS Information Centre. *Statistics on Obesity, Physical Activity and Diet: England, 2010*. Available at: www.ic.nhs.uk/webfiles/publications/opad10/Statistics_on_Obesity_Physical_Activity_and_Diet_England_2010.pdf. Accessed November 2010.

Naimi TS, Brown DW, Brewer RD, et al. Cardiovascular risk factors and confounders among non-drinking and moderate-drinking U.S. adults. *American Journal of Preventive Medicine*, 2005;28(4):369–73.

National Eating Disorder Information Centre website. Available at: www.nedic.ca. Accessed November 2010.

National Eating Disorder Information Centre. *Definitions*. Available at: www.nedic.ca/knowthefacts/definitions.shtml. Accessed September 2010.

National Heart, Lung and Blood Institute. *Clinical Guidelines on the Identification, Evaluation and Treatment of Overweight and Obesity in Adults*. Available at: www.nhlbi.nih.gov/guidelines/obesity/ob_gdlns.pdf. Accessed December 2010.

National Heart, Lung and Blood Institute. *Practical Guide to the Identification, Evaluation and Treatment of Overweight and Obesity in Adults*. Available at: www.nhlbi.nih.gov/guidelines/obesity/prctgd_c.pdf. Accessed November 2010.

National Institute of Diabetes and Digestive and Kidney Diseases website. Available at: www.niddk.nih.gov. Accessed September 2010.

National Institute of Health website. Available at: www.nih.gov. Accessed November 2010.

National Task Force on the Prevention and Treatment of Obesity. Medical care for obese patients: Advice for health care professionals. *American Family Physician*, 2002;1:65(1):81–88.

National Task Force on the Prevention and Treatment of Obesity. Overweight, obesity, and health risk. *Archives of Internal Medicine*, 2000;160(7):898–904.

Nestle Nutrition website. Available at: www.nutrition.nestle.ca. Accessed October 2010.

Neumark-Sztainer D, van den Berg P, Hannan PJ, Story M. Self-weighing in adolescents: Helpful or harmful? Longitudinal associations with body weight changes and disordered eating. *Journal of Adolescent Health*, 2006;39(6):811–18.

Neven K, Dymek M, leGrange, D, et al. The effects of Roux-en-Y gastric bypass surgery on body image. *Obesity Surgery*, 2002;12(2):265–69.

Norris J. Struggling for normality following gastroplasty. *Bariatric Nursing and Surgical Patient Care*, 2009;4(2):95–101.

Obesityhelp.ca website. Available at: www.obesityhelp.ca. Accessed September 2010.

The Obesity Society website. Available at: www.obesity.org. Accessed October 2010.

Odom J, Zalesin KC, Washington TL, et al. Behavioral predictors of weight regain after bariatric surgery. *Obesity Surgery*, 2010;20(3):349–56.

Office for National Statistics. *Population Estimates*. Available at: www.statistics.gov.uk/cci/nugget.asp?id=6. Accessed October 2010.

Office of Health Economics. *Shedding the Pounds: Obesity Management, NICE Guidance and Bariatric Surgery in England*. Available at: www.ohe.org/lib/liDownload/692/OHE_Spreads.pdf?CFID=2533930CFTOKEN=21002187. Accessed November 2010.

Omichinski L. *Non-Diet Weight Management: A Lifestyle Approach to Health and Fitness*, 5th ed. Ashland, OR: Nutrition Dimension, Inc., 2007.

Ontario Bariatric Network website. Available at: www.ontariobariatricnetwork.ca. Accessed January 2011.

Pepsi. *Pepsi Product Facts*. Available at: www.pepsiproductfacts.com/infobycategory.php?pc=p1062&t=1026&print=1&i=ingrdnt&s=8. Accessed September 2010.

Prochaska JO, DiClemente CC. Transtheoretrical therapy: Toward a more integrative model of change. *Psychotherapy: Therapy, Research and Practice*, 1982;19(3):276–88.

Public Health Agency of Canada website. Available at: www.phac-aspc.gc.ca. Accessed December 2010.

Public Health Agency of Canada. *The Benefits of Physical Activity*. Available at: www.phac-aspc.gc.ca/alw-vat/intro/key-cle-eng.php. Accessed October 2010.

Raper NR, Cronin FJ, Exler J. Omega-3 fatty acid content of the US food supply. *Journal of the American College of Nutrition*, 1992;11(3):304–8.

Rubino F, Kaplan LM, Schauer PR, Cumming DE; Diabetes Surgery Summit Delegates. The Diabetes Surgery Summit consensus conference: Recommendations for the evaluation and use of gastrointestinal surgery to treat type 2 diabetes mellitus. *Annals of Surgery*, 2010;251(3):399–405.

Schauer PR, Ikramuddin S, Gourash W, et al. Outcomes after laparoscopic Roux-en-Y gastric bypass for morbid obesity. *Annals of Surgery*, 2000;232(4):515–29.

Shah W, Cannon C. *Craving Change: Facilitator's Manual*. Calgary: Shah Cannon, 2008.

Shikora SA, Kim JJ, Tarnoff ME, et al. Laparoscopic Roux-en-Y gastric bypass: Results and learning curve of a high-volume academic program. *Archives of Surgery*, 2005;140(4):362–67.

Sjöström L. Bariatric surgery and reduction in morbidity and mortality: Experiences from the SOS study. *International Journal of Obesity*, 2008;32(7):S93–S97.

Sjöström L, Lindroos AK, Peltonen M, et al. Lifestyle, diabetes, and cardiovascular risk factors 10 years after bariatric surgery. *The New England Journal of Medicine*, 2004;351(26):2683–93.

Sjöström L, Narbro K, Sjöström CD, et al. Effects of bariatric surgery on mortality in Swedish obese subjects. *The New England Journal of Medicine*, 2007;357(8):741–52.

Slim Band Toronto Laparoscopic Band Surgery website. Available at www.slimbandtoronto.com/. Accessed December 2010.

Stewart KE, Olbrisch ME, Bean MK. Back on track: Confronting post-surgical weight gain. *Bariatric Nursing and Surgical Patient Care*, 2010;5(2):179–85.

Stice E, Cameron RP, Killen JD, et al. Naturalistic weight-reduction efforts prospectively predict growth in relative weight and onset of obesity among female adolescents. *Journal of Consulting and Clinical Psychology*, 1999;67(6):967–74.

Still CD, Benotti P, Wood CG, et al. Outcomes of preoperative weight loss in high-risk patients undergoing gastric bypass surgery. *Archives of Surgery*, 2007;142(10):994–98.

Surgical Weight Loss Centre website. Available at www.obesitysurgery.ca. Accessed September 2010.

Sutton D, Raines DA. Health-related quality of life: Physical and mental functioning after bariatric surgery. *Bariatric Nursing and Surgical Patient Care*, 2008;3(4):271–77.

Sutton D, Raines DA. Perception of health and quality of life after bariatric surgery. *Bariatric Nursing and Surgical Patient Care*, 2007;2(3):193–98.

Syin D, Magnuson T, Flum D, et al. Pregnancy outcomes after bariatric surgery. *Bariatric Nursing and Surgical Patient Care*, 2007;2(2):113–18.

Thonney B, Pataky Z, Badel S, et al. The relationship between weight loss and psychosocial functioning among bariatric surgery patients. *The American Journal of Surgery*, 2010;199(2):183–88.

Tice JA, Karliner L, Walsh J, et al. Gastric banding or bypass? A systematic review comparing the two most popular bariatric procedures. *The American Journal of Medicine*, 2008;121(10):885–93.

Toronto Minimally Invasive Surgery Group website. Available at: www.misgroup.ca. Accessed September 2010.

Tortora GJ, Grabowski SR. *Principles of Anatomy and Physiology*, 9th ed. New York: John Wiley & Sons, Inc., 2000.

Tyler RD, Lidor AO. Ulcer occurrence in the Roux-en-Y gastric bypass patient. *Bariatric Nursing and Surgical Patient Care*, 2006;1(1):47–52.

Tyler RD, Rowen L, Bloch MJ, et al. Postdischarge issues with postbariatric surgery. *Bariatric Nursing and Surgical Patient Care*, 2010;5(1):3–13.

U.S. Food and Drug Administration website. Available at: www.fda.gov. Accessed September 2010.

UW Health website. Available at http://www.uwhealth.org/. Accessed December 2010.

Vincent RP, le Roux CW. Changes in gut hormones after bariatric surgery. *Clinical Endocrinology*, 2008;69(2):173–79.

Virji A, Murr MM. Caring for patients after bariatric surgery. *American Family Physician*, 2006;73(8):1403–8.

Wansick B. *Mindless Eating*. New York: Bantam Dell, 2007.

Weight Awareness website. Available at: www.weightawareness.com. Accessed December 2010.

Whitlock G, Lewington S, Sherliker P, et al. Body-mass index and cause-specific mortality in 900,000 adults: Collaborative analyses of 57 prospective studies. *Lancet*, 2009;373(9669):1083–96.

World Health Organization website. Available at: www.who.int. Accessed September 2010.

Ybarra J, Sánchez-Hernández J, Gich I, et al. Unchanged hypovitaminosis D and secondary hyperparathyroidism in morbid obesity after bariatric surgery. *Obesity Surgery*, 2005;15(3):330–35.

Yeager SF. Role of the dietitian in a multidisciplinary bariatric program. *Bariatric Nursing and Surgical Patient Care*, 2008;3(2):107–16.

Library and Archives Canada Cataloguing in Publication

Ekserci, Sue
    The complete weight-loss surgery guide & diet program : includes 150 delicious & nutritious recipes : everything you need to know for bariatric surgery / Sue Ekserci with Laz Klein.

Includes index.
ISBN 978-0-7788-0273-0

    1. Obesity—Surgery. 2. Weight loss. 3. Low-fat diet—Recipes. I. Klein, Laz. II. Title.

RD540.E47 2011   617.4'3   C2011-903185-X

Index